Healthy and Safe Environments across Occupational and Environmental Contexts

Healthy and Safe Environments across Occupational and Environmental Contexts

Guest Editors

Carlos Alberto Alves Carvalhais
Joana Carvalho dos Santos
Cristiana Maria Matos da Costa Pereira

MDPI
Basel • Beijing • Wuhan • Barcelona • Belgrade • Novi Sad • Cluj • Manchester

Guest Editors
Carlos Alberto Alves Carvalhais
Environmental Health Department
School of Health of Polytechnic Institute of Porto
Porto
Portugal

Joana Carvalho dos Santos
Environmental Health Department
School of Health of Polytechnic Institute of Porto
Porto
Portugal

Cristiana Maria Matos da Costa Pereira
Department of Health Protection
Laboratoire National de Santé
Dudelange
Luxembourg

Editorial Office
MDPI AG
Grosspeteranlage 5
4052 Basel, Switzerland

This is a reprint of the Special Issue, published open access by the journal *Environments* (ISSN 2076-3298), freely accessible at: https://www.mdpi.com/journal/environments/special_issues/23P75513WP.

For citation purposes, cite each article independently as indicated on the article page online and as indicated below:

Lastname, A.A.; Lastname, B.B. Article Title. *Journal Name* **Year**, *Volume Number*, Page Range.

ISBN 978-3-7258-5567-4 (Hbk)
ISBN 978-3-7258-5568-1 (PDF)
https://doi.org/10.3390/books978-3-7258-5568-1

Contents

About the Editors

Carlos Alberto Alves Carvalhais

Carlos Alberto Alves Carvalhais holds a degree in Environmental Health from the School of Health of the Polytechnic Institute of Porto (ESS|P.Porto), a master's degree in Occupational Safety and Hygiene Engineering from the Faculty of Engineering of the University of Porto, and a PhD in Occupational Health and Safety from the University of Porto. He also has postgraduate experience in Radiation Protection and Safety from University College of Dublin and ESS|P.Porto and postgraduate experience in Chemical Toxicology from the Polytechnic University of Catalunia (Spain). After graduating, he developed professional and scientific activity in occupational and environmental health in the Air and Occupational Health Unit of the National Institute of Health Dr. Ricardo Jorge. He also has experience in the area of quality, environment and safety management in the industry. Currently, he is an Assistant Professor at ESS|P.PORTO, teaching in the Environmental Health BSc degree program and in the Safety and Hygiene in Organizations master's degree program. He has also supervised several master's and doctoral research projects in his field. He is an integrated researcher at the RISE - Health Research Network, specifically at the Center for Translational Health and Medical Biotechnology Research (T.BIO), and a collaborator researcher at the HBMEx: Human biomonitoring for Environmental Exposure and Risk Lab from ITR. He has been developing research on topics related to occupational health and safety, indoor environments and OSHE management, of which results have been awarded. He is the author of several publications, articles published in international journals with peer reviews, book chapters, and full articles in international indexed conference proceedings. He also has several communications that have been presented at national and international conferences.

Joana Carvalho dos Santos

Joana Carvalho dos Santos is currently a Professor at the Environmental Health Department of the School of Health, Polytechnic University of Porto (ESS|P. PORTO). She is presently the coordinator of the Bachelor's degree in Environmental Health and the President of the Pedagogical Council of ESS|P.PORTO. She is also a researcher at the Center for Translational Health and Medical Biotechnology Research, ESS | P. PORTO, and at the Biomechanics and Health Unit of the Institute of Science and Innovation in Mechanical and Industrial Engineering (INEGI/LAETA). She received her PhD in Occupational Health and Safety from the Faculty of Engineering, University of Porto (Cum Laude distinction), with a thesis focused on understanding the development of fatigue (including mental fatigue) in real work conditions (assembly work). Her scientific research has been developed in the domains of Ergonomics and Human Factors, Occupational Fatigue, Occupational Health, Safety and Hygiene. Currently, her main interest is the risk management and health outcomes of human–robot collaboration (HRC) workplaces. She has been a principal investigator and team member in several research projects (e.g., WINWORL [Interreg fund]; ActionSAFE [FCT funded], ASA [Contract funded], NeoNoise, PELE project, COBOSHe, among others) and has published papers in international peer-reviewed journals, book chapters, and conference proceedings. Over the years, her research has been awarded, and in 2023 her scientific merit was publicly recognized by the Polytechnic University of Porto through the PAPRE program. She has also supervised and co-supervised several MSc and PhD theses.

Cristiana Maria Matos da Costa Pereira

Cristiana Maria Matos da Costa Pereira is a researcher with expertise in environmental health, microbiology, toxicology, and public health. She graduated in Biology from the University of Porto in 1998 and obtained her PhD in Metabolism—Clinic and Experimentation from the Faculty of Medicine of the University of Porto in 2017, with distinction, with a thesis on oxidative stress and DNA damage as contributors to inflammatory bowel disease. She was an Auxiliary Researcher at the National Institute of Health Dr. Ricardo Jorge (INSA) and currently works at the Environmental Hygiene and Human Biological Monitoring Unit, Department of Health Protection from Laboratoire National de Santé (Luxembourg), and has been an integrated researcher at the Institute of Public Health of the University of Porto (ISPUP) since 2012. Her career includes previous roles in clinical microbiology, quality control, and virology research. Her scientific activity spans a broad range of topics, with a particular focus on indoor air quality and its impact on respiratory health, microbiological risk assessment, the development of self-disinfecting surfaces, and the role of oxidative stress and DNA damage in chronic diseases. She has published more than 30 peer-reviewed articles in specialized journals and contributed as co-author to numerous collaborative studies with national and international partners. She has also supervised master's and doctoral research projects. Cristiana has been actively involved in national and European research projects, including participation in COST Actions and international scientific networks, enhancing the dissemination and impact of her work. She has received several distinctions for her research, notably the Arnaldo Sampaio Award for the best public health investigation in Portugal (2014–2016) and the Young Investigator Award in 2005.

Preface

This Reprint brings together contributions that address the complex interactions between occupational and environmental health, with the shared goal of promoting safe and sustainable living and working conditions. Its scope spans diverse contexts, from industrial settings to community environments, highlighting both traditional hazards and emerging risks that affect human well-being.

The purpose of this Reprint is to provide readers with an integrated view of how scientific evidence can inform practice and policy in order to reduce exposures, prevent disease, and foster resilience. Motivated by the growing convergence of occupational and environmental challenges, the collection underscores the value of cross-disciplinary perspectives, innovative research, and applied solutions.

The Reprint is intended for a broad audience, including researchers, practitioners, and policymakers who are engaged in public health, and environmental and occupational health and safety. It may also serve as a reference for educators and students seeking to understand the evolving landscape of risks and interventions in this field.

By gathering these studies under a unified framework, we hope to contribute to a better understanding of how shared determinants of health can be addressed collectively, and to inspire new collaborations that strengthen the link between evidence and action.

Carlos Alberto Alves Carvalhais, Joana Carvalho dos Santos, and Cristiana Maria Matos da Costa Pereira
Guest Editors

environments MDPI

Editorial

Healthy and Safe Environments Across Occupational and Environmental Contexts: A Holistic Perspective

Carlos Carvalhais [1,2,*], Cristiana C. Pereira [2,3,4] and Joana Santos [1,5]

1 RISE-Health, Center for Translational Health and Medical Biotechnology Research (TBIO), ESS, Polytechnic of Porto, Rua Doutor António Bernardino de Almeida, No. 400, 4200-072 Porto, Portugal; jds@ess.ipp.pt
2 ITR/EPIUnit—Instituto de Saúde Pública, Universidade do Porto, Rua das Taipas, No. 135, 4050-600 Porto, Portugal; cristiana.costapereira@lns.etat.lu
3 Environmental Hygiene and Human Biological Monitoring Unit, Department of Health Protection, Laboratoire National de Santé, 1, rue Louis Rech, Dudelange, L-3555 Luxembourg, Luxembourg
4 Environmental Health Department, National Institute of Health, Rua Alexandre Herculano, No. 321, 4000-055 Porto, Portugal
5 Associated Laboratory for Energy, Transports and Aeronautics (PROA/LAETA), Faculty of Engineering, University of Porto, 4200-465 Porto, Portugal
* Correspondence: caa@ess.ipp.pt

Introduction

According to the World Health Organization (WHO), "good health depends on clean air, a stable climate, and a preserved natural environment, as well as access to adequate water, sanitation, and hygiene. It also requires protection from harmful radiation, unsafe chemical management, and unhealthy working conditions. A healthy environment could prevent nearly a quarter of the global disease burden" [1]. In line with this, environmental health is defined as the science that "addresses all the physical, chemical, and biological factors external to a person, and all the related factors impacting behaviors. It encompasses the assessment and control of those environmental factors that can potentially affect health. It is targeted towards preventing disease and creating health-supportive environments" [2].

Complementing this perspective, occupational health is defined as "an area of work in public health to promote and maintain the highest degree of physical, mental, and social well-being of workers in all occupations" [3]. Achieving safe and healthy workplaces requires sustained interaction between scientific evidence and policymaking. To illustrate this, the International Labour Organization (ILO) and the WHO outline five major categories of occupational risks: biological; physical; ergonomics and work design; psychosocial factors and job-related stress; and chemical hazards [4].

In recent years, however, shifts in the nature of work have generated new risks that impact both physical and mental health, while also deepening health inequalities within and between nations [5]. Although occupational health historically developed as a separate domain from environmental health, growing evidence highlights their convergence. In many cases, hazards in the workplace and in the general environment stem from the same sources, making common approaches to risk control both feasible and effective [6,7]. Indeed, environmental and occupational health hazards—whether biological, chemical, physical (including radiological), biomechanical, or psychosocial—share the potential to cause severe consequences, from injuries and acute toxic exposures to chronic conditions such as cancer, respiratory, and cardiovascular diseases [6,7].

The convergence of these challenges has never been more evident. Climate change, industrial development, and urbanization have intensified exposures that affect not only workers but also entire communities, underscoring the urgency of integrated approaches to environmental and occupational health [8]. This Special Issue, "Healthy and Safe Environments across Occupational and Environmental Contexts", was conceived as a timely response to these challenges—aiming to promote a cross-sectoral dialogue and evidence-based strategies for protecting human health in a wide variety of settings.

This Special Issue is a valuable opportunity to reflect on the overarching theme and to share our perspective as Guest Editors. Our primary intention was to provide a platform for advancing research that bridges the boundaries between occupational safety and environmental health. We encouraged submissions that embraced innovation, explored interconnections across disciplines, and addressed real-world complexities in exposure assessment, risk communication, health promotion, and policy design.

We are pleased to present eight high-quality contributions that illustrate the thematic richness and relevance of this Special Issue.

Several papers deepen our understanding of the subtle, long-term health effects of environmental pollutants. In their umbrella review, Fiore et al. examine the link between air pollution and breast cancer, revealing consistent associations with NO_2 and particulate matter exposures and reinforcing the urgency of integrating cancer prevention strategies into environmental health policy. Similarly, Badanta et al. focus on sustainability in healthcare systems, highlighting hospitals not only as care providers but also as potential sources of environmental degradation. Their review proposes pathways toward greener, more resilient healthcare infrastructure.

Two other studies explore the implications of endocrine-disrupting chemicals (EDCs) on women's health. Moon et al. present a prospective cohort study linking EDC exposure to perinatal depression, while Caporossi et al. provide case–control evidence of associations between phthalates, bisphenol A, and infertility, particularly in relation to endocrine dysfunction and recurrent pregnancy loss. These studies remind us that environmental exposures are intimately connected to reproductive and mental health, and that vulnerable populations—especially women—require targeted protection.

The occupational dimension of this Special Issue is equally compelling. In an industrial context, Carvalhais et al. identify stress vulnerability and perceived occupational noise as significant predictors of burnout, calling for integrated psychosocial and physical risk management approaches. Worker safety in highly specialized environments is addressed by Flori et al., who examine the unique exposure risks in high-field nuclear magnetic resonance spectroscopy laboratories—a less studied but growing concern in scientific and research institutions.

Health promotion is also explored from an organizational and cultural perspective. Garzillo et al. assesses the adherence to healthy lifestyles among young workers in a Mediterranean context and underscores the need for differentiated interventions, particularly addressing nutritional education and gender-sensitive approaches to physical activity, to improve long-term well-being and reduce health risks. Meanwhile, Saccardo et al. presents a retrospective study examining the relationship between air quality and Ear, Nose, and Throat (ENT) emergencies during the COVID-19 pandemic, revealing the persistent impact of environmental factors even amid heightened public health protections.

Altogether, the studies featured in this Special Issue illustrate the diversity of environmental and occupational contexts, the variety of health outcomes they affect, and the range of scientific methodologies being applied to study them. What binds them together is a shared recognition: that ensuring healthy and safe environments requires interdisciplinary collaboration, systems thinking, and a proactive approach to both research and intervention.

Looking forward, we recommend that future research continue to explore synergistic effects across occupational and environmental exposures, particularly in underrepresented populations and emerging sectors. It is also essential to strengthen surveillance systems and harmonize exposure assessment methodologies to enable comparability and to support effective policy implementation. Bridging the gap between scientific evidence and actionable policy must remain a key priority. We hope this Special Issue will serve as a reference and stimulus for both established and early-career researchers committed to advancing health, equity, and sustainability across disciplines.

Conflicts of Interest: The authors declare no conflict of interest.

List of Contributions:

1. Badanta, B.; Porcar Sierra, A.; Fernández, S.T.; Rodríguez Muñoz, F.J.; Pérez-Jiménez, J.M.; Gonzalez-Cano-Caballero, M.; Ruiz-Adame, M.; de-Diego-Cordero, R. Advancing Environmental Sustainability in Healthcare: Review on Perspectives from Health Institutions. *Environments* **2025**, *12*, 9. https://doi.org/10.3390/environments12010009.
2. Fiore, M.; Palella, M.; Ferroni, E.; Miligi, L.; Portaluri, M.; Marchese, C.A.; Mensi, C.; Civitelli, S.; Tanturri, G.; Mangia, C. Air Pollution and Breast Cancer Risk: An Umbrella Review. *Environments* **2025**, *12*, 153. https://doi.org/10.3390/environments12050153.
3. Moon, N.; Heo, S.J.; Kim, J.H. Associations of Exposure to 24 Endocrine-Disrupting Chemicals with Perinatal Depression and Lifestyle Factors: A Prospective Cohort Study in Korea. *Environments* **2025**, *12*, 15. https://doi.org/10.3390/environments12010015.
4. Caporossi, L.; Viganò, P.; Paci, E.; Capanna, S.; Alteri, A.; De Rosa, M.; Pigini, D.; Partenzi, E.; Papaleo, B. Evidence About the Possible Role of Phthalates and Bisphenol A in Recurrent Pregnancy Loss and Endocrine Dysfunctions: A Case–Control Study. *Environments* **2025**, *12*, 38. https://doi.org/10.3390/environments12020038.
5. Flori, A.; Acri, G.; D'Avanzo, M.A.; Mattozzi, M.; Hartwig, V. Worker Safety in High-Field NMR Spectroscopy Laboratories: Challenges and Risk Assessment. *Environments* **2025**, *12*, 113. https://doi.org/10.3390/environments12040113.
6. Garzillo, E.M.; Corvino, A.R.; Porciello, G.; Guida, D.; Spasiano, M.; Miraglia, N.; Lamberti, M. Young Workers and Lifestyles in a Mediterranean Cultural Context: What Is the Contribution of Occupational Health Promotion? *Environments* **2025**, *12*, 147. https://doi.org/10.3390/environments12050147.
7. Saccardo, T.; Masetto, E.; Biancoli, E.; Colombo, A.R.; Daloiso, A.; Deretti, A.; Benvegnù, F.; Crivellaro, M.A.; Marani, M.; Nicolai, P.; et al. Impact of Environmental Pollutants on Otorhinolaryngological Emergencies in the COVID-19 Era. *Environments* **2025**, *12*, 115. https://doi.org/10.3390/environments12040115.
8. Carvalhais, C.; Ribeiro, L.A.; Pereira, C.C. Unveiling Stress Vulnerability and Occupational Noise Perception as Burnout Predictors: Results of an Exploratory Study in Industrial Environments. *Environments* **2025**, *12*, 208. https://doi.org/10.3390/environments12060208.

References

1. World Health Organization. Health Topics: Environmental Health. 2025. Available online: https://www.who.int/health-topics/environmental-health#tab=tab_1 (accessed on 28 July 2025).
2. Bircher, J.; Kuruvilla, S. Defining health by addressing individual, social, and environmental determinants: New opportunities for health care and public health. *J. Public Health Policy* **2014**, *35*, 363–386. [CrossRef]
3. World Health Organization. Health Topics: Occupational Health. 2025. Available online: https://www.who.int/health-topics/occupational-health (accessed on 28 July 2025).
4. Xu, H.; Zhang, M.; Hudson, A. Occupational Health Protection for Health Workers in China with Lessons Learned from the UK: Qualitative Interview and Policy Analysis. *Saf. Health Work* **2021**, *12*, 304–310. [CrossRef]
5. Pega, F.; Momen, N.C.; Abubakar, A.H.A.; Al-Emam, R.; Hassan, M.N.; Howard, J.; Hussein, S.H.; Iavicoli, S.; Kevi, S.K.; Kgalamono, S.M.; et al. Monitoring Workers' Health: Focus on Rights, Determinants, and Equity. *Lancet* **2023**, *402*, 1306–1308. [CrossRef]
6. Tulchinsky, T.H.; Varavikova, E.A. Environmental and Occupational Health. In *The New Public Health*, 3rd ed.; Academic Press: San Diego, CA, USA, 2014; pp. 471–533. [CrossRef]

7. Yassi, A.; Kjellström, T. Linkages Between Environmental and Occupational Health. In *Environmental Health Hazards (Part VII)*; International Labour Organization ILO Encyclopaedia of Occupational Health and Safety: Geneva, Switzerland, 2011; Section "Linkages Between Environmental and Occupational Health".
8. Costello, A.; Abbas, M.; Allen, A.; Ball, S.; Bell, S.; Bellamy, R.; Friel, S.; Groce, N.; Johnson, A.; Kett, M.; et al. Managing the Health Effects of Climate Change. *Lancet* **2009**, *373*, 1693–1733. [CrossRef] [PubMed]

environments

MDPI

Systematic Review

Air Pollution and Breast Cancer Risk: An Umbrella Review

Maria Fiore [1,2], Marco Palella [2,3,*], Eliana Ferroni [2,4], Lucia Miligi [2,5], Maurizio Portaluri [6], Cristiana Alessandra Marchese [2,7], Carolina Mensi [2,8], Serenella Civitelli [2,9], Gabriella Tanturri [2,7] and Cristina Mangia [2,10,*]

1 Department of Medical, Surgical Sciences and Advanced Technologies "G.F. Ingrassia", University of Catania, 95123 Catania, Italy; mfiore@unict.it
2 Gender Epidemiology Working Group, AIE—Associazione Italiana di Epidemiologia, 00147 Rome, Italy; eliana.ferroni@azero.veneto.it (E.F.); carolina.mensi@unimi.it (C.M.); serenella.civitelli@unisi.it (S.C.)
3 Medical Specialization School in Hygiene and Preventive Medicine, 95123 Catania, Italy
4 Epidemiological Service Veneto Region, 35131 Padua, Italy
5 Institute for Cancer Research, Prevention and Clinical Network (ISPRO) Foundation, 50139 Florence, Italy
6 SC Radioterapy, ASST Papa Giovanni XXIII, 24127 Bergamo, Italy; brimapo@gmail.com
7 Italian Association of Women Doctors (Associazione Italiana Donne Medico), 10100 Turin, Italy
8 Occupational Health Unit, Fondazione IRCCS Ca' Granda Ospedale Maggiore Policlinico, 20122 Milan, Italy
9 Department of Medical, Surgical and Neuroscience Sciences, University of Siena, 53100 Siena, Italy
10 CNR ISAC, National Research Council, Institute of Sciences of Atmosphere and Climate, 73100 Lecce, Italy
* Correspondence: marco.palella@aoec.it (M.P.); cristina.mangia@cnr.it (C.M.)

Abstract: Breast cancer (BC) is a major global health challenge, responsible for one in four cancer diagnoses and one in six cancer-related deaths worldwide. It is the most frequently diagnosed cancer among women and the primary cause of cancer-related deaths in most countries. Recent studies have suggested a potential link between exposure to ambient air pollutants—such as nitrogen dioxide (NO_2) and particulate matter (PM_{10} and $PM_{2.5}$)—and an increased risk of breast cancer. However, the existing evidence remains inconclusive. This umbrella review, conducted according to PRISMA guidelines, aimed to evaluate the strength and reliability of epidemiological evidence concerning this association. All seven meta-analyses included in this review reported a relative risk greater than 1 for exposure to the three pollutants, though findings varied in terms of heterogeneity and publication bias. Notably, the overall analysis indicates that exposure to both NO_2 and $PM_{2.5}$ may be associated with an increased risk of breast cancer incidence, while the evidence linking $PM_{2.5}$ exposure to breast cancer mortality appears to be weaker. The most vulnerable groups were identified as premenopausal European women exposed to NO_2 and PM_{10}, as well as individuals in developed countries exposed to $PM_{2.5}$. Further research is necessary to examine PM composition and refine exposure assessment methodology. Given the widespread impact of breast cancer as the most common invasive malignancy, incorporating this outcome into environmental health research on air pollution is essential. A clearer understanding of these associations could support more targeted environmental interventions. Importantly, the available evidence suggests that breast cancer prevention can be addressed not only through personal lifestyle changes but also through broad public health policies focused on reducing NO_2, PM_{10} and $PM_{2.5}$ levels.

Keywords: air pollution; female breast cancer; particulate matter; nitrogen dioxide

1. Introduction

Breast cancer (BC) continues to represent a significant public health concern due to its high prevalence, accounting for roughly 11.6% of all cancer diagnoses worldwide [1,2]. The development of BC is influenced by a complex interplay of factors, as there are several types of breast cancer, each with different pathophysiological mechanisms [3,4]. Epidemiological studies have reported various risk factors associated with the development or progression of BC. These include hereditary and genetic factors, such as an individual or family history of BC and/or ovarian cancer, and inherited mutations (i.e., BRCA1, BRCA2, and other BC susceptibility genes). Other important risk factors include early age at menarche, late age at menopause, nulliparity, late age at first birth, obesity, and smoking [5,6], while breastfeeding and physical activity are recognized as protective factors [7–9]. Additionally, the International Agency for Research on Cancer (IARC) has highlighted some environmental and lifestyle-related risk factors, such as alcohol consumption, diethylstilbestrol exposure, hormonal therapies (including combined estrogen–progestin contraceptives and menopausal treatments), and ionizing radiation (X-rays and gamma rays) [10]. Recent studies have increasingly associated environmental pollutants—particularly endocrine-disrupting chemicals (EDCs) like dioxins and phthalates—with early breast development, breastfeeding difficulties, and a heightened risk of breast cancer due to their ability to interfere with the endocrine system and mammary gland development [11–15].

An emerging area of investigation is the potential relationship between ambient air pollution and breast cancer. While current findings vary across studies [16–25], a notable increase in BC cases in U.S. women between 1986 and 2002 has been partly attributed to greater exposure to emissions from traffic and industrial sources [26]. The biological plausibility of a potential connection between air pollution and BC is supported by the International Agency for Research on Cancer (IARC)'s classification of outdoor air pollution as a human carcinogen [27]. Given that approximately 80% of the global urban population is exposed to air pollution levels that exceed the recommended limits set by the World Health Organization (WHO) [28], further exploration of this potential association is crucial. Research has primarily concentrated on three pollutants—nitrogen dioxide (NO_2), and particulate matter (PM_{10} and $PM_{2.5}$)—as potential contributors to BC risk. This work aims to systematically assess the available literature using the umbrella review approach, which synthesizes findings from existing reviews to clarify areas of agreement, identify methodological limitations, and highlight directions for future investigation [29,30].

2. Materials and Methods

2.1. *Umbrella Review Methods*

Umbrella reviews, as described by Aromataris et al. [29], aggregate and re-analyze findings from existing systematic reviews to identify potential biases, areas of consensus, and gaps in the literature. As noted by Fusar-Poli [30], this approach offers a higher-level synthesis that enhances the interpretation and relevance of evidence, supporting more informed clinical and policy decisions.

The current umbrella review was conducted in accordance with the Preferred Reporting Items for Systematic Reviews and Meta-Analyses (PRISMA) guidelines [31,32], in line with a priori protocol agreed upon by all authors and registered in PROSPERO (CRD42023395494).

2.2. *Objective, Inclusion Criteria, and Exclusion Criteria*

2.2.1. Review Question

This review seeks to determine whether exposure to air pollution is associated with an increased risk of BC incidence and mortality. Specifically, it examines the potential association between BC risk and exposure to nitrogen dioxide (NO_2) and to particulate matter (PM_{10} and $PM_{2.5}$).

2.2.2. Objective

The primary objective of this review is to assess the quality and reliability of existing evidence pertaining to the associations between exposure to NO_2, PM_{10}, and $PM_{2.5}$ and the risk of BC incidence and mortality.

2.2.3. Inclusion Criteria

Meta-analyses investigating the association between air pollution exposure and BC incidence or mortality in women, based on observational studies, were considered. The inclusion criteria were structured according to the Population, Exposure, Comparator, and Outcome (PECO) framework. The specific PECO criteria used for selecting meta-analyses are detailed below.

Participants:

Women in the general population who are at risk of developing BC.

Exposures and comparator:

Meta-analyses considering the exposure to the three pollutants PM_{10}, $PM_{2.5}$, and NO_2, using various exposure assessment models, and comparing different concentration levels.

Outcomes:

Incidence and mortality risks reported using statistical measures such as the pooled relative risk (RR).

2.2.4. Exclusion Criteria

The following types of studies were excluded: commentary, letters, non-English language studies, studies that did not report relevant BC outcomes, and studies that did not include a meta-analysis.

A study was classified as a meta-analysis if it met the following criteria:

- It clearly detailed the methodology used for systematic review;
- It provided details on the search strategy employed;
- It identified relevant primary studies from at least one database (e.g., PubMed OR Embase);
- It performed a quality appraisal of the include primary studies.

2.3. Search Strategy and Data Extraction

A comprehensive search was conducted in the PubMed (MEDLINE) and Embase databases from inception to December 2024. The search strategy was designed around the key terms "breast cancer" and "air pollutants" and was limited to meta-analyses with a search filter in the title or abstract fields. Table S1 provides the detailed search strategy.

Study selection was independently performed by two authors (CM and CAM), ensuring a rigorous screening process, while data extraction was performed in pairs by all authors (CM and MPo, MPa and MF, LM and SC, EF and CM, and CaM and GT). Extracted data included the following variables: first author, year of publication, study design, total population, number of events, age of the participants, country, confounders, pollutant increase, effect size with the corresponding 95% confidence interval (CI), exposure models, pollutants, exposure time, heterogeneity, and publication bias. We also discuss histological type, TNM stage, hormonal receptors, and menopausal status in the selected studies. To assess the extent of overlap among primary studies listed in each review, a citation matrix was constructed, and the Corrected Covered Area (CCA) was calculated. This metric quantifies the proportion of shared studies across various meta-analyses, providing a standardized measure of redundancy [33]. The formula for the CCA is as follows:

$$CCA = (N - r)/(rc - r)$$

where N represents the total number of citations of primary studies (including repeated citations), r is the count of primary studies, and c is the number of meta-analyses considered. The CCA is then classified as minimal (<5%), moderate (5–10%), or high (>10%), based on the proportion of overlap among studies [33].

2.4. Meta-Analytical Methods Used by the Authors of the Included Studies

To ensure a thorough assessment of the methodologies employed in the meta-analyses included in this umbrella review, we examined several key aspects: stated objectives and research questions, search strategy, eligibility criteria, data extraction process, quality assessment, statistical analysis (effect size measurement, model selection, heterogeneity, and publication bias), sensitivity analysis, registration and protocol adherence, PRISMA reporting, and ethical considerations.

2.5. Quality of Assessment

Two researchers (MP and MF) evaluated the methodological quality of each included meta-analysis using the AMSTAR 2 tool [34]. This 16-item checklist assesses key aspects of meta-analysis, with seven items, marked with an asterisk, designated as critical domains due to their significant impact on overall validity (Table S2). These items may be modified by the authors according to their perspectives on the article under review. In particular, we decided to classify domain 8 (Did the review authors describe the included studies in adequate detail) as 'critical', instead of domain 7 (Did the review authors provide a list of excluded studies and justify the exclusions?) of the original list, considering domain 8 a more appropriate measure of the quality of the studies.

Each criterion was evaluated based on whether it was fully met or only partially met. The overall assessment of methodological quality was determined by considering the extent to which criteria were satisfied. If a review exhibited multiple non-critical weaknesses, confidence in its findings was considered lower, which could result in a reclassification from moderate to low confidence. The confidence ratings are summarized in Table 1 [34].

Table 1. Rating overall confidence in the results of the review [34].

Rating	Description
High	No or one non-critical weakness: the meta-analysis provides an accurate and comprehensive summary of the results of the available studies that address the question of interest.
Moderate	More than one non-critical weakness *: the meta-analysis has more than one weakness but no critical flaws; it may provide an accurate summary of the results of the available studies that were included in the review.
Low	One critical flaw with or without non-critical weaknesses: the review has a critical flaw and may not provide an accurate and comprehensive summary of the available studies that address the question of interest.
Critically low	More than one critical flaw with or without non-critical weaknesses: the review has more than one critical flaw and should not be relied on to provide an accurate and comprehensive summary of the available studies.

* Multiple non-critical weaknesses diminish confidence in the review, and it is appropriate to move the overall appraisal down from moderate to low confidence.

2.6. Evaluation of the Strength of Evidence

The strength of the evidence was initially classified into four categories—strong, moderate, modest, and weak—based primarily on the percentage of meta-analyses reporting positive associations, grouped as follows: strong: ≥75%; moderate: ≥50–75%; modest: ≥25–50%; and weak: <25% [35].

This initial classification was then subject to potential downgrading by 1 level based on 3 additional criteria: number of cases (less or greater than 1000); level of heterogeneity, measured using the I^2 statistic (with thresholds at 40%, 60%, and 80% for increasing heterogeneity); and presence of publication bias, assessed via Egger's test ($p > 0.10$ = low risk; $p = 0.05–0.10$ = moderate risk; and $p < 0.05$ = high risk) or using the trim-and-fill method. Criteria are summarized in Table 2.

Table 2. Criteria used to evaluate the strength of evidence.

Evidence	Positive Association	Cases	Heterogeneity I^2	Publication Bias
Strong	≥75%	>1000	0–40%	Absent: Egger's test $p > 0.10$ or Negligible difference in case of trim-and-fill
Moderate	≥50–75%	>1000	41–60%	Possible: Egger's test $p = 0.05–<0.10$
Modest	≥25–<50%	<1000	61–80%	High: Egger's test $p \leq 0.05$
Weak	0–<25%	<1000	81–100%	High: Egger's test $p \leq 0.05$

The strength of the association was based on the pooled relative risks (RRs) from multiple meta-analyses and classified as follows: very strong (RR > 5), strong (RR > 2), moderate (RR > 1.5), modest (RR > 1.2), and weak (RR > 1). In accordance with the American Statistical Association's recommendations, a positive relative risk (RR) with a lower confidence interval limit between 0.70 and 1.00 was considered a potential trend warranting further investigation [36–38].

3. Results

3.1. Search Strategy Outcome

The complete process of article collection, screening, and eligibility assessment is shown in Figure 1. The initial search identified 40 studies. After eliminating duplicates, 34 studies remained and were screened based on their title and abstract. Of these, 15 were excluded for not meeting the inclusion criteria, leaving 19 full-text articles that were considered potentially eligible for inclusion. Of these, eight studies were not meta-analyses, one study was a mapping review, two studies had no inherent topic, and one study had no data stratified for sex. Finally, seven meta-analyses were included in this umbrella review: [39–45]. Excluded articles and the reasons for exclusion are reported in Table S3.

3.2. Quality Assessment and Bias

The seven studies evaluated received scores ranging from 10.5 to 14 based on the number of positive/yes ratings. Specifically, five studies were classified as having "moderate" quality, one as "low" quality, and another as "critically low" quality (Table 3). Additionally, all confounding factors considered within each study were analyzed and systematically categorized (Table S4). Regarding publication bias, Gabet et al., 2021 [39], Guo et al., 2021 [40], and Wei et al., 2021 [43] used a funnel plot, an Egger's test and trim-and-fill analysis to investigate publication bias. Zhang et al., 2019 [41], Praud et al., 2023 [44], and Arif et al., 2024 [45] used a funnel plot and an Egger's test, while Yu et al., 2021 [42] used only a funnel plot.

3.3. Associations Between NO_2, PM_{10}, and $PM_{2.5}$ Exposure and Breast Cancer

Tables 4 and 5 summarize the key characteristics of the seven studies examining the associations between exposure to these three pollutants and breast cancer incidence and mortality, respectively. Table S5 summarizes the primary studies included in each meta-analysis for individual pollutants and outcomes, along with their corresponding CCA index. Tables S6–S8 provide a summary of the increases in pollutant levels, the exposure assessment models used, sensitivity analyses, heterogeneity, and potential publication bias for the meta-analyses included in this umbrella review, categorized by NO_2, $PM_{2.5}$, and PM_{10}, respectively.

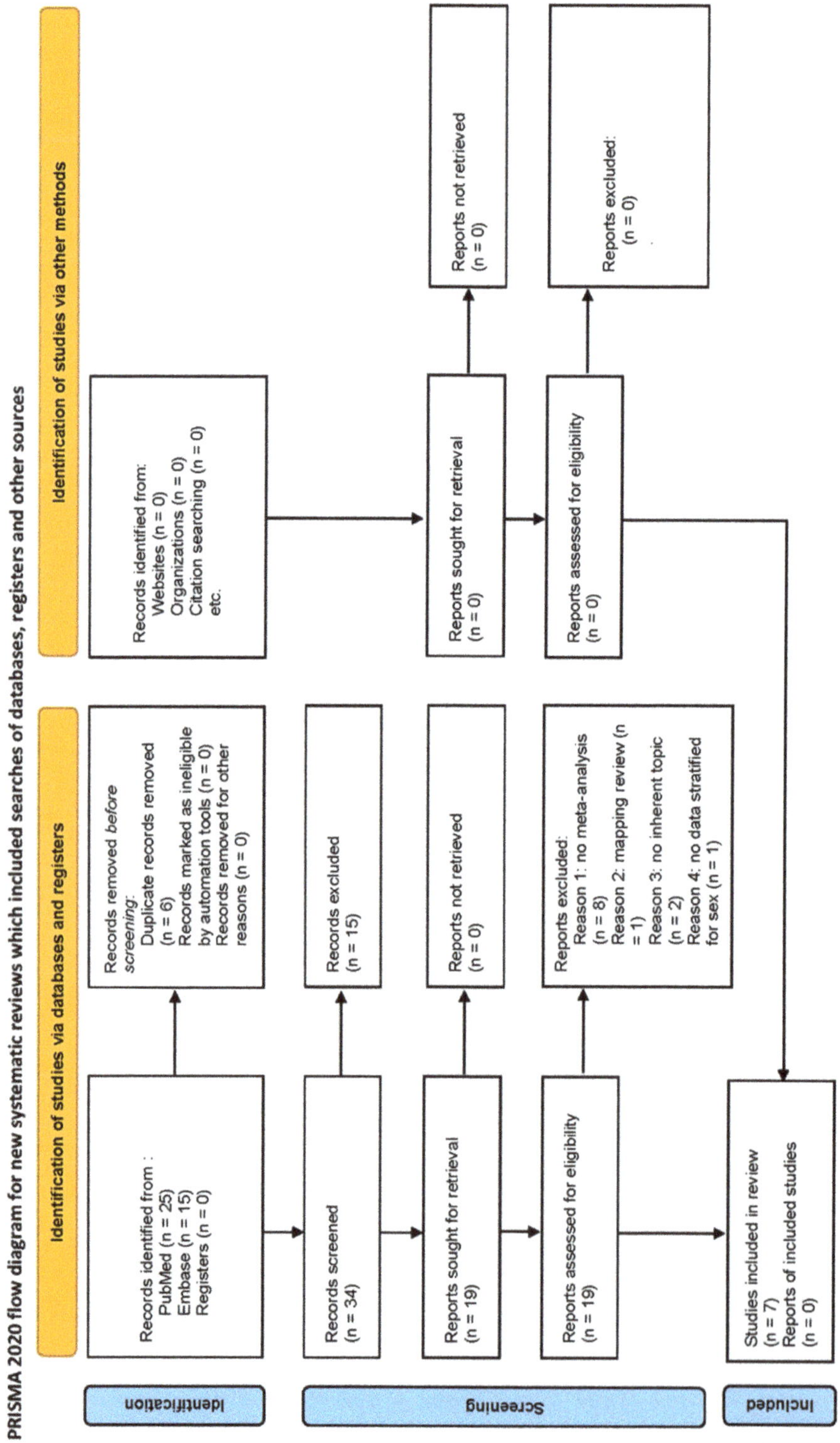

Figure 1. PRISMA flow chart describing the selection of included articles. Adapted by Page et al. 2021 [32].

Table 3. Quality assessment and risk of bias in meta-analysis using AMSTAR 2 [34].

	Gabet et al., 2021 [39]	Guo et al., 2021 [40]	Zhang et al., 2019 [41]	Yu et al., 2021 [42]	Wei et al., 2021 [43]	Praud et al., 2023 [44]	Arif et al., 2024 [45]
1. Did the research questions and inclusion criteria for the review include the components of PICO/PECOS?	Yes	Yes	Yes	Yes	Yes	Yes	Yes
2. * Did the report of the review contain an explicit statement that the review methods were established prior to the conduct of the review and did the report justify any significant deviations from the protocol?	Yes	Yes	Yes	Partial Yes	Yes	Yes	Partial Yes
3. Did the review authors explain their selection of the study designs for inclusion in the review?	Yes	No	Yes	Yes	Yes	Yes	Yes
4. * Did the review authors use a comprehensive literature search strategy?	No	Yes	Yes	Yes	Yes	Yes	Yes
5. Did the review authors perform study selection in duplicate?	Yes	No	No	Yes	Yes	Yes	Yes
6. Did the review authors perform data extraction in duplicate?	No	Yes	Yes	Yes	No	No	No
7. Did the review authors provide a list of excluded studies and justify the exclusions?	No	No	No	No	No	No	No
8. * Did the review authors describe the included studies in adequate detail?	Yes	Yes	Yes	Yes	Yes	Yes	Yes
9. * Did the review authors use a satisfactory technique for assessing the risk of bias (RoB) in individual studies that were included in the review?	Yes	Yes	Yes	Yes	Yes	Yes	Yes
10. Did the review authors report on the sources of funding for the studies included in the review?	Yes	Yes	Yes	Yes	Yes	No	No
11. * If meta-analysis was performed, did the review authors use appropriate methods for statistical combination of results?	Yes	Yes	Yes	Yes	Yes	Yes	Yes
12. * If meta-analysis was performed, did the review authors assess the potential impact of RoB in individual studies on the results of the meta-analysis or other evidence synthesis?	Yes	Yes	Yes	Yes	Yes	Yes	No
13. * Did the review authors account for RoB in primary studies when interpreting/discussing the results of the review?	Yes	Yes	Yes	Yes	Yes	Yes	No
14. Did the review authors provide a satisfactory explanation for, and discussion of, any heterogeneity observed in the results of the review?	Yes	Yes	Yes	No	Yes	Yes	Yes
15. * If they performed quantitative synthesis, did the review authors carry out an adequate investigation of publication bias (small study bias) and discuss its likely impact on the results of the review?	Yes	Yes	Yes	Yes	Yes	Yes	Yes
16. Did the review authors report any potential sources of conflict of interest, including any funding they received for conducting the review?	No	No	No	No	No	Yes	Yes
Total of yes	13/16 (81.2%)	13/16 (81.2%)	14/16 (87.5%)	14/16 (87.5%)	14/16 (87.5%)	13/16 (81.2%)	10.5/16
Rating overall confidence	Low	Moderate	Moderate	Moderate	Moderate	Moderate	Critically low

The domains considered critical are identified using an asterisk.

Table 4. Associations between NO_2, PM_{10}, and $PM_{2.5}$ exposure and BC incidence.

Pollutant	Author, Year	Design of Included Studies	Total Population	Age (Years)	Country	Effect Size RR (95% CI)	Heterogeneity I^2 *	Publication Bias **
NO_2	Gabet et al., 2021 [39]	6 cohort, 4 case-control	3,914,690	25–75	1 Germany, 2 Sweden, 5 Canada, 2 Denmark, 2 France, 1 Netherlands, 1 UK, 1 Spain, 2 Italy, 1 Norway, 2 USA, 1 Austria	1.03 (1.01–1.05)	24	0.018
	Wei et al., 2021 [43]	11 cohort, 3 case-control	4,002,546	35–85	3 Denmark, 4 USA, 1 Europe, 1 Germany, 1 Israel, 5 Canada	1.02 (1.01–1.04)	46.8	0.024
	Praud et al., 2023 [44]	8 cohort, 5 case-control	128,618	Not reported	3 USA, 5 Canada, 1 Denmark, 2 France, 1 Germany, 1 Europe	1.02 (1.00–1.03)	16.9	0.27
PM_{10}	Zhang et al., 2019 [41]	8 cohort	592,369	25–65+	5 USA, 2 Denmark, 1 Netherlands, 1 UK, 1 Italy, 1 Norway, 1 Germany	1.05 (0.98–1.12)	72.7	Not Reported
	Yu et al., 2021 [42]	4 cohort	2,107,018	0–90	1 Denmark, 1 USA, 1 Germany	1.05 (0.93–1.19)	68	0.030
	Gabet et al., 2021 [39]	1 case-control, 5 cohort	1,326,524	0–90	1 France, 1 Germany, 1 Sweden, 2 Denmark, 1 Netherlands, 1 UK, 1 Italy, 1 Norway, 3 USA, 1 Austria	1.06 (0.99–1.13)	27.6	0.41
	Guo et al., 2021 [40]	1 case-control, 8 cohort	2,552,761	0–90	5 USA, 1 Canada, 2 Denmark, 1 Italy	1.03 (0.98–1.09)	65.1	0.009
	Wei et al., 2021 [43]	7 cohort	2,290,241	0–90	4 USA, 1 Germany, 1 Denmark, 1 Europe	1.04 (0.98–1.10)	70.3	0.06
	Arif et al., 2024 [45]	10	Not reported	Not reported	4 Europe, 4 Americas	1.14 (0.97–1.30)	84.0	0.00
$PM_{2.5}$	Yu et al., 2021 [42]	6 cohort	2,871,705	25–85	1 Denmark, 1 USA, 3 Canada	1.03 (0.93–1.13)	63	0.020
	Wei et al., 2021 [43]	11 cohort	11,755,200	0–90	2 Denmark, 6 USA, 1 Europe (Sweden, Norway, Italy, UK, Netherlands, Austria), 3 Canada	1.03 (0.99–1.06)	8.2	0.00023
	Gabet et al., 2021 [39]	1 case-control, 6 cohort	2,848,486	25–85	1 France, 1 Sweden, 2 Canada, 2 Denmark, 1 Netherlands, 1 UK, 1 Italy, 1 Norway, 3 USA, 1 Austria	1.01 (0.93–1.11)	37.4	0.72
	Guo et al., 2021 [40]	11 cohort, 1 case-control, 1 ecological, 1 cross-sectional	6,643,972	25–85	7 USA, 2 Canada, 2 China, 2 Denmark, 1 Italy, 1 Japan	1.04 (0.98–1.10)	17,4	0,293
	Zhang et al., 2019 [41]	11 cohort, 2 ecological	994,551	25–>65	1 Canada, 6 USA, 1 Sweden, 2 Denmark, 1 Netherlands, 1 UK, 1 Austria, 1 France, 3 Italy, 1 Spain, 1 Germany, 1 China, 1 Puerto Rico, 1 Taiwan, 1 Japan	1.02 (0.93–1.11)	30.6	0.218
	Arif et al., 2024 [45]	14	Not reported	Not reported	4 Europe, 7 Americas	1.05 (0.98–1.12)	55.7	0.00

* I^2 test interpretation: 0–40%: might not be important, 41–60%: may be moderate, 61–80%: may be substantial, 81–100%: may be considerable. ** Egger's test *p*-value: *p*-value < 0.05 indicates the presence of publication bias.

Table 5. Associations between PM_{10} and $PM_{2.5}$ exposure and BC mortality.

Pollutant	Author, Year	Study Design	Total Population (nr)	Cases	Age (Years)	Country	Effect Size RR (95% CI)	Heterogeneity I^2 *	Publication Bias **
$PM_{2.5}$	Yu et al., 2021 [42]	4 cohort	756,393	7895	0–90	3 USA, 1 Hong Kong	1.18 (0.81–1.73)	70	0.02
	Zhang et al., 2019 [41]	5 cohort, 2 ecological	913,779	5439	25–65+	1 Canada, 6 USA, 1 Sweden, 2 Denmark, 1 Netherlands, 1 UK, 1 Austria, 1 France, 3 Italy, 1 Spain, 1 Germany, 1 China, 1 Puerto Rico, 1 Taiwan, 1 Japan	1.17 (1.05–1.30)	73.1	0.122
	Guo et al., 2021 [40]	3 cohort, 1 case-control, 1 ecological, 1 cross-sectional	692,257	51,661	25 to 85	7 USA, 2 Canada, 2 China, 2 Denmark, 1 Italy, 1 Japan	1.20 (0.92–1.48)	52.5	0.12
	Arif et al., 2024 [45]	Not reported	Not reported	Not reported	Not reported	Not reported	1.17 (1.07–1.27)	55.2	0.04
PM_{10}	Zhang et al., 2019 [41]	cohort/case-control	264,064		25–55+	USA	1.11 (1.02–1.21)	0.0	
	Guo et al., 2021 [40]	cohort/case-control	264,064		25–55+	USA	1.07 (0.93–1.20)	56.4	Not NA

* I^2 test interpretation: 0–40%: might not be important, 41–60%: may be moderate, 61–80%: may be substantial, 81–100%: may be considerable. ** Egger's test *p*-value: *p*-value < 0.05 indicates the presence of publication bias.

3.3.1. NO_2 Exposure and BC Incidence

The association between NO_2 exposure and BC incidence is addressed in only three of the seven selected studies: Gabet et al. [39], Wei et al. [43], and Praud et al. [44]. All three studies reported a positive association with relative risks (RRs) of 1.03 (95% CI: 1.01–1.05), 1.02 (95% CI: 1.02–1.04), and 1.015 (95% CI: 1.003–1.028), respectively, per 10 $\mu g/m^3$ NO_2 increase. The meta-analyses included 16 primary studies [46–61] showing a very high level of overlap (CCA = 66%) [33] and heterogeneity ranging from 16% to 46.8%.

Wei et al. [43] conducted four subgroup analyses based on study design, geographical region, menopausal status, and estrogen/progesterone receptor (ER/PR) status. Risk was higher in case-control studies and among Asian populations. No differences in risk were observed based on hormonal receptor status. In other subgroup analyses, risk estimates remained unchanged, while heterogeneity was lower among studies conducted in North America and Europe, as well as in postmenopausal women and receptor-positive and receptor-negative groups. Gabet et al. [39] also conducted multiple subgroup analyses, showing stable association across study design, population characteristics, level of adjustment, and analytical approaches. Variations emerged depending on how exposure was characterized. Risk estimates ranged from 1.01 in studies using residential history for exposure assessment to 1.06 in studies involving participants recruited from 2000 onward and were higher in premenopausal women (1.04, 95% CI 0.94–1.16). Regarding hormone receptor status, the relative risk (RR) was 1.045 (0.980–1.114) for estrogen-receptor-positive/progesterone-receptor-positive (ER+/PR+) tumors and 0.987 (0.885–1.101) for estrogen-receptor-negative/progesterone-receptor-negative (ER−/PR−) tumors. Similarly, Praud et al. [44] found an increased risk among European populations and ER+/PR+ tumors, with negligible heterogeneity. Sensitivity analyses are detailed in Table S6.

The overall findings suggest a moderate positive association between NO_2 exposure and BC incidence, despite substantial study overlap.

3.3.2. PM_{10} Exposure and BC Incidence

The association between PM_{10} exposure and BC incidence is addressed in six studies. The reported relative risks (RRs) across studies were as follows: 1.06 (95% CI: 0.99–1.13) [39], 1.03 (95% CI: 0.98–1.09) [40], 1.05 (95% CI: 0.98–1.12) [41], 1.05 (95% CI: 0.93–1.19) [42], 1.04 (95% CI: 0.98–1.10) [43], and 1.14 (95% CI: 0.97–1.30) [45]. All six meta-analyses reported a positive association with the lower confidence interval limit exceeding 0.93, well above the 0.70 threshold suggested by the American Statistical Association to indicate a positive trend [36]. The meta-analyses included nine primary studies [25,46,47,49,52,56,58,62,63] showing a very high level of overlap (CCA =56%) [33] and high heterogeneity (from 27.6% to 84.0%). Five studies conducted subgroup analyses to explore heterogeneity (Table S7). Zhang et al. [41] performed three subgroup analyses, adjusting for invasive breast cancer and estrogen/progesterone receptor status. No significant differences in risk estimates were observed, though heterogeneity decreased across all subgroups. Wei et al. [43] analyzed factors such as study design, geographic location, menopausal status, and estrogen/progesterone receptor status, with the European population showing higher risk (RR = 1.16, 95% CI: 1.07–1.25). Gabet et al. [39] performed extensive subgroup analyses, noting reductions in both risk estimates and heterogeneity when considering major reproductive factors, residential history, hormone-receptor-positive cases, menopausal status, North American cohorts, and studies using home addresses for exposure assessment. Increased heterogeneity was reported for hormone-receptor-negative cases. Studies published since 2000, and those using modelling for exposure assessment, reported higher risk estimates alongside increased heterogeneity. Guo et al. [40] observed higher risk estimates in studies with follow-up periods shorter than 11 years and greater heterogeneity in studies conducted in North America, and in those published before 2017. Arif et al. [45] reported a higher risk measure in European studies compared to those from the Americas with low heterogeneity (<0.01%). Yu et al. [42] did not perform subgroup analyses. The overall findings suggest a weak positive trend between PM_{10} exposure and BC incidence, highlighting the necessity of further research.

3.3.3. $PM_{2.5}$ Exposure and BC Incidence

The association between $PM_{2.5}$ exposure and BC incidence is addressed in six of the seven selected meta-analyses. These studies reported relative risk (RR) estimates of 1.03 (95% CI: 0.93–1.13) [39], 1.01 (95% CI: 0.93–1.11) [40], 1.042 (95% CI: 0.987–1.108) [41], 1.02 (95% CI: 0.93–1.11) [42], 1.03 (95% CI: 0.99–1.06) [43], and 1.05 (95% CI: 0.98–1.12) [45]. All studies reported a positive association, with the lower bound of the confidence interval exceeding 0.93—well above the 0.70 threshold suggested by the American Statistical Association [36]. The meta-analyses included 18 primary studies [22,25,46–49,56,58–60,62–68] showing high overlap (CCA = 38%) and heterogeneity between 8.2% and 55.7%.

Five studies conducted subgroup analyses (Table S7). Zhang et al. [41] performed three subgroup analyses, examining invasive breast cancer and estrogen/progesterone receptor status. Their results indicated similar risk estimates across subgroups, with a reduction in heterogeneity. Wei et al. [43] conducted four subgroup analyses, considering study design, geographic region, menopausal status, and receptor type. While risk estimates remained stable, heterogeneity decreased in some cases, particularly among European populations and receptor status subgroups. Gabet et al. [39] reported lower risk estimates and reduced heterogeneity for reproductive factors, residential history, hormonal status, and North American populations. Both risk estimates and heterogeneity increased in studies conducted in Europe and in those using exposure modeling and home address data. Guo et al. [40] analyzed subgroups based on follow-up duration (greater or less than 11 years), geographic region, and publication period (before or after 2017). They found no significant changes in risk estimates but observed lower heterogeneity in studies with follow-up periods exceeding 11 years, those conducted in North America, and those published before 2017. Arif et al. [45] reported lower risk estimates in the Americas but higher heterogeneity compared to Europe. Yu et al. [42] did not perform any subgroup analyses. The overall findings suggest a positive moderate potential trend between $PM_{2.5}$ exposure and BC incidence, pointing to the need for additional studies and more in-depth analysis in future work.

3.3.4. $PM_{2.5}$ Exposure and BC Mortality

The association between $PM_{2.5}$ exposure and BC mortality is addressed in only four of the seven selected studies [40–42,45]. The meta-analyses reported relative risk (RR) estimates of 1.20 (95% CI: 0.92–1.48) [40], 1.17 (95% CI: 1.05–1.30) [41], 1.18 (95% CI: 0.81–1.73) [42], and 1.17 (95% CI: 1.07–1.27) [45]. Two meta-analyses reported a positive association, with the lower bound of the confidence interval exceeding 1. In the other two studies, the lower bounds exceeded 0.81—higher than the threshold of 0.70 suggested by the American Statistical Association [36]. The meta-analyses included 10 primary studies, [49,63,69–76] with high overlap (CCA = 30%) and heterogeneity from 52.5% to 73.1%.

Subgroup analyses were conducted in only two studies [41,42] and details are reported in Table S7. Zhang et al. [41] found increased risk in cohort studies and higher exposure levels, though heterogeneity remained high (Table S4). Guo et al. [40] reported higher risk in studies with shorter follow-up periods and in developing countries, while heterogeneity increased with longer follow-up durations (>11 years), older publications, and in Asian cohorts and research from developing countries. Yu et al. [42] and Arif et al. [45] did not conduct subgroup analyses.

Overall, findings suggest a positive modest trend between $PM_{2.5}$ exposure and BC mortality, highlighting the necessity for additional studies.

3.3.5. PM_{10} Exposure and BC Mortality

Only two meta-analyses [40,41] evaluated the relationship between PM_{10} exposure and BC mortality, both including the same two primary studies [69,70], but assigning them different weights in the pooled relative risk estimates. The two meta-analyses reported an RR of 1.11 (95% CI: 1.02–1.21) with no heterogeneity (I^2 = 0%) and an RR of 1.07 (95% CI: 0.93–1.20) with moderate heterogeneity (I^2 = 56.4%), respectively. The association between PM_{10} exposure and BC mortality was classified as "weak". Guo et al. [40] performed subgroup analyses, noting higher risks with shorter follow-up periods and earlier publication dates, but found no major differences in other subgroups. Zhang et al. [41] did not perform subgroup analyses due to lack of heterogeneity. Given the limited number of studies, further investigation is needed.

4. Discussion

This umbrella review synthesizes evidence on the associations between exposure to nitrogen dioxide (NO_2), fine particulate matter ($PM_{2.5}$), and coarse particulate matter (PM_{10}) and the risk of breast cancer (BC) incidence and mortality in women. All included meta-analyses reported pooled relative risks (RRs) greater than 1 for each pollutant–outcome pair, with lower bounds of confidence intervals (CIs) exceeding 0.70, although with varying levels of heterogeneity. Among the pollutants examined, NO_2 showed sufficiently conclusive evidence of a weak positive association with BC incidence. For $PM_{2.5}$ and PM_{10}, the findings suggest a positive trend for both incidence and mortality outcomes, with the trend being more pronounced for $PM_{2.5}$ and incidence. The most vulnerable groups included premenopausal European women exposed to NO_2 and PM_{10} and individuals in developed countries exposed to $PM_{2.5}$. A recent cohort study in the U.S. study [77] found an 8% increase in estrogen-receptor-positive BC per 10 $\mu g/m^3$ increase in $PM_{2.5}$.

The carcinogenic effects of NO_2 may be driven by both direct and indirect mechanisms. NO_2 exposure has been associated with reduced DNA methylation, which can alter gene expression and contribute to genomic instability—a key factor in cancer progression [78]. Epigenomic studies have identified lower DNA methylation levels in blood samples years before BC diagnosis [79]. Additionally, as a major component of vehicle emissions and other high-temperature fossil fuel combustion, NO_2 can be a marker of traffic-related and industrial air pollution, including harmful substances like heavy metals, PAHs, and benzene, which have known genotoxic, mutagenic, and endocrine-disrupting effects [80–88], supporting the association between NO_2 exposure and breast cancer risk. Accordingly, the IARC classifies diesel emissions as carcinogenic (Group 1) and gasoline exhaust as possibly carcinogenic (Group 2B) [89]. The carcinogenic potential of particulate matter (PM) is less defined due to variations in composition and particle size, which depend on emission sources and regional air quality [90]. Certain PM components—black carbon, elemental carbon, and sulfates—are recognized as risk factors [65,91,92], along with airborne metals like mercury, cadmium, and lead, which are linked to increased postmenopausal BC risk [93–95].

Epidemiological and toxicological studies suggest two key mechanisms for PM-related cancer risk: (1) oxidative stress from reactive oxygen species (ROS), causing DNA damage [96,97] and (2) inflammation, with the release of cytokines like TNF-α and IL-1α that may promote tumor progression [98]. Furthermore, evidence indicates a dose–response relationship between PM exposure, elevated C-reactive protein (CRP) levels, and breast cancer risk [99]. Finally, BC mortality is influenced not only by environmental exposures but also by healthcare-related factors such as delays in diagnosis, limited treatment access, and barriers to early detection.

Strengths and Limitations

This umbrella review presents several strengths. To our knowledge, a comprehensive synthesis evaluating the links between NO_2, $PM_{2.5}$, and PM_{10} exposure and breast cancer risk has not yet been conducted. By providing a broad perspective on air pollution as a public health concern, this review highlights its potential role in breast cancer, the most commonly diagnosed malignancy worldwide, with incidence peaking between the ages of 60 and 70. A rigorous methodology was applied, including a structured literature search across two scientific databases, independent study selection and data extraction by two researchers, and quality assessment using AMSTAR 2.

However, some limitations exist. First, the included meta-analyses exhibited considerable heterogeneity, which weakens causal inferences. This variability stems from differences in geographic regions, time periods, data collection methods, and exposure assessments. While subgroup analyses attempted to address this issue, they remained limited by their reliance on general study characteristics. More refined stratifications—such as histologic and molecular subtypes, mammographic breast density, occupational history, and individual-level exposure data—were unavailable, as these factors were not considered in the original studies. This heterogeneity is further complicated by physiological changes that occur during critical periods of mammary tissue development and hormone signaling, such as puberty, pregnancy, and menopause. These stages, known as windows of susceptibility (WOS), may represent heightened vulnerability to chemical exposures. Assessing the impact of such exposures during these critical windows is essential for accurately evaluating their contributions to breast cancer risk [100–104]. Understanding pollutant impacts during these periods is essential for effective prevention [99–104]. A further limitation is the high overlap among the included meta-analyses, as reflected by the high Corrected Covered Area (CCA) index (30–66%). This overlap indicates that the synthesized evidence is not entirely independent. Although alternative methods like network meta-analysis or excluding redundant reviews are suggested [105], we included all of them due to their unique subgroup analyses. Still, this highlights the need for more primary studies.

Another concern pertains to how exposure is measured. Estimating individual exposure to air pollution is a key challenge in environmental health research, especially in regions with multiple pollution sources and uneven pollutant distribution. The accuracy of these estimates can vary depending on the method used—for instance, whether data come from air quality monitoring stations, land-use regression (LUR) models, or other modeling techniques. In addition, differences in the length and timing of exposure assessments between studies can introduce inconsistencies. These variations may lead to exposure misclassification, which can influence the reliability of the results and complicate comparisons across studies [106]. Many studies assessed only one pollutant, ignoring potential combined effects, and few analyzed PM composition, even though toxicity varies by component [107,108]. Furthermore, most meta-analyses assumed a linear relationship between air pollution and BC risk, without exploring potential nonlinear effects. Residual confounding is also a concern, as not all studies adjusted for socioeconomic, behavioral, or genetic factors. Lastly, publication bias may influence results. Although funnel plots and Egger's tests were used, three authors also applied trim-and-fill methods, excluding smaller studies to estimate adjusted summary effects based on larger ones [39,40,43].

5. Conclusions

This umbrella review highlights the growing evidence that air pollution, particularly exposure to nitrogen dioxide (NO_2), fine particulate matter ($PM_{2.5}$), and coarse particulate matter (PM_{10}), may increase the risk of both breast cancer incidence and mortality in women, though findings varied in terms of heterogeneity and publication bias. The most vulnerable groups were identified as premenopausal European women exposed to NO_2 and PM_{10}, as well as individuals in developed countries exposed to $PM_{2.5}$.

Given that breast cancer remains the most frequently diagnosed invasive malignancy and the second leading cause of cancer-related deaths among women worldwide, it is imperative that future environmental epidemiological research prioritize breast cancer as a critical health outcome when assessing the effects of air pollution.

In particular, further studies are needed to investigate the impact of multi-pollutant exposures and their combined effects on breast cancer risk. Additionally, identifying specific components of PM, such as black carbon, elemental carbon, and various metals, that may drive carcinogenic risks, is crucial. It is also important to assess breast cancer risk across different histologic and molecular subtypes, as the effects of environmental pollutants may vary in their carcinogenicity across different types of cancer. Furthermore, the existing evidence base is adequate to support breast cancer prevention strategies encompassing both individual lifestyle modifications and public health policies and environmental regulations designed to decrease NO_2, $PM_{10,}$ and $PM_{2.5}$ concentrations.

Supplementary Materials: The following supporting information can be downloaded at https://www.mdpi.com/article/10.3390/environments12050153/s1: Table S1: Search strategy in PubMed and Embase; Table S2: AMSTAR2 check list. Table S3: Excluded articles and reasons. Table S4: Confounders included in the study analysis. Table S5: Primary studies included in each review. Table S6: Sensitivity analysis and publication bias for NO_2 exposure. Table S7: Sensitivity analysis and publication bias for PM2.5 exposure. Table S8: Sensitivity analysis and publication bias for PM10 exposure.

Author Contributions: Conceptualization: C.M. (Cristina Mangia) and E.F.; Writing—original draft: M.F., M.P. (Marco Palella), L.M. and M.P. (Maurizio Portaluri); Writing—review and editing: C.A.M., C.M. (Carolina Mensi), S.C., G.T. and C.M. (Cristina Mangia); Supervision: C.M. (Cristina Mangia). All authors have read and agreed to the published version of the manuscript.

Funding: This research received no external funding.

Conflicts of Interest: The authors declare no conflicts of interest.

Abbreviations

The following abbreviations are used in this manuscript:

BC Breast cancer

References

1. Bray, F.; Laversanne, M.; Sung, H.; Ferlay, J.; Siegel, R.L.; Soerjomataram, I.; Jemal, A. Global cancer statistics 2022: GLOBOCAN estimates of incidence and mortality worldwide for 36 cancers in 185 countries. *CA Cancer J. Clin.* **2024**, *74*, 229–263. [CrossRef] [PubMed]
2. Filho, A.M.; Laversanne, M.; Ferlay, J.; Colombet, M.; Piñeros, M.; Znaor, A.; Parkin, D.M.; Soerjomataram, I.; Bray, F. The GLOBOCAN 2022 cancer estimates: Data sources, methods, and a snapshot of the cancer burden worldwide. *Int. J. Cancer* **2025**, *156*, 1336–1346. [CrossRef]
3. Kohler, B.A.; Sherman, R.L.; Howlader, N.; Jemal, A.; Ryerson, A.B.; Henry, K.A.; Boscoe, F.P.; Cronin, K.A.; Lake, A.; Noone, A.M.; et al. Annual report to the nation on the status of cancer, 1975–2011, featuring incidence of breast cancer subtypes by race/ethnicity, poverty, and state. *J. Natl. Cancer Inst.* **2015**, *107*, djv048. [CrossRef] [PubMed]

4. Hiatt, R.A.; Porco, T.C.; Liu, F.; Balke, K.; Balmain, A.; Barlow, J.; Braithwaite, D.; Diez-Roux, A.V.; Kushi, L.H.; Moasser, M.M.; et al. A multilevel model of postmenopausal breast cancer incidence. *Cancer Epidemiol. Biomark. Prev.* **2014**, *23*, 2078–2092. [CrossRef]
5. Scala, M.; Bosetti, C.; Bagnardi, V.; Possenti, I.; Specchia, C.; Gallus, S.; Lugo, A. Dose-response relationships between cigarette smoking and breast cancer risk: A systematic review and meta-analysis. *J. Epidemiol.* **2023**, *33*, 640–648. [CrossRef] [PubMed]
6. Cohen, S.Y.; Stoll, C.R.; Anandarajah, A.; Doering, M.; Colditz, G.A. Modifiable risk factors in women at high risk of breast cancer: A systematic review. *Breast Cancer Res.* **2023**, *25*, 45. [CrossRef] [PubMed]
7. De Cicco, P.; Catani, M.V.; Gasperi, V.; Sibilano, M.; Quaglietta, M.; Savini, I. Nutrition and Breast Cancer: A Literature Review on Prevention, Treatment and Recurrence. *Nutrients* **2019**, *11*, 1514. [CrossRef]
8. Migliavacca Zucchetti, B.; Peccatori, F.A.; Codacci-Pisanelli, G. Pregnancy and Lactation: Risk or Protective Factors for Breast Cancer? *Adv. Exp. Med. Biol.* **2020**, *1252*, 195–197. [CrossRef] [PubMed]
9. Kudiarasu, C.; Lopez, P.; Galvão, D.A.; Newton, R.U.; Taaffe, D.R.; Mansell, L.; Fleay, B.; Saunders, C.; Fox-Harding, C.; Singh, F. What are the most effective exercise, physical activity and dietary interventions to improve body composition in women diagnosed with or at high-risk of breast cancer? A systematic review and network meta-analysis. *Cancer* **2023**, *129*, 3697–3712. [CrossRef] [PubMed]
10. *IARC Monographs on the Identification of Carcinogenic Hazards to Humans: Night Shift Work 2020*; IARC: Lyon, France, 2020; Volume 124.
11. Rutkowska, A.Z.; Szybiak, A.; Serkies, K.; Rachoń, D. Endocrine disrupting chemicals as potential risk factor for estrogen-dependent cancers. *Pol. Arch. Med. Wewn.* **2016**, *126*, 562–570. [CrossRef] [PubMed]
12. Rodgers, K.M.; Udesky, J.O.; Rudel, R.A.; Brody, J.G. Environmental chemicals and breast cancer: An updated review of epidemiological literature informed by biological mechanisms. *Environ. Res.* **2018**, *160*, 152–182. [CrossRef] [PubMed]
13. Ahern Thomas, P.; Timothy, A.B.; Lash, L.; Cronin-Fenton, D.P.; Ulrichsen, S.P.; Christiansen, P.M.; Cole, B.F.; Tamimi, R.M.; Sørensen, H.T.; Damkier, P. Phthalate exposure and breast cancer incidence: A Danish nationwide cohort study. *J. Clin. Oncol.* **2019**, *37*, 1800–1809. [CrossRef]
14. Kay, J.E.; Cardona, B.; Rudel, R.A.; Vandenberg, L.N.; Soto, A.M.; Christiansen, S.; Birnbaum, L.S.; Fenton, S.E. Chemical Effects on Breast Development, Function, and Cancer Risk: Existing Knowledge and New Opportunities. *Curr. Environ. Health Rpt.* **2022**, *9*, 535–562. [CrossRef] [PubMed]
15. du Plessis, M.; Fourie, C.; Stone, W.; Engelbrecht, A.M. The impact of endocrine disrupting compounds and carcinogens in wastewater: Implications for breast cancer. *Biochimie* **2023**, *209*, 103–115. [CrossRef]
16. White, A.; Teitelbaum, S.; Stellman, S.; Beyea, J.; Steck, S.; Mordukhovich, I.; McCarty, K.; Ahn, J.; Rossner, P.; Santella, R.; et al. Indoor air pollution exposure from use of indoor stoves and fireplaces in association with breast cancer: A case-control study. *Environ. Health* **2014**, *13*, 108. [CrossRef] [PubMed]
17. White, A.J.; Sandler, D.P. Indoor wood-burning stove and fireplace use and breast cancer in a prospective cohort study. *Environ. Health Perspect.* **2017**, *125*, 077011. [CrossRef] [PubMed]
18. Garcia, E.; Hurley, S.; Nelson, D.O.; Hertz, A.; Reynolds, P. Hazardous air pollutants and breast cancer risk in California teachers: A cohort study. *Environ. Health* **2015**, *14*, 14. [CrossRef]
19. Cheng, I.; Yang, J.; Tseng, C.; Wu, J.; Conroy, S.M.; Shariff-Marco, S.; Gomez, S.L.; Whittemore, A.S.; Stram, D.O.; Le Marchand, L.; et al. Outdoor ambient air pollution and breast cancer survival among California participants of the Multiethnic Cohort Study. *Environ. Int.* **2022**, *161*, 107088. [CrossRef]
20. White, A.J. Invited Perspective: Air Pollution and Breast Cancer Risk: Current State of the Evidence and Next Steps. *Environ. Health Perspect.* **2021**, *129*, 51302. [CrossRef]
21. Zeinomar, N.; Oskar, S.; Kehm, R.D.; Sahebzeda, S.; Terry, M.B. Environmental exposures and breast cancer risk in the context of underlying susceptibility: A systematic review of the epidemiological literature. *Environ. Res.* **2020**, *187*, 109346. [CrossRef]
22. Terre-Torras, I.; Recalde, M.; Díaz, Y.; de Bont, J.; Bennett, M.; Aragón, M.; Cirach, M.; O'Callaghan-Gordo, C.; Nieuwenhuijsen, M.J.; Duarte-Salles, T. Air pollution and green spaces in relation to breast cancer risk among pre and postmenopausal women: A mega cohort from Catalonia. *Environ. Res.* **2022**, *214*, 113838. [CrossRef] [PubMed]
23. De Guzman, R.; Schiller, J. Air pollution and its impact on cancer incidence, cancer care and cancer outcomes. *BMJ Oncol.* **2025**, *4*, e000535. [CrossRef]
24. Tippila, J.; Wah, N.L.S.; Akbar, K.A.; Bhummaphan, N.; Wongsasuluk, P.; Kallawicha, K. Ambient Air Pollution Exposure and Breast Cancer Risk Worldwide: A Systematic Review of Longitudinal Studies. *Int. J. Environ. Res. Public Health* **2024**, *21*, 1713. [CrossRef]
25. Hart, J.E.; Bertrand, K.A.; DuPre, N.; James, P.; Vieira, V.M.; Tamimi, R.M.; Laden, F. Long-term particulate matter exposures during adulthood and risk of breast cancer incidence in the Nurses' Health Study II prospective cohort. *Cancer Epidemiol. Biomark. Prev.* **2016**, *25*, 1274–1276. [CrossRef]
26. Wei, Y.; Davis, J.; Bina, W.F. Ambient air pollution is associated with the increased incidence of breast cancer in, U.S. *Int. J. Environ. Health Res.* **2012**, *22*, 12–21. [CrossRef] [PubMed]

27. IARC Working Group on the Evaluation of Carcinogenic Risks to Humans. Definition of outdoor air pollution. In *Outdoor Air Pollution;* International Agency for Research on Cancer: Lyon, France, 2016.
28. World Health Organization. *Ambient Air Pollution: A Global Assessment of Exposure and Burden of Disease;* WHO: Geneva, Switzerland, 2016.
29. Aromataris, E.; Fernandez, R.; Godfrey, C.M.; Holly, C.; Khalil, H.; Tungpunkom, P. Summarizing systematic reviews: Methodological development, conduct and reporting of an umbrella review approach. *JBI Evid. Implement.* **2015**, *13*, 132–134. [CrossRef] [PubMed]
30. Fusar-Poli, P.; Radua, J. Ten simple rules for conducting umbrella reviews. *BMJ Ment. Health* **2018**, *21*, 95–100. [CrossRef]
31. Moher D, Liberati A, Tetzlaff J, Altman DG Preferred reporting items for systematic reviews and meta-analyses: The PRISMA statement. *BMJ* **2009**, *339*, b2535. [CrossRef]
32. Page, M.J.; Moher, D.; Bossuyt, P.M.; Boutron, I.; Hoffmann, T.C.; Mulrow, C.D.; Shamseer, L.; Tetzlaff, J.M.; Akl, E.A.; Brennan, S.E.; et al. PRISMA 2020 explanation and elaboration: Updated guidance and exemplars for reporting systematic reviews. *BMJ* **2021**, *372*, n 160. [CrossRef]
33. Pieper, D.; Antoine, S.L.; Mathes, T.; Neugebauer, E.A.; Eikermann, M. Systematic review finds overlapping reviews were not mentioned in every other overview. *J. Clin. Epidemiol.* **2014**, *67*, 368–375. [CrossRef]
34. Shea, B.J.; Reeves, B.C.; Wells, G.; Thuku, M.; Hamel, C.; Moran, J.; Moher, D.; Tugwell, P.; Welch, V.; Kristjansson, E.; et al. AMSTAR 2: A critical appraisal tool for systematic reviews that include randomised or non-randomised studies of healthcare interventions, or both. *BMJ* **2017**, *358*, j4008. [CrossRef]
35. de Bont, J.; Jaganathan, S.; Dahlquist, M.; Persson, Å.; Stafoggia, M.; Ljungman, P. Ambient air pollution and cardiovascular diseases: An umbrella review of systematic reviews and meta-analyses. *J. Intern. Med.* **2022**, *291*, 779–800. [CrossRef] [PubMed]
36. Wasserstein, R.L.; Schirm, A.L.; Lazar, N.A. Moving to a World Beyond "$p < 0.05$". *Am. Stat.* **2020**, *73*, 1–19.
37. Ioannidis, J.P. The importance of predefined rules and prespecified statistical analyses: Do not abandon significance. *JAMA* **2019**, *321*, 2067–2068. [CrossRef] [PubMed]
38. Onyije, F.M.; Olsson, A.; Baaken, D.; Erdmann, F.; Stanulla, M.; Wollschlaeger, D.; Schuez, J. Environmental risk factors for childhood acute lymphoblastic leukemia: An umbrella review. *Cancers* **2022**, *14*, 382. [CrossRef]
39. Gabet, S.; Lemarchand, C.; Guénel, P.; Slama, R. Breast Cancer Risk in Association with Atmospheric Pollution Exposure: A Meta-Analysis of Effect Estimates Followed by a Health Impact Assessment. *Environ. Health Perspect.* **2021**, *129*, 57012. [CrossRef]
40. Guo, Q.; Wang, X.; Gao, Y.; Zhou, J.; Huang, C.; Zhang, Z.; Chu, H. Relationship between particulate matter exposure and female breast cancer incidence and mortality: A systematic review and meta-analysis. *Int. Arch. Occupupational Environ. Health* **2021**, *94*, 191–201. [CrossRef]
41. Zhang, Z.; Yan, W.; Chen, Q.; Zhou, N.; Xu, Y. The relationship between exposure to particulate matter and breast cancer incidence and mortality: A meta-analysis. *Medicine* **2019**, *98*, e18349. [CrossRef]
42. Yu, P.; Guo, S.; Xu, R.; Ye, T.; Li, S.; Sim, M.R.; Abramson, M.J.; Guo, Y. Cohort studies of long-term exposure to outdoor particulate matter and risks of cancer: A systematic review and meta-analysis. *Innovation* **2021**, *2*, 100143. [CrossRef]
43. Wei, W.; Wu, B.J.; Wu, Y.; Tong, Z.T.; Zhong, F.; Hu, C.Y. Association between long-term ambient air pollution exposure and the risk of breast cancer: A systematic review and meta-analysis. *Environ. Sci. Pollut. Res. Int.* **2021**, *28*, 63278–63296. [CrossRef]
44. Praud, D.; Deygas, F.; Amadou, A.; Bouilly, M.; Turati, F.; Bravi, F.; Xu, T.; Grassot, L.; Coudon, T.; Fervers, B. Traffic-Related Air Pollution and Breast Cancer Risk: A Systematic Review and Meta-Analysis of Observational Studies. *Cancers* **2023**, *15*, 927. [CrossRef] [PubMed] [PubMed Central]
45. Arif, I.; Adams, M.D.; Johnson, M.T.J. A meta-analysis of the carcinogenic effects of particulate matter and polycyclic aromatic hydrocarbons. *Environ. Pollut.* **2024**, *351*, 123941. [CrossRef] [PubMed]
46. Andersen, Z.J.; Ravnskjær, L.; Andersen, K.K.; Loft, S.; Brandt, J.; Becker, T.; Ketzel, M.; Hertel, O.; Lynge, E.; Bräuner, E.V. Long-Term Exposure to Fine Particulate Matter and Breast Cancer Incidence in the Danish Nurse Cohort Study. *Cancer Epidemiol. Biomark. Prev. Publ. Am. Assoc. Cancer Res. Cosponsored Am. Soc. Prev. Oncol.* **2017**, *26*, 428–430. [CrossRef]
47. Andersen, Z.J.; Stafoggia, M.; Weinmayr, G.; Pedersen, M.; Galassi, C.; Jørgensen, J.T.; Oudin, A.; Forsberg, B.; Olsson, D.; Oftedal, B.; et al. Long-Term Exposure to Ambient Air Pollution and Incidence of Postmenopausal Breast Cancer in 15 European Cohorts within the ESCAPE Project. *Environ. Health Perspect.* **2017**, *125*, 107005. [CrossRef]
48. Bai, L.; Shin, S.; Burnett, R.T.; Kwong, J.C.; Hystad, P.; van Donkelaar, A.; Goldberg, M.S.; Lavigne, E.; Weichenthal, S.; Martin, R.V.; et al. Exposure to Ambient Air Pollution and the Incidence of Lung Cancer and Breast Cancer in the Ontario Population Health and Environment Cohort. *Int. J. Cancer* **2019**, *146*, 2450–2459. [CrossRef]
49. Cheng, I.; Tseng, C.; Wu, J.; Yang, J.; Conroy, S.M.; Shariff-Marco, S.; Li, L.; Hertz, A.; Gomez, S.L.; Le Marchand, L.; et al. Association between Ambient Air Pollution and Breast Cancer Risk: The Multiethnic Cohort Study. *Int. J. Cancer* **2020**, *146*, 699–711. [CrossRef]

50. Cohen, G.; Levy, I.; Yuval; Kark, J.D.; Levin, N.; Witberg, G.; Iakobishvili, Z.; Bental, T.; Broday, D.M.; Steinberg, D.M.; et al. Chronic Exposure to Traffic-Related Air Pollution and Cancer Incidence among 10,000 Patients Undergoing Percutaneous Coronary Interventions: A Historical Prospective Study. *Eur. J. Prev. Cardiol.* **2018**, *25*, 659–670. [CrossRef] [PubMed]
51. Crouse, D.L.; Goldberg, M.S.; Ross, N.A.; Chen, H.; Labrèche, F. Postmenopausal Breast Cancer Is Associated with Exposure to Traffic-Related Air Pollution in Montreal, Canada: A Case-Control Study. *Environ. Health Perspect.* **2010**, *118*, 1578–1583. [CrossRef] [PubMed]
52. Datzmann, T.; Markevych, I.; Trautmann, F.; Heinrich, J.; Schmitt, J.; Tesch, F. Outdoor Air Pollution, Green Space, and Cancer Incidence in Saxony: A Semi-Individual Cohort Study. *BMC Public. Health* **2018**, *18*, 715. [CrossRef]
53. Goldberg, M.S.; Labrèche, F.; Weichenthal, S.; Lavigne, E.; Valois, M.-F.; Hatzopoulou, M.; Van Ryswyk, K.; Shekarrizfard, M.; Villeneuve, P.J.; Crouse, D.; et al. The Association between the Incidence of Postmenopausal Breast Cancer and Concentrations at Street-Level of Nitrogen Dioxide and Ultrafine Particles. *Environ. Res.* **2017**, *158*, 7–15. [CrossRef]
54. Goldberg, M.S.; Villeneuve, P.J.; Crouse, D.; To, T.; Weichenthal, S.A.; Wall, C.; Miller, A.B. Associations between Incident Breast Cancer and Ambient Concentrations of Nitrogen Dioxide from a National Land Use Regression Model in the Canadian National Breast Screening Study. *Environ. Int.* **2019**, *133*, 105182. [CrossRef] [PubMed]
55. Hystad, P.; Villeneuve, P.J.; Goldberg, M.S.; Crouse, D.L.; Johnson, K. Canadian Cancer Registries Epidemiology Research Group Exposure to Traffic-Related Air Pollution and the Risk of Developing Breast Cancer among Women in Eight Canadian Provinces: A Case-Control Study. *Environ. Int.* **2015**, *74*, 240–248. [CrossRef]
56. Lemarchand, C.; Gabet, S.; Cénée, S.; Tvardik, N.; Slama, R.; Guénel, P. Breast Cancer Risk in Relation to Ambient Concentrations of Nitrogen Dioxide and Particulate Matter: Results of a Population-Based Case-Control Study Corrected for Potential Selection Bias (the CECILE Study). *Environ. Int.* **2021**, *155*, 106604. [CrossRef]
57. Raaschou-Nielsen, O.; Andersen, Z.J.; Hvidberg, M.; Jensen, S.S.; Ketzel, M.; Sørensen, M.; Hansen, J.; Loft, S.; Overvad, K.; Tjønneland, A. Air Pollution from Traffic and Cancer Incidence: A Danish Cohort Study. *Environ. Health Glob. Access Sci. Source* **2011**, *10*, 67. [CrossRef] [PubMed]
58. Reding, K.W.; Young, M.T.; Szpiro, A.A.; Han, C.J.; DeRoo, L.A.; Weinberg, C.; Kaufman, J.D.; Sandler, D.P. Breast cancer risk in relation to ambient air pollution exposure at residences in the Sister Study cohort. *Cancer Epidemiol. Biomark. Prev.* **2015**, *24*, 1907–1909. [CrossRef] [PubMed]
59. White, A.J.; Keller, J.P.; Zhao, S.; Carroll, R.; Kaufman, J.D.; Sandler, D.P. Air Pollution, Clustering of Particulate Matter Components, and Breast Cancer in the Sister Study: A U.S.-Wide Cohort. *Environ. Health Perspect.* **2019**, *127*, 107002. [CrossRef]
60. White, A.J.; Gregoire, A.M.; Niehoff, N.M.; Bertrand, K.A.; Palmer, J.R.; Coogan, P.F.; Bethea, T.N. Air Pollution and Breast Cancer Risk in the Black Women's Health Study. *Environ. Res.* **2021**, *194*, 110651. [CrossRef]
61. Amadou, A.; Praud, D.; Coudon, T.; Deygas, F.; Grassot, L.; Dubuis, M.; Faure, E.; Couvidat, F.; Caudeville, J.; Bessagnet, B.; et al. Long-Term Exposure to Nitrogen Dioxide Air Pollution and Breast Cancer Risk: A Nested Case-Control within the French E3N Cohort Study. *Environ. Pollut.* **2022**, *317*, 120719. [CrossRef]
62. Shin, M.; Kim, O.J.; Yang, S.; Choe, S.A.; Kim, S.Y. Different mortality risks of long-term exposure to particulate matter across different cancer sites. *Int. J. Environ. Res. Public. Health* **2022**, *19*, 3180. [CrossRef]
63. Coleman, N.C.; Burnett, R.T.; Ezzati, M.; Marshall, J.D.; Robinson, A.L.; Pope, C.A., III. Fine particulate matter exposure and cancer incidence: Analysis of SEER cancer registry data from 1992–2016. *Environ. Health Perspect.* **2020**, *128*, 107004. [CrossRef]
64. Villeneuve, P.J.; Goldberg, M.S.; Crouse, D.L.; To, T.; Weichenthal, S.A.; Wall, C.; Miller, A.B. Residential exposure to fine particulate matter air pollution and incident breast cancer in a cohort of Canadian women. *Environ. Epidemiol.* **2018**, *2*, e021. [CrossRef]
65. Poulsen, A.H.; Hvidtfeldt, U.A.; Sørensen, M.; Pedersen, J.E.; Ketzel, M.; Brandt, J.; Geels, C.; Christensen, J.H.; Raaschou-Nielsen, O. Air pollution with NO_2, $PM_{2.5}$, and elemental carbon in relation to risk of breast cancer– a nationwide case-control study from Denmark. *Environ. Res.* **2023**, *216*, 11474. [CrossRef]
66. Prada, D.; Baccarelli, A.A.; Terry, M.B.; Valdéz, L.; Cabrera, P.; Just, A.; Kloog, I.; Caro, H.; García-Cuellar, C.; Sánchez-Pérez, Y.; et al. Long-term PM2.5 exposure before diagnosis is associated with worse outcome in breast cancer. *Breast Cancer Res. Treat.* **2021**, *188*, 525–533. [CrossRef]
67. To, T.; Zhu, J.; Villeneuve, P.J.; Simatovic, J.; Feldman, L.; Gao, C.; Williams, D.; Chen, H.; Weichenthal, S.; Wall, C.; et al. Chronic disease prevalence in women and air pollution—A 30-year longitudinal cohort study. *Environ. Int.* **2015**, *80*, 26–32. [CrossRef] [PubMed]
68. Huang, Y.J.; Lee, P.H.; Chen, L.C.; Lin, B.C.; Lin, C.; Chan, T.C. Relationships among green space, ambient fine particulate matter, and cancer incidence in Taiwan: A 16-year retrospective cohort study. *Environ. Res.* **2022**, *212*, 113416. [CrossRef] [PubMed]
69. DuPré, N.C.; Hart, J.E.; Holmes, M.D.; Poole, E.M.; James, P.; Kraft, P.; Laden, F.; Tamimi, R.M. Particulate matter and traffic-related exposures in relation to breast cancer survival. *Cancer Epidemiol. Biomarkers Prev.* **2019**, *2*, 751–759. [CrossRef] [PubMed]
70. Hu, H.; Dailey, A.B.; Kan, H.; Xu, X. The effect of atmospheric particulate matter on survival of breast cancer among US females. *Breast Cancer Res. Treat.* **2013**, *139*, 217–226. [CrossRef]

71. Hung, L.J.; Chan, T.F.; Wu, C.H.; Chiu, H.F.; Yang, C.Y. Traffic air pollution and risk of death from ovarian cancer in Taiwan: Fine particulate matter (PM2.5) as a proxy marker. *J. Toxicol. Environ. Health A* **2012**, *75*, 174–182. [CrossRef] [PubMed]
72. Iwai, K.; Mizuno, S.; Miyasaka, Y.; Mori, T. Correlation between suspended particles in the environmental air and causes of disease among inhabitants: Cross-sectional studies using the vital statistics and air pollution data in Japan. *Environ. Res.* **2005**, *99*, 106–117. [CrossRef]
73. Turner, M.C.; Krewski, D.; Diver, W.R.; Pope CA3rd Burnett, R.T.; Jerrett, M.; Marshall, J.D.; Gapstur, S.M. Ambient air pollution and cancer mortality in the Cancer Prevention Study II. *Environ. Health Perspect.* **2017**, *125*, 087013. [CrossRef]
74. Wong, C.M.; Tsang, H.; Lai, H.K.; Thomas, G.N.; Lam, K.B.; Chan, K.P.; Zheng, Q.; Ayres, J.G.; Lee, S.Y.; Lam, T.H.; et al. Cancer mortality risks from long-term exposure to ambient fine particle. *Cancer Epidemiol. Biomark. Prev.* **2016**, *25*, 839–845. [CrossRef] [PubMed]
75. Cheng, I.; Yang, J.; Tseng, C.; Wu, J.; Shariff-Marco, S.; Park, S.L.; Conroy, S.M.; Inamdar, P.P.; Fruin, S.; Larson, T.; et al. Traffic-related air pollution and lung cancer incidence: The California Multiethnic Cohort Study. *Am. J. Respir. Crit. Care Med.* **2022**, *206*, 1008–1018. [CrossRef] [PubMed]
76. Yu, P.; Xu, R.; Li, S.; Coelho, M.S.Z.S.; Saldiva, P.H.N.; Sim, M.R.; Abramson, M.J.; Guo, Y. Associations between long-term exposure to PM2.5 and site-specific cancer mortality: A nationwide study in Brazil between 2010 and 2018. *Environ. Pollut.* **2022**, *302*, 119070. [CrossRef]
77. White, A.J.; Fisher, J.A.; Sweeney, M.R.; Freedman, N.D.; Kaufman, J.D.; Silverman, D.T.; Jones, R.R. Ambient fine particulate matter and breast cancer incidence in a large prospective US cohort. *JNCI J. Natl. Cancer Inst.* **2024**, *116*, 53–60. [CrossRef]
78. Plusquin, M.; Guida, F.; Polidoro, S.; Vermeulen, R.; Raaschou-Nielsen, O.; Campanella, G.; Hoek, G.; Kyrtopoulos, S.A.; Georgiadis, P.; Naccarati, A.; et al. DNA methylation and exposure to ambient air pollution in two prospective cohorts. *Environ. Int.* **2017**, *108*, 127–136. [CrossRef] [PubMed]
79. van Veldhoven, K.; Polidoro, S.; Baglietto, L.; Severi, G.; Sacerdote, C.; Panico, S.; Mattiello, A.; Palli, D.; Masala, G.; Krogh, V.; et al. Epigenome-wide association study reveals decreased average methylation levels years before breast cancer diagnosis. *Clin. Epigenetics* **2015**, *7*, 67. [CrossRef]
80. Li, S.; Liao, X.; Ma, R.; Deng, N.; Wu, H.; Zhang, Z.; Chen, L.; Wang, Q.; Liao, Q.; Li, Q.; et al. Effects of Co-Exposure to Benzene, Toluene, and Xylene, Polymorphisms of microRNA Genes, and Their Interactions on Genetic Damage in Chinese Petrochemical Workers. *Toxics* **2024**, *12*, 821. [CrossRef]
81. Mordukhovich, I.; Beyea, J.; Herring, A.H.; Hatch, M.; Stellman, S.D.; Teitelbaum, S.L.; Richardson, D.B.; Millikan, R.C.; Engel, L.S.; Shantakumar, S.; et al. Vehicular traffic-related polycyclic aromatic hydrocarbon exposure and breast cancer incidence: The Long Island Breast Cancer Study Project (LIBCSP). *Environ. Health Perspect.* **2016**, *124*, 30–38. [CrossRef]
82. Agudo, A.; Peluso, M.; Munnia, A.; Lujan-Barroso, L.; Barricarte, A.; Amiano, P.; Navarro, C.; Sanchez, M.J.; Quiros, J.R.; Ardanaz, E.; et al. Aromatic DNA adducts and breast cancer risk: A case-cohort study within the EPIC-Spain. *Carcinogenesis* **2017**, *38*, 691–698. [CrossRef] [PubMed]
83. Lee, K.H.; Shu, X.O.; Gao, Y.T.; Ji, B.T.; Yang, G.; Blair, A.; Rothman, N.; Zheng, W.; Chow, W.H.; Kang, D. Breast cancer and urinary biomarkers of polycyclic aromatic hydrocarbon and oxidative stress in the Shanghai Women's Health Study. *Cancer Epidemiol. Biomark. Prev.* **2010**, *19*, 877–883. [CrossRef]
84. Plísková, M.; Vondrácek, J.; Vojtesek, B.; Kozubík, A.; Machala, M. Deregulation of cell proliferation by polycyclic aromatic hydrocarbons in human breast carcinoma MCF-7 cells reflects both genotoxic and nongenotoxic events. *Toxicol. Sci.* **2004**, *83*, 246–256. [CrossRef] [PubMed]
85. Gammon, M.D.; Santella, R.M.; Neugut, A.I.; Eng, S.M.; Teitelbaum, S.L.; Paykin, A.; Levin, B.; Terry, M.B.; Young, T.L.; Wang, L.W.; et al. Environmental toxins and breast cancer on Long Island. *I. Polycycl. Aromat. Hydrocarb. DNA Adducts Cancer Epidemiol. Biomark. Prev.* **2002**, *11*, 677–685.
86. Rundle, A.; Tang, D.L.; Hibshoosh, H.; Estabrook, A.; Schnabel, F.; Cao, W.F.; Grumet, S.; Perera, F.P. The relationship between genetic damage from polycyclic aromatic hydrocarbons in breast tissue and breast cancer. *Carcinogenesis* **2000**, *21*, 1281–1289. [CrossRef]
87. Korsh, J.; Shen, A.; Aliano, K.; Davenport, T. Polycyclic aromatic hydrocarbons and breast cancer: A review of the literature. *Breast Care* **2015**, *10*, 316–318. [CrossRef]
88. Madrigal, J.M.; Pruitt, C.N.; Fisher, J.A.; Liao, L.M.; Graubard, B.I.; Gierach, G.L.; Silverman, D.T.; Ward, M.H.; Jones, R.R. Carcinogenic industrial air pollution and postmenopausal breast cancer risk in the National Institutes of Health AARP Diet and Health Study. *Environ. Int.* **2024**, *191*, 108985. [CrossRef] [PubMed]
89. Benbrahim-Tallaa, L.; Baan, R.A.; Grosse, Y.; Lauby-Secretan, B.; El Ghissassi, F.; Bouvard, V.; Guha, N.; Loomis, D.; Straif, K.; International Agency for Research on Cancer Monograph Working Group. Carcinogenicity of diesel-engine and gasoline-engine exhausts and some nitroarenes. *Lancet Oncol.* **2012**, *13*, 663–664. [CrossRef]

90. González, L.T.; Pérez-Rodríguez, M.; Rodríguez, F.L.; Mancilla, Y.; Acuña-Askar, K.; Campos, A.; Luis, A.; González, P.; Vidaurri, L.G.S.; Zapata, A.A.; et al. Insights from the combined bulk chemical and surface characterization of airborne PM10 on source contributions and health risk: The case of three Mexican cities. *Air Qual. Atmos. Health* **2023**, *16*, 1455–1477. [CrossRef]
91. Hvidtfeldt, U.A.; Chen, J.; Rodopoulou, S.; Strak, M.; de Hoogh, K.; Andersen, Z.J.; Bellander, T.; Brandt, J.; Fecht, D.; Forastiere, F.; et al. Breast cancer incidence in relation to long-term low-level exposure to air pollution in the ELAPSE pooled cohort. *Cancer Epidemiol. Biomark. Prev.* **2023**, *32*, 105–113. [CrossRef]
92. Song, Y.; Yang, L.; Kang, N.; Wang, N.; Zhang, X.; Liu, S.; Li, H.; Xue, T.; Ji, J. Associations of incident female breast cancer with long-term exposure to $PM_{2.5}$ and its constituents: Findings from a prospective cohort study in Beijing, China. *J. Hazard. Mater.* **2024**, *473*, 134614. [CrossRef]
93. Kresovich, J.K.; Erdal, S.; Chen, H.Y.; Gann, P.H.; Argos, M.; Rauscher, G.H. Metallic air pollutants and breast cancer heterogeneity. *Environ. Res.* **2019**, *177*, 108639. [CrossRef]
94. Liu, R.; Nelson, D.O.; Hurley, S.; Hertz, A.; Reynolds, P. Residential exposure to estrogen disrupting hazardous air pollutants and breast cancer risk: The California Teachers Study. *Epidemiology* **2015**, *26*, 365–373. [CrossRef]
95. White, A.J.; O'Brien, K.M.; Niehoff, N.M.; Carroll, R.; Sandler, D.P. Metallic air pollutants and breast cancer risk in a nationwide cohort study. *Epidemiology* **2019**, *30*, 20–28. [CrossRef]
96. Farahzadi, R.; Valipour, B.; Fathi, E.; Pirmoradi, S.; Molavi, O.; Montazersaheb, S.; Sanaat, Z. Oxidative stress regulation and related metabolic pathways in epithelial-mesenchymal transition of breast cancer stem cells. *Stem Cell Res. Ther.* **2023**, *14*, 342. [CrossRef] [PubMed] [PubMed Central]
97. Mazzuferi, G.; Bacchetti, T.; Islam, M.O.; Ferretti, G. High density lipoproteins and oxidative stress in breast cancer. *Lipids Health Dis.* **2021**, *20*, 143. [CrossRef] [PubMed] [PubMed Central]
98. Bahiraee, A.; Ebrahimi, R.; Halabian, R.; Aghabozorgi, A.S.; Amani, J. The role of inflammation and its related microRNAs in breast cancer: A narrative review. *J. Cell Physiol.* **2019**, *234*, 19480–19493. [CrossRef] [PubMed]
99. Chan, D.S.; Bandera, E.V.; Greenwood, D.C.; Norat, T. Circulating C-Reactive Protein and Breast Cancer Risk-Systematic Literature Review and Meta-analysis of Prospective Cohort Studies. *Cancer Epidemiol. Biomarkers Prev.* **2015**, *24*, 1439–1449. [CrossRef] [PubMed]
100. Terry, M.B.; Michels, K.B.; Brody, J.G.; Byrne, C.; Chen, S.; Jerry, D.J.; Malecki, K.M.; Martin, M.B.; Miller, R.L.; Neuhausen, S.L.; et al. Environmental exposures during windows of susceptibility for breast cancer: A framework for prevention research. *Breast Cancer Res.* **2019**, *21*, 96. [CrossRef]
101. Board on Health Sciences Policy, Committee on Breast Cancer, The Scientific Evidence, Research Methodology, & Future Directions. *Breast Cancer and the Environment: A Life Course Approach*; National Academies Press: Washington, DC, USA, 2012.
102. Cohn, B.A.; Cirillo, P.M.; Terry, M.B. DDT and breast cancer: Prospective study of induction time and susceptibility windows. *JNCI J. Natl. Cancer Inst.* **2019**, *111*, 803–810. [CrossRef]
103. Nie, J.; Beyea, J.; Bonner, M.R.; Han, D.; Vena, J.E.; Rogerson, P.; Vito, D.; Muti, P.; Trevisan, M.; Edge, S.B.; et al. Exposure to traffic emissions throughout life and risk of breast cancer: The Western New York Exposures and Breast Cancer (WEB) study. *Cancer Causes Control.* **2007**, *18*, 947–955. [CrossRef]
104. Smotherman, C.; Sprague, B.; Datta, S.; Braithwaite, D.; Qin, H.; Yaghjyan, L. Association of air pollution with postmenopausal breast cancer risk in UK Biobank. *Breast Cancer Res.* **2023**, *25*, 83. [CrossRef]
105. Lunny, C.; Pieper, D.; Thabet, P.; Kanji, S. Managing overlap of primary study results across systematic reviews: Practical considerations for authors of overviews of reviews. *BMC Med. Res. Methodol.* **2021**, *21*, 140. [CrossRef]
106. Duboeuf, M.; Amadou, A.; Coudon, T.; Grassot, L.; Ramel-Delobel, M.; Faure, E.; Salizzoni, P.; Gulliver, J.; Severi, G.; Mancini, F.R.; et al. Long-term exposure to air pollution at residential and workplace addresses and breast cancer risk: A case-control study nested in the French E3N-Générations cohort from 1990 to 2011. *Eur. J. Cancer.* **2024**, *210*, 114293. [CrossRef] [PubMed]
107. Lewis-Michl, E.L.; Melius, J.M.; Kallenbach, L.R.; Ju, C.L.; Talbot, T.O.; Orr, M.F. Breast cancer risk and residence near industry or traffic in Nassau and Suffolk Counties, Long Island, New York. *Arch. Environ. Health An. Int. J.* **1996**, *51*, 255–265. [CrossRef] [PubMed]
108. Giampiccolo, C.; Amadou, A.; Coudon, T.; Praud, D.; Grassot, L.; Faure, E.; Couvidat, F.; Severi, G.; Mancini, F.R.; Fervers, B.; et al. Multi-pollutant exposure profiles associated with breast cancer risk: A Bayesian profile regression analysis in the French E3N cohort. *Environ. Int.* **2024**, *190*, 108943. [CrossRef]

environments

MDPI

Systematic Review

Advancing Environmental Sustainability in Healthcare: Review on Perspectives from Health Institutions

Bárbara Badanta [1,2], Anabel Porcar Sierra [1], Saray Torner Fernández [1], Francisco Javier Rodríguez Muñoz [1], José Miguel Pérez-Jiménez [1,2,3,*], María Gonzalez-Cano-Caballero [4,*], Manuel Ruiz-Adame [5,6] and Rocío de-Diego-Cordero [1,2]

1 Department of Nursing, Schools of Nursing, Physiotherapy and Podiatry, University of Seville, 41009 Seville, Spain; bbadanta@us.es (B.B.); anabelporcarsierra@gmail.com (A.P.S.); saraytorner01@gmail.com (S.T.F.); paco6502@gmail.com (F.J.R.M.); rdediego2@us.es (R.d.-D.-C.)

2 Research Group CTS1149: Integral and Sustainable Health: Bio-Psycho-Social, Cultural and Spiritual Approach for Human Development, 41009 Seville, Spain

3 Anaesthesiology and Resuscitation Clinical Management Unit, University Hospital Virgen Macarena, 41009 Sevilla, Spain

4 Department of Nursing, Faculty of Health Sciences, University of Granada, 18071 Granada, Spain

5 Biosanitary Research Institute Granada, ibs.Granada, 18012 Granada, Spain; mruizadame@ugr.es

6 Faculty of Social and Legal Sciences (Campus Melilla), University of Granada, 52005 Melilla, Spain

* Correspondence: jpjimenez@us.es (J.M.P.-J.); mariagcc@ugr.es (M.G.-C.-C.); Tel.: +34-654114336 (J.M.P.-J.)

Abstract: Hospitals play a key role in promoting sustainable and healthy living. Few studies have taken this perspective into account. Therefore, we explored the role of hospital institutions in the development and implementation of sustainability strategies linked to the provision of health services. Applying the PRISMA guidelines, we conducted a systematic review of the PubMed, Scopus, CINAHL, PsycINFO and Web of Science databases and the references of the resulting articles in Mendeley Desktop v1.19.8. Articles peer-reviewed between 2016 and 2023 were eligible if they analyzed sustainable healthcare, activities derived from services provided and professional involvement. From the 27 articles that constituted the final sample, two themes were identified: (a) environmental sustainability in healthcare and (b) involvement of healthcare professionals in environmental sustainability. Proposals for sustainable actions to reduce the environmental impact of healthcare related to the use of natural resources, sustainable food, sustainable transport and waste management were reviewed. The role of healthcare workers, their attitudes and perceptions of sustainability and global health improvement were investigated. Reducing health pollution involves addressing excessive or inappropriate consumption of resources and minimizing the environmental footprint of healthcare activities. The different contexts reveal the heterogeneity of the sustainability interventions existing in the healthcare industry, both in terms of subject matter and in terms of the number of publications from each country.

Keywords: development strategies; green hospital; healthcare sector; sustainable development

1. Introduction

The World Health Organization (WHO) has declared that climate change presents a threat to human health in terms of death and illness from increasingly extreme weather events, such as heatwaves, storms and floods; the disruption of food systems and an increase in vector-borne diseases. Between 2030 and 2050, climate change is expected to cause approximately 250,000 additional deaths per year from undernutrition, malaria, diarrhea and heat stress alone. Furthermore, it is undermining many of the social determinants of good health, such as livelihoods, equality, access to healthcare and functioning of health systems and social support structures [1]

Healthcare and, more specifically, hospitals, play a crucial role in contributing to environmental deterioration, since they generate pathological, pharmaceutical, chemical and radioactive waste, posing significant health risks [2]). Health activities in Western countries such as Canada emit thousands or millions of tons of greenhouse gases and other pollutants each year, which has resulted in the annual loss of 23,000 disability-adjusted life years [3].

The future quality of health services in terms of climate resilience and environmental sustainability is directly related to support health systems to leapfrog to cheaper, cleaner and more reliable solutions, while decarbonizing high-emitting health systems [1].

Some strategies to mitigate the environmental and health impact generated by the provision of health services are being carried out in several dimensions. Firstly, it is worth highlighting the modernization of facilities with new technologies and the design and construction of ecological hospitals through thermal (electrical energy savings and solar protection), acoustic (patient comfort and no noise pollution) and lighting strategies (i.e., openings in building facades) [4]. Several studies have determined that the introduction of elements to provide greater interior thermal comfort (i.e., an increase in relative humidity) reduces the load on air conditioning systems [5,6]). In fact, the results of the first study reflected that increasing indoor relative humidity by 10% reduced the cooling load and energy consumption by 24.9% in green hospitals compared to conventional hospitals.

Secondly, the implementation of sustainable measures can be driven by political and management commitments. In fact, new business models are emerging for pharmaceutical companies, where innovation is a key element in improving sustainable development, especially in the field of green technologies [7]. To achieve this, regulatory frameworks and management plans as well as awareness among managers and health professionals are necessary. Results from several studies show that the corporate responsibility of a proactive manager or leader with high environmental values positively influences (39%) the pro-environmental behavior of healthcare professionals [8,9]). In addition, various authors support training in sustainable development, climate change or gas emissions, among others, to increase knowledge that can be reflected in the clinical practice of health professionals, in the generation of scientific data and in the proposal of new policies [10,11]

Finally, healthcare sustainability science also explores dimensions of resource consumption and environmental emissions associated with healthcare activities. Previous studies have shown that some proposals include the inclusion of new forms of care, such as telemedicine, which would contribute to a reduction in carbon emissions [12,13], the development of life cycle inventory databases for medical devices and drugs and revision of infection control standards driving non-evidence-based uptake of single-use disposable devices [14]. More simply, health education can itself be an ally of sustainability. In this way, advising more physical activity in parks, bicycling or walking, as well as reducing the consumption of prepared foods not only encourages more healthy active lifestyles but could also help reduce air pollution and the use of plastics.

Reducing pollution from healthcare involves addressing excessive or inappropriate consumption of resources and minimizing the environmental footprint of healthcare activities. Efforts to achieve these measures will result in higher-value care and better population health [15]. Therefore, given the active role that hospital institutions must develop to achieve global health and the direct relationship between sustainability initiatives and the well-being of the population, this work aims to explore the role of hospital institutions in the development and implementation of sustainability strategies linked to the provision of health services.

2. Materials and Methods

2.1. Study Design

A systematic review following the PRISMA (Preferred Reporting Items for Systematic Reviews and Meta-Analyses) guidelines [16] (Supplementary Materials) was conducted using five electronic databases: PubMed, Scopus, CINAHL, PsycINFO and Web of Science. The searches were performed by two researchers independently between December 2023 and January 2024, using the following Boolean expression, slightly adapted for each database: ("green hospital" OR "healthcare sector" OR "healthcare institution*" OR "sustainable hospital*") AND ("agenda 2030" OR "eco-friendly" OR "pro-environmental" OR "sustainable development" OR "sustainability development goals" OR "sustainability strategy" OR sustainab*).

2.2. Inclusion and Exclusion Criteria

Articles were included if they investigated sustainability issues related to healthcare and were (a) peer-reviewed articles published between 2016 and 2023 and (b) quantitative, qualitative or mixed-design studies. No language restrictions were applied. Articles were excluded if they were editorials, conference proceedings, opinion essays, literature reviews or books or if they did not address environmental sustainability in the healthcare sector. Studies that focused on policies and regulations regarding health environmental sustainability, as well as sustainability measures applied to health infrastructures, were also excluded.

2.3. Study Selection and Data Extraction

After the search, 1575 publications matching the search criteria were included as references in the software Mendeley Desktop v1.19.8. The screening procedure was carried out by two researchers independently, aiming to identify relevant studies based on the inclusion and exclusion criteria. First, duplicate publications were removed (n = 548); then, the reviewers screened 1027 articles by title and abstract. Two hundred and twenty-four full-text articles were screened by two researchers, and if there was a disagreement, another reviewer was consulted. After reading the full-text articles, our final sample included 27 studies. The flowchart is included in Figure 1.

Finally, the following items were extracted for each study: authors, country, year of publication, study objective, research design, sample characteristics and major findings (Appendix A). The summary tables were thoroughly reviewed by all reviewers independently, with critical discussions of the extracted data.

To develop the themes for this systematic review, a thematic analysis approach was used [17]. Two reviewers involved in the searches, screening, article evaluation and data extraction organized descriptive labels, focusing on emerging or persistent concepts and similarities or differences in the role of hospital institutions in the development and implementation of sustainability strategies linked to health service delivery. The coded data from each paper were examined and compared with the data from all the other studies. Finally, the different categories were gathered (grouped) into the following two themes: (a) environmental sustainability in healthcare and (b) engaging health professionals in environmental sustainability.

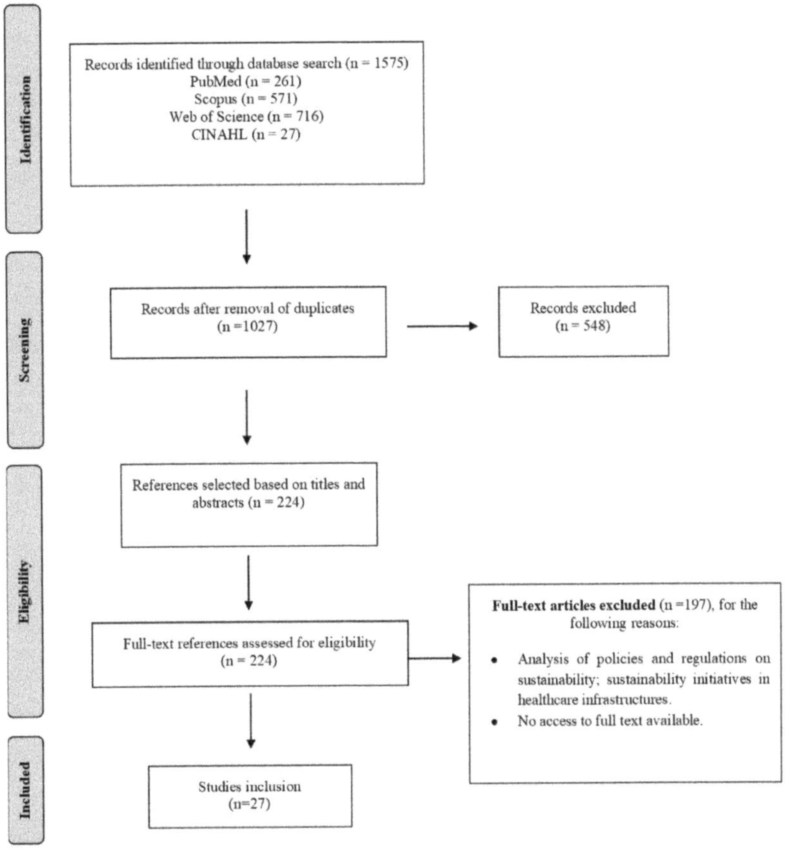

Figure 1. Flowchart for article selection in this systematic review. From Page MJ, McKenzie JE, Bossuyt PM, Boutron I, Hoffmann TC, Mulrow CD, et al. The PRISMA 2020 statement: an updated guideline for reporting systematic reviews. *BMJ* 2021;372:n71. doi: 10.1136/bmj.n71. For more information, visit www.prisma-statement.org (accessed on 10 June 2024) [16].

3. Results

The results below show the main characteristics of the studies included in this review, as well as a qualitative analysis of the content based on the themes established by the authors.

Characteristics of the Included Studies

A total of 27 articles were included in the final step of the systematic review; 70% of them were published in the last three years (n = 19). Seventy percent of the studies were conducted in Europe and Asia (n = 10; 37% and n = 9; 33%), followed by the Americas (n = 4; 14%) and Australia (n = 2; 8%).

Most of the articles selected for this review investigated sustainability strategies in healthcare systems (n = 14; 51.8%). In addition, some publications focused on analyzing environmental damage caused by healthcare activity and identified facilitators and barriers to the implementation of sustainability measures (n = 9; 33.3%), and some addressed the role of healthcare professionals in the implementation of these measures (n = 8; 29.6%). Most studies' respondents were healthcare workers from public hospitals (n = 15; 68%), of those studies, four (18%) included management and leadership professionals. Other participants were medical students, food chain staff and health industry workers (n = 3; 13%). The full characteristics of the selected studies are shown in Appendix A; a scheme (Figure 2) reflecting the dynamics of environmental impact of medical activities and proposed measures to reduce such impact, as well as a qualitative analysis of the results, are presented below.

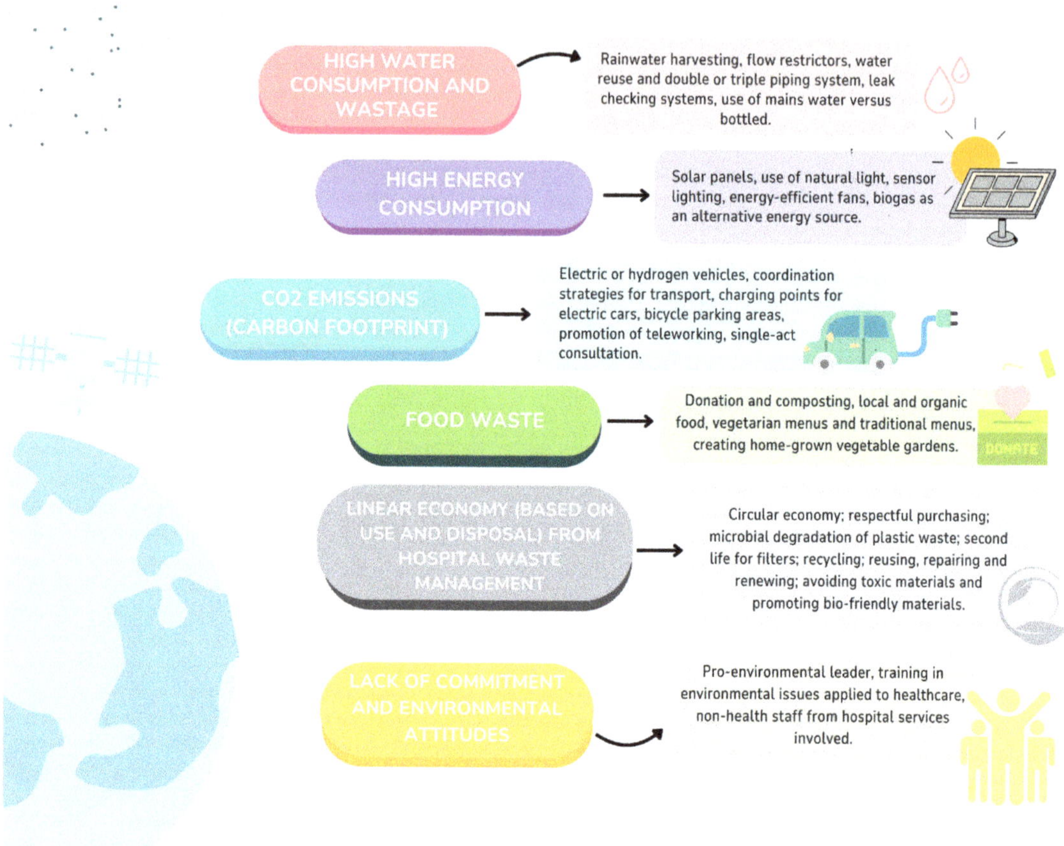

Figure 2. Dynamics of environmental impact of medical activities and measures to reduce it.

Theme 1. Environmental sustainability in healthcare

The detection of a greater environmental impact of the activities of healthcare institutions has been linked to air conditioning; the use of electromedical material for diagnosis; surgical procedures; pharmaceutical products and single-use products such as sterile gloves, gowns, masks or syringes, as well as the transfer of patients themselves to receive healthcare [18,19]. Based on analyses of these forms of damage, various actions in favor of sustainable healthcare stand out.

Promoting sustainable practices in the use of energy and natural resources and in reducing the carbon footprint: Using solar panels and natural light, sensor lighting, energy-efficient fans, biogas and biodiesel, rainwater collection and water treatment were different strategies implemented to achieve a reduction of up to 30% in hospital consumption [20]. Other measures also stand out: checking for leaks in the piping system, using flow restrictors, recycling water and using a double or triple piping system (cold water, hot water and reticulation of non-potable water) [21]. Finally, a study also showed that patient care procedures such as anesthesia could in-corporate climate benefits in pediatrics [22].

Encouraging sustainable transport: Some hospitals have opted to use electric or hydrogen vehicles instead of diesel, create a transport coordination role, install charging points in parking lots for electric cars and create better and larger bicycle parking areas. In addition, the promotion of teleworking has been analyzed as a measure to limit travel and pollution, and to this end, awareness of the importance of sustainable transport for staff and patients has been promoted [23] This is also helped by single-act consultations, where the patient is seen by all professionals involved on the same day (decreasing transport and therefore up to 35% of emissions) [24].

Sustainable food: On the one hand, this review highlights the waste of food in health services and the need to create measures to avoid food waste, such as the reduction of waste by reusing both edible and inedible waste (i.e., donation) [25] and composting. On the other hand, the consumption of local and organic food is encouraged [25,26], as well as implementing vegetarian menus and traditional menus, creating home-grown vegetable gardens [26] and using mains water instead of bottled water in canteens [21]. As an example, the cost of bottled water consumption in a hospital canteen for about 200 people is about €14,000. In contrast, the installation of a microfiltration system in the drinking water supply network plus the water consumed would cost €2800, which would translate into savings of around €11,200 per year [21].

Adopting sustainable practices in waste management: According to some authors [21,27], one hospital produces about 10.58 kg/person/month of non-hazardous waste and 5.26 kg/month of potentially infectious waste. Of this, 62% is not segregated (40% textiles, 20% paper, 17% plastic). It is therefore necessary to promote the separation of waste in order to recycle; promote respectful purchasing (i.e., avoiding composite packaging of needles reduces unsorted waste by 3%); encourage a change in clinical practice to reduce the use of materials [21,28].; reuse, repair and renew (bases of the circular economy) [29]; avoid toxic materials and promote bio-friendly materials and renewable sources [28].

Currently, the linear economy (based on use and disposal) is the most widespread [27]. Achieving a circular economy will require measures such as changes in protocols; staff training; clear instructions from companies on how to recycle material after use; smaller and more recyclable packaging [21,27] or promotion of the segregation of waste in a way that allows its subsequent reuse. A proposed example of creating strategies that include members of society in the functioning of the hospital circular economy consists of cooperatives that allow citizens to take charge of the segregation and sorting of materials, so that they can use them to create recycled objects such as purses, bags or packages, which they can then display or sell at a craft fair [30].

Another specific strategy contemplates microbial degradation as the most sustainable and economical option for the treatment of plastic waste [31] or the possibility of giving a second life to dialysis filters, which can be used as water filters [25]

Theme 2. The involvement of healthcare professionals in environmental sustainability

The studies included in this review have analyzed different attitudes and perceptions of health professionals towards sustainability as well as factors that influence them.

Deng et al. [8] observed that healthcare staff with pro-environmental values significantly tended to favor reducing hospitals' carbon footprint through actions such as the rational use of energy, switching off electrical equipment that is not being used or using recyclable materials. According to Xu et al. [32], the figure of a pro-environmental and sustainability-minded leader could have an influence of around 40% on workers. In addition to this, this leader figure also had a mediating character between the pro-environmental attitudes of healthcare workers and corporate social responsibility in 47% of cases [8], highlighting the positive moderation of female leaders [33]. Another study states that a leader with strong environmental values favors better management of energy expenditure by workers during their clinical activity. For example, up to 90% of the costs of air conditioning can be reduced [9].

In this way, knowledge acquired through training is highlighted as a key factor [8,34–36], which can be extrapolated to future professionals, that is, nursing and medical students. As an example, students from a medical school in Bristol were sent to a SusQI (sustainability in quality improvement) workshop, with the aim of identifying challenges in translating knowledge into practice. Institutional inertia was found to affect their confidence in suggesting changes, and only a minority perceived sustainable healthcare as more than their professional role [37].

Despite the interest of healthcare providers in promoting sustainable measures, several perceived barriers were mentioned, of which the following should receive particular attention: lack of interest on the part of the healthcare facility, difficulty and effort involved in implementing strategies, cost and lack of training [26,27,38]. Regarding renewables, they mentioned that the major impediment to increasing the supply of renewables consisted of the limitations due to the state-level electricity contract and the prices/costs of renewables [39]. However, decreasing the environmental footprint, improving community health, reducing costs, composting and involving non-health staff from other hospital services are perceived as enablers.

4. Discussion

To evaluate the contribution of this review, an analysis of existing similar works was conducted beforehand. The review of other systematic review studies did not reveal a perspective equivalent to that addressed in this work, which has focused on offering a comprehensive literature review to provide a broad perspective on the current state of knowledge, specifically centered on the attitude of healthcare institutions towards implementing environmental care measures within their organizations and the importance of the involvement of healthcare professionals in the application of such measures. This review paper specifically aims to synthesize the state of knowledge concerning the role of hospital institutions in the development and implementation of sustainability strategies related to healthcare service delivery and reducing pollutant emissions such as chemical, radioactive or greenhouse gases and other harmful substances. It also explores the extent to which hospital management prioritizes environmental harm reduction through facility design, technology adoption and the influence of an environmentally oriented organizational culture within the healthcare sector.

Although certain reviews have addressed issues related to the role of healthcare managers, such as those by van Schie [40] and McCauley et al. [41], these studies lack the broad, synthesizing approach undertaken in this review. The systematic reviews published in recent years, although abundant, primarily focus in most cases on environmental improvements in the management of specific healthcare services, such as surgery [42], radiology [43], gastroenterology [44] or radiology departments [45].

Regarding the included works, it is noteworthy that 70% of the papers included in the review were published in the last three years, predominantly in Europe, indicating the cultural influence underlying the prevalence of such policies. Furthermore, the reviewed literature reveals no controversies or opposing viewpoints regarding the necessity of implementing measures to improve hospital management practices. However, while studies such as those of Barbero and Pallaro [25], Cakmak and Yol [46] and Dagenais et al. [38] highlighted the importance of organizational involvement, others, such as that of Boussuge-Roze et al. [27], revealed that healthcare professionals surveyed across

42 countries perceived a lack of interest from the hospitals (59%) and insufficient training (37%) in the implementation of new procedures. The relevance of programs involving staff in environmental care is underscored by other systematic literature reviews with a narrower focus on specific services, such as the review by Huo et al. [47], which pertains to surgical services.

An intriguing aspect regarding potential areas for knowledge expansion lies in the economic evaluation of the benefits derived from implementing waste reduction strategies and improving environmental management in healthcare facilities. While the reviewed studies mention economic advantages, including those from a circular economy perspective, no comprehensive economic analysis supporting these claims has been conducted. This topic is only partially addressed in the literature review conducted by Davies et al. [48].

Implications for Clinical Practice

The results of this study provide a starting point to help create a model for healthcare facility management that contributes to global health and the development of green hospitals. For nurses, in particular, this review is a call to action within the decision-making competencies of the management bodies of healthcare institutions and health systems. Considering the breadth of services offered by nurses, proposals for environmentally sustainable healthcare can emerge. Furthermore, the results highlight the need for sustainability training from academic to continuing education courses and multidisciplinary collaborative work.

Another implication would be the possibility of involving other managers and policymakers in refining regulations that motivate the environmental participation of the centers, that is, that the people who provide healthcare would have the political and regulatory support needed to contribute to the achievement of the 2030 Agenda.

Finally, we must address the implications for citizens. Firstly, by reducing environmental pollution and promoting the use of preventive and health-promoting practices, sustainable practices can help prevent disease and improve the quality of life of the population. Secondly, reducing resource consumption and improving efficiency in service delivery can make health services more accessible and affordable to society. Lastly, reducing energy and water consumption contributes to a healthier and safer environment. In other words, the implementation of sustainable healthcare systems has important implications in terms of improving the quality of healthcare, reducing healthcare costs and environmental impact and promoting a culture of sustainability.

5. Limitations

The present review has some limitations that should be highlighted. It is possible that not all available information has been found, as many hospital sustainability initiatives or approaches may be part of hospital policies, regulations and/or projects that have not been disseminated at a scientific level. However, very broad descriptors and five electronic databases were applied to ensure the greatest number of available resources. A broader review of the gray literature, as well as a review of calls for projects and data from ministries related to health and the environment or from healthcare organizations or systems themselves, would likely be productive in future lines of research. Finally, although this work highlights the assessment of unexplored aspects of the problem, it has the limitations of a review, that is, the absence of proven novelties. To this end, this group of authors, as part of the SUSTAinsHealth project, is carrying out interviews with a qualitative approach regarding environmental sustainability strategies in the health sector that could be replicated in different countries.

6. Conclusions

The health system is increasingly adopting 'green' hospital services, which emphasize the environmental and social impacts of institutional operations. Hospitals play a pivotal role in evaluating and mitigating the environmental footprint of healthcare activities. This study identified a range of sustainable initiatives grounded in a circular economy framework, encompassing sustainable practices in energy and natural resource use, eco-friendly transport solutions, sustainable food procurement and comprehensive waste management strategies. Furthermore, the findings underscore the critical role of committed leadership and the pro-environmental attitudes of managers and healthcare professionals, which act as catalysts to foster more sustainable and environmentally conscious healthcare practices. This highlights the necessity of integrating environmental stewardship into the strategic and operational frameworks of healthcare systems, positioning hospitals as key players in promoting ecological sustainability within their communities.

Supplementary Materials: The following supporting information can be downloaded at: https://www.mdpi.com/article/10.3390/environments12010009/s1.

Author Contributions: Conceptualization, B.B. and R.d.-D.-C.; methodology, B.B.; formal analysis, B.B. and M.G.-C.-C.; investigation, B.B., J.M.P.-J., M.G.-C.-C., M.R.-A., A.P.S., S.T.F. and F.J.R.M.; resources, B.B., J.M.P.-J., M.R.-A., A.P.S., S.T.F. and F.J.R.M.; data curation, B.B. and R.d.-D.-C.; writing—original draft preparation, B.B., R.d.-D.-C., J.M.P.-J., M.G.-C.-C., M.R.-A., A.P.S., S.T.F. and F.J.R.M.; writing—review and editing, B.B., R.d.-D.-C., J.M.P.-J., M.G.-C.-C., M.R.-A., A.P.S., S.T.F. and F.J.R.M.; supervision, B.B. and R.d.-D.-C. All authors have read and agreed to the published version of the manuscript.

Funding: This work is related to the project "Development of a Model with an Ethical and Gender Perspective for the Implementation of Sustainability Measures in Healthcare Centres and Institutions" (SUSTAinsHealth). It was funded in 2024 by the VII Own Research Plan—V.1C Program to stimulate areas with research needs and emerging research activity (Vice-Rectorate for Research of the University of Seville). VIIPPIT-2023-V.1—Programme for the Stimulation of Areas with Research Needs and Emerging Research Activity. Modality C. SOL2024-30413.

Data Availability Statement: The data that support the findings of this study are available upon request from the corresponding authors.

Conflicts of Interest: The authors declare no conflicts of interest.

Appendix A

Table A1. Results of the Systematic Review.

Reference	Objective	Methodology	Main Findings	Theme
Abhilash, 2022 [31] (India)	To analyze the means of treatment and/or disposal of plastic waste in the hospital setting during the COVID-19 pandemic.	Qualitative narrative analysis of degradation methods for plastic polymers.	The microbial degradation of plastic waste (degradation of plastic polymers and production of bio-based polymers) was found to be the most cost-effective and least ecotoxic method compared to other methods such as chemical disinfection; dissolution of plastic polymers to recover pigments or other polymers and thermal processes, most notably pyrolysis (use of thermal energy to break the chemical bonds in polymers).	Environmental sustainability in healthcare

Table A1. *Cont.*

Reference	Objective	Methodology	Main Findings	Theme
Barbero and Pallaro, 2017 [25] (Italy)	To discuss the potential of applying a systemic design (SD) approach for sustainable healthcare.	Qualitative study using a systemic design (SD) approach	The SD methodology is presented for enhanced material and energy production processes in the healthcare industry, thus reducing energy expenditure. Several examples of the use of this system include "communication design" (e.g., raising awareness about local food consumption, improving the circular economy, and protecting the environment), "NUF portable filters" (reusing dialysis filters to purify water in other low-income countries), "recovery of hospital food waste" (preventing food waste generation and promoting its reuse in hospitals by educating staff and users) and "eco-dialysis" (exploring the relationship between the components of dialysis devices to optimize material and energy flow, thus creating an efficient and sustainable system adapted to patient needs).	Environmental sustainability in healthcare
Boussuge-Roze et al., 2022 [27] (Various countries)	To investigate the current practice and expectations of European cardiac electro-physiology (EP) centers in terms of environmental sustainability, with a focus on EP catheters.	Quantitative study (online survey) Sample: N = 278 public hospital workers from 42 countries. Gender: 76% men Average age: 43 years.	A total of 72% of the healthcare professionals surveyed say that a linear economy of disposable catheters and packaging is still in place. Possible solutions include changes through protocols, educating professionals, clear instructions from companies after use of the material for recycling, reusing catheters after the necessary regulatory measures and using recyclable and smaller packaging. Overall, 82% of respondents showed interest in performing sustainable work, identifying the main barriers as the lack of interest from the hospital (59%), the complexity of the measures (48%), the effort required to change practices (47%), cost (33%) and lack of training (37%).	Engaging health professionals in environmental sustainability
Burch and McGain, 2021 [39] (Australia)	To identify points of view of healthcare leaders about the carbon footprint, sources of energy and barriers in the field of health.	Qualitative study (interviews) Sample: N = 13 Victorian public healthcare chief executive officers	Most participants acknowledged the importance of climate change and were cognizant of its negative impact. In addition, they had a consensus regarding the significant role of leadership in prompting environmental sustainability in the health public sector. Currently, however, support for renewable electricity is, for the most part, an aspiration and not perceived as a priority, although electricity accounts for 7% of total carbon emissions in Australia. The main perceived barriers to increasing renewable energy supply were limitations due to state-level electricity contracts and the costs of renewable energy resources.	Engaging health professionals in environmental sustainability

Table A1. *Cont.*

Reference	Objective	Methodology	Main Findings	Theme
Cakmak and Yol, 2019 [46] (Türkiye)	To create awareness of optimizing energy while maintaining quality in the provision of health services in medical devices.	Quantitative study calculating the energy density of hospital equipment. Sample: N = 1 hospital in Turkey	The medical devices that consume the most energy were radiological imaging, angiography, nuclear medicine, biosafety cabinets, autoclaves, incubators and operating rooms. The majority of this consumption was due to laser devices. Large medical imaging equipment accounted for 38% of the hospital's energy consumption, followed by nuclear medicine at 15%. Energy-saving strategies include reducing standby power levels, using hibernation and shortening startup times on high-power devices.	Environmental sustainability in healthcare
Carino et al., 2021 [26] (Various countries)	To explore the perspectives of hospital food supply chain staff on sustainable practices in food provision, identifying existing barriers and enablers and gathering recommendations for future implementation of sustainable foodservice practices.	Qualitative (semi-interview structure) Sample: N = 46 participants from across the food supply chain for patients Gender: 65% women	Strategies were identified to achieve sustainable food services, such as purchasing organic and local food, composting, vegetarian menus, use of traditional foods and creation of vegetable gardens. Innovation, education of society and environmental professionals and the creation of government regulations were highlighted as facilitators for sustainable food practices. Barriers included strict infection control standards and requirements, restrictions in current waste disposal contracts and the lack of a food sustainability policy.	Environmental sustainability in healthcare
Cockrell et al., 2022 [13] (USA)	To evaluate the environmental impact of implementing telehealth.	Quantitative (Retrospective cohort study at a pediatric surgical care center) Sample: N = 60,773 face-to-face meetings and 10,626 telehealth meetings	The incorporation of telehealth in preanesthesia and pediatric surgery clinics resulted in significant reductions in CO_2 emissions. Telehealth resulted in 1477 patient-km saved and a 312-ton reduction in CO_2 emissions. It was also shown that the greater the distance from home to the hospital, the greater the use of telehealth.	Environmental sustainability in healthcare

Table A1. *Cont.*

Reference	Objective	Methodology	Main Findings	Theme
Dagenais et al., 2022 [38] (Canada)	To analyze the barriers and facilitators to implementing sustainable menu practices (SMPs) in Quebec healthcare institutions.	Qualitative study (interviews) Sample: N = 17 foodservice managers from healthcare institutions	The barriers encountered were perceived to a greater extent than the facilitators. These include the complexity of implementation due to the lack of adaption to all institutional contexts, which is related to the lack of support from these organizations and the perception of high cost. This highlights the need for greater collaboration and communication between all actors in the hospital food system. The highlighted facilitators include a reduction in the ecological footprint, contribution to improving community health, the possibility of composting, cost reduction, a reduction in subcontracting, centralization of the kitchen and the involvement of kitchen staff in sustainable development.	Environmental sustainability in healthcare
Deng et al., 2022 [8] (Pakistan)	To examine the relationship between a hospital's corporate social responsibility (CSR) initiatives and employees' pro-environmental behavior with the mediating effect of environmentally specific transformational leadership (ESTL).	Quantitative study (self-administered survey) Sample: N = 239 employees of the Lahore Hospital (39% position) leadership and 66% between 1 and 5 years of work experience). Gender: 58.39% men Age: 89% between 22 and40 years	Leaders embracing environmental sustainability and CSR have a transformational role and significantly influence the pro-environmental attitudes of healthcare workers (manifested as pro-environmental behavior, or PEB), thus facilitating the development of sustainability measures. The ESTL not only directly influences PEB but also acts as a mediator between the PEB and CSR of healthcare workers in 47% of cases. Furthermore, a positive relationship was observed between altruistic values and greater involvement of staff in the initiatives. Thus, the promotion of these values through training was recommended.	Engaging health professionals in environmental sustainability
Eckelman et al., 2018 [3] (Canada)	To estimate the life cycle emissions and associated environmental impacts and secondary health damage produced by the Canadian healthcare system.	Qualitative study Economic–environmental–epidemiological analysis to compare medical expenses with emissions of greenhouse gases and other pollutants.	Greenhouse gas emissions in the Canadian health industry are mainly due to hospital activities, pharmaceutical products and medical services. Canadian healthcare activities accounted for 33 million tons of greenhouse gas emissions and more than 200,000 tons of other pollutant emissions, resulting in an estimated annual loss of 23,000 disability-adjusted life years due to exposure to these pollutants.	Environmental sustainability in healthcare

Table A1. *Cont.*

Reference	Objective	Methodology	Main Findings	Theme
Fang et al., 2022 [34] (China)	To review the experiences acquired in nosocomial environments around the world related to healthcare waste management.	Quantitative study (survey) Sample: N = 416 Hospital workers and managers in Shanghai.	A key factor in achieving sustainable waste management is environmental education of staff. Other strategies include conducting an orderly environmental inventory, planning and executing the placement of materials with reuse of everything possible, reducing wastage of energy (turning off electrical appliances when not in use, rational use of air conditioning) and materials and reducing power systems (electrical, thermal, etc.).	Environmental sustainability in healthcare
Geethika and Devi, 2022 [20] (India)	To measure the ecological costs, using carbon foot-printing and operational costs, of a 250-bed multi-specialty hospital with basic green hospital compliance.	Mixed study Participant observation, discussion groups and data obtained from the hospital database. Sample: N = 250-bed multi-specialty hospital	The service with the highest cost and energy consumption (up to 80%) for any hospital is air conditioning. The factors that generate the largest carbon footprint during hospital practices are electricity consumption (17,000 tons of CO_2/year) and the biomedical waste generated (723 tons of CO_2). Some sustainable ecological tools that have been used are as follows: - Use of solar energy (145 solar panels) and natural light; - Combined heat and power system; - Low-consumption ceiling fans; - Motion-sensor lighting; - Local suppliers; - Use of biogas and biodiesel; - Rainwater harvesting and on-site water treatment. These measures reduced the hospital's operating costs by 30%.	Environmental sustainability in healthcare
Hunfeld et al., 2023 [19] (Netherland)	To perform a material flow analysis in an academic intensive care unit and to obtain information on mass, carbon footprint, agricultural land occupation and water usage and to determine so-called "environmental hotspots" in the ICU.	Mixed study Material flow analysis by combining data analysis, measurements, desk research and interviews with staff members Sample: N = 1 ICU at Erasmus MC hospital in Rotterdam (56 mixed surgical and non-surgical beds)	The environmental impact per patient admitted to the ICU was 17 kg of solid waste, 12 kg of CO_2 eq, 300 L of water use and 4 m^2 of agricultural land occupation per day. Five single-use products were identified as the elements with the greatest environmental impact in terms of resource use and waste generation: non-sterile gloves, isolation gowns, bed protectors, surgical masks and syringes (including packaging).	Environmental sustainability in healthcare

Table A1. *Cont.*

Reference	Objective	Methodology	Main Findings	Theme
Irianti, 2016 [29] (Australia)	To gain information about methods and technology used in hospital waste management that can be adopted by Indonesian hospitals.	Qualitative study In-depth interviews and observation Sample: Hospital personnel of HWM practices in The Royal Brisbane and Women's Hospital (Australia).	The proposed hospital waste management is based on the division of waste into four groups (clinical, cytotoxic, recyclable and general waste) and focuses on the incorporation of the '3 Rs' (reduce, recycle and reuse), the segregation of sources, color-coded collection to minimize the production of medical waste and the development of a leadership figure to minimize illnesses and accidents related to waste management.	Environmental sustainability in healthcare
Marsden et al., 2021 [37] (United Kingdom)	To evaluate a training workshop on improving sustainability for clinical practice.	Qualitative study (5 focus groups) Sample: N = 17 third-year medical students at Bristol Medical School who participated in a SusQI (sustainability in quality improvement) workshop	Although the workshop motivated students and gave them skills they wanted to use in the future to improve quality, they expressed that there were multiple barriers to translating what they had learned into actual practice. Thus, although the workshop was successful in restructuring students' perceptions of sustainability, it was not enough, as some students were constrained by the social and cultural contexts of their clinical practice settings. Medical students who applied their learning to the clinical workplace were internally motivated and self-determined but needed time and opportunities to complete projects. Other students were cautious about disrupting established hierarchies and practices or were frustrated by institutional inertia. These barriers impacted their confidence in suggesting or achieving change. A minority saw sustainable healthcare as beyond their professional role.	Engaging health professionals in environmental sustainability
Narayanan et al., 2022 [22] (UK)	To compare the differences in the carbon footprint of inhalational anesthesia and total intravenous anesthesia (TIVA) when used in children.	Quantitative study Mathematical simulation models to compare four pediatric anesthesia techniques in children weighing 5, 10, 20, 30, 40 and 50 kg	TIVA with propofol and remifentanil had a smaller carbon footprint during a typical 60 min anesthetic process (1.26 kg of carbon dioxide equivalents [CO_2 eq] for a 20 kg child) than IV induction. followed by maintenance by inhalation (2.58 kg CO_2 eq) and inhalation induction and maintenance (2.98 kg CO_2 eq). Inhalation induction followed by IV maintenance alone had a lower carbon footprint than inhalation induction and maintenance when used in longer procedures (>77 min for children 5–20 kg; >105 min for children 30–50 kg). All in all, IV anesthesia had climate benefits in pediatrics. However, when used after inhalation induction, the benefits were only achieved in longer procedures.	Environmental sustainability in healthcare

Table A1. *Cont.*

Reference	Objective	Methodology	Main Findings	Theme
Peng et al., 2022 [9] (Pakistan)	To improve the energy-specific pro-environmental behavior (EPEB) of hospital employees in an environmentally specific servant leadership (ESL) framework.	Quantitative study Surveys where the variables ESL, EPEB, GSE and GPOS were measured by adapting items from different sources Sample: N = 316 healthcare professionals. Sex: 63% males Age: between 22 and 65 years	The statistical results of the study showed that a servant leadership style with high environmental values (i.e., leaders who prefer environmental benefits to economic ones) has a positive influence on pro-environmental behavior specifically related to energy use by healthcare professionals during the performance of their duties, as employees learn from their leadership and improve their attitudes toward the environment due to the greater perception of support from the organization for implementing ecological initiatives (for instance, without this influence, the energy consumption due to air conditioning increases by 90%). Similarly, the energy consumption behavior of hospital employees improved due to different organizational factors, including leadership style and support for green initiatives.	Engaging health professionals in environmental sustainability
Power et al., 2021 [24] (Ireland)	To estimate the carbon footprint of a single intravitreal injection in a hospital-based intravitreal service.	Quantitative study Calculation of greenhouse gas emissions using the hybrid lifecycle analysis technique (Data on materials procurement, patient travel to and from the hospital and building energy use were used for this calculation)	The carbon emissions associated with an intravitreal injection were 13.68 kg CO_2 eq. This equates to 82,100 kg CO_2 eq annually per ophthalmological service. - Patient journeys: 10.49 kg CO_2 eq per injection (77% of emissions); - Materials procurement: 2.54 kg CO_2 eq (19%); - Building energy use: 0.65 kg CO_2 eq (4% of total emissions). Several aspects were identified that could help reduce emissions, such as bilateral injections on the same day, which would reduce emissions by 35% (less patient travel). Eliminating items considered dispensable from injection packs (povidone–iodine forceps, hand towels, 2 mL syringe, etc.) would reduce emissions by approximately 0.56 kg per injection, i.e., an annual saving of 3360 kg CO_2 eq for an average hospital. No savings were identified in energy use.	Environmental sustainability in healthcare

Table A1. *Cont.*

Reference	Objective	Methodology	Main Findings	Theme
Puška et al., 2022 [23] (Bosnia and Herzegovin)	To suggest a model for the selection of healthcare waste incinerators in secondary healthcare institutions in Bosnia and Herzegovina.	Qualitative study Study in four phases: selection of experts to create a questionnaire to evaluate incinerator alternatives, establishing the weight of the criteria selected in the previous phase, ranking of incinerators and sensitivity analysis and examination of the results. Sample: N = 3 experts examined 6 incinerators	Based on fuel consumption and environmental impact, alternative A2 (I8-M50) best meets the objectives, followed by alternative A1 (I8-M40). Small incinerators have less impact on the environment than larger ones because they consume less fuel and destroy less waste. Their community acceptance is better; they take up less space and are less expensive compared to large incinerators. They can also be installed in populated areas because they do not generate significant air pollution. The study showed that the most important criterion according to the experts' assessment is the technical criterion, followed by the economic and environmental criteria, with the social criterion (acceptance of the incinerator by the community) being the least important.	Environmental sustainability in healthcare
Ryan-Forgarty et al., 2016 [36] (Ireland).	To explain and evaluate a systems-based action framework designed to create synergies between both regulatory requirements and voluntary initiatives, supported by government agencies and NGOs, so as to best meet environmental impact mitigation objectives.	Qualitative study Review of programs and actions on waste management and energy consumption. Sample: Cork University Hospital Programs: Green Campus; Eco-Schools; EPA Green Health; Global Network of Green Hospitals Healthy; Public Sector Energy Efficiency Program	This implementation resulted in the mitigation of existing impacts and a commitment to continuous improvement. Environmental education programs, especially action- and reward-based programs, proved successful in providing a systematic approach that facilitates environmental action and education. The researchers acted as advisors and highlighted the seven steps of the program, namely, creating an environmental committee, conducting an environmental study, developing an action plan, monitoring and evaluation (using sustainability indicators), reporting and engagement, linking to on-campus learning and developing a green charter (to ensure continuity).	Environmental sustainability in healthcare

Table A1. *Cont.*

Reference	Objective	Methodology	Main Findings	Theme
Simpson et al., 2022 [35] (United Kingdom)	To scope, identify and appraise the effectiveness of proposed actions relevant to air quality across all areas of operational management at the Queen Elizabeth Hospital Birmingham.	Mixed study Semi-structured interviews and questionnaire to score 79 actions identified in the qualitative phase Sample: 32 experts in areas of interest for the project	The actions with the greatest impact on improving air quality were as follows: - Improve the efficiency of activities that are executed remotely; - Create the role of transportation coordinator to help reduce the impact of employee travel and transportation; - Convert the fleet to electric or hydrogen fuel to replace diesel trucks and vans; - Establish real optimal levels of teleworking and guide the sustainable use of transport to establish new habits; - Implement 'auto-off' periods for non-essential information technology equipment; - Incorporate sustainability into procurement processes by rewarding low-impact and low-emission supply chains; - Install charging points for electric vehicles in the parking lot; - Evaluate the capacity of bicycle courier logistics; - Collect patient and visitor travel data through registration systems; - Integrate sustainable transportation into the patient mindset; - Create and promote a 'sustainability in health management' module with the education department; - Create more and better secure bicycle storage.	Environmental sustainability in healthcare
Scavarda et al., 2019 [30] (Brazil)	To analyze the central sterilization department and the storage of materials in the health supply chain in a Brazilian private health institution and propose a management framework.	Literature review and analysis of the supply chain of materials that make up surgical kits in a healthcare institution (observing the processing of approximately 400 surgical kits from 50 hip arthroplasty surgical procedures). Sample: private health institution in Rio de Janeiro with 200 beds and 11 operating rooms	The proposed healthcare supply chain management framework addresses four materials. It advocates strategies to sell cardboard for packaging to recycling cooperatives, which could save USD 132,000 at the end of one year. Paperboard also provides craftsman cooperatives with other possibilities for conversion into several other products, such as earring, bracelet and necklace boxes. In relation to plastics, a reduction in their use is encouraged, including incineration, reducing the release of toxins. Furthermore, the sale of plastic may reduce the costs of nonwoven sterile barrier systems, thereby allowing reverse logistics of these products to be implemented in the supply chain.	Environmental sustainability in healthcare

Table A1. Cont.

Reference	Objective	Methodology	Main Findings	Theme
Vaccari et al., 2017 [21] (Italy)	To examine approaches to more sustainable management of waste and water consumption in a healthcare facility.	Quantitative study Sample: N = 1, Gardone Val Trompia Hospital in Brescia, Italy.	Some of the highlighted proposals are as follows: - Technological practices: modification of plants or supply procedures. - Behavioral practices: changing staff and patient water usage habits (i.e., using fresh water instead of bottled water in the dining room). - Healthcare solid waste management: the hospital produces 10.58 kg/person/month of non-hazardous waste and 5.26 kg/month of potentially infectious waste. A high level of unsorted waste was observed (62%), mainly textiles (40%), paper (20%) and plastics (17%). Given the high consumption of paper and plastics, there is a possibility of recovering their value provided they can be segregated, waste can be selectively collected, and recycling is increased. On the other hand, efforts must be made to change clinical practices by using fewer materials and incorporating the use of environmentally friendly materials.	Environmental sustainability in healthcare
Vishwakarma et al., 2022 [28] (India)	To investigate the relationship among the indicators of stakeholder involvement, sustainable supply chain practices, sustainable performance and the circular economy and its effect on attaining sustainability at large.	Quantitative study Questionnaires to identify SHSCP, HSI, SHP and CHE practices. Sample: N = 145 participants (60.68% hospital staff and 39.32% healthcare industry stakeholders)	A positive relationship was confirmed among the circular economy, the supply chain, the participation of people interested in healthcare and sustainability measures (statistically significant relationships between HSI and SHSCP; HSI and SHP; SHSCP and SHP; SHSCP and CHE and SHP and CHE. Some of the proposals include repairing, reusing and renewing resources; reducing biomedical waste and the use of toxic materials; extending the useful life of products; and making greater use of bio-friendly products and renewable sources. In addition, the circular economy was promoted as a mechanism to streamline consumption and increase digitalization.	Engaging health professionals in environmental sustainability

Table A1. *Cont.*

Reference	Objective	Methodology	Main Findings	Theme
Wei et al., 2021 [33] (China, Pakistan and Romania)	To reduce the environmental footprint of a hospital by promoting its employees' environment-specific behavior via corporate social responsibility (CSR) and ethical leadership (EL).	Quantitative study Survey Sample: N = 489 staff surveys from the hospital (61.76% health workers and 38.24% general administration) Gender: 56.85% men Age: 42.55% from 20 to 30 years, 46.01% from 31 to 50 and 11.6% over 50	The respondents confirmed that they were motivated to participate in different activities related to environmental behavior in response to the commitment to corporate social responsibility (CSR) by this organization ($\beta1 = 0.426$; $p < 0.05$). Therefore, to reduce the environmental footprint of institutions, policies are needed that redefine the CRS of institutions, and they need to understand the importance of CRS. A positive relationship was observed between EL and CRS ($\beta2 = 0.388$; $p < 0.05$), as well as between EL and employee pro-environmental behavior ($\beta3 = 0.32$; $p < 0.05$). An ethical leader must communicate to the employee the importance of improving the environmental footprint. The overall environmental performance of organizations is enhanced through the voluntary commitment of their employees. In the presence of such leadership, employees increase their environmental commitment to a higher level, stimulating their pro-environmental behavior ($\beta4 = 0.128$, $p < 0.05$). Finally, both male and female leaders positively moderated the indirect relationship between CSR and pro-environmental behavior, but this moderation was stronger among female leaders.	Engaging health professionals in environmental sustainability
Weisz et al., 2020 [18] (Austria and Germany)	To identify areas for sustainability improvement in healthcare systems and break down carbon emissions attributable to this care.	Quantitative study Multi-regional input–output analysis for carbon emissions by healthcare providers. Sample: healthcare systems in Austria and Germany	Austria's healthcare carbon footprint was 6.8 million tonnes of CO_2 in 2014 (14% less than in 2005, thanks to the use of renewable energy). Hospitals contributed 32% of emissions, with 48 tCO_2 per bed per year. Emissions were mainly produced by purchases of medical goods and services (36%), pharmaceuticals (19%) and energy consumption (31%). CO_2 emissions from patient transport also increased by 15%, demonstrating the need for improved planning. The six main areas of intervention in sustainability are direct energy use, product alternatives, prevention of inefficiencies in the health system (e.g., rational use of pharmaceuticals), changes in medical treatments, changes in national planning of health service delivery and transformation of the healthcare system towards promotion.	Environmental sustainability in healthcare

Table A1. *Cont.*

Reference	Objective	Methodology	Main Findings	Theme
Xu et al., 2022 [22] (Pakistan)	To analyze the attitude and the pro-environmental behavior (PEB) of healthcare professionals through corporate social responsibility (CSR) and green organizational practices in the health sector of an emerging economy.	Quantitative study Survey Sample: N = 441 health professionals Sex: 58% men (256) and 42% women (185) Age: from 18 to 65 years	CSR activities were shown to positively influence employees' pro-environmental behavior ($\beta1 = 0.493$; $p < 0.01$) and promote the adoption of green practices in organizations ($\beta2 = 0.362$; $p < 0.01$). Furthermore, the results indicated that the implementation of green organizational practices fosters employees' green behavior ($\beta3 = 0.183$; $p < 0.01$). Healthcare professionals with pro-environmental, altruistic values favor a reduction in the carbon footprint of a hospital ($\beta4 = 0.276$, $p < 0.01$) through actions such as rational energy use, turning off electrical equipment when not in use and using recyclable and reusable materials. Therefore, it was suggested that the hospital re-evaluate its hiring procedure to select these types of professionals, as they will help the hospital's sustainability to a greater extent. Similarly, HE demonstrates the importance of personal values and the corporate responsibility of managers to be proactive in environmental sustainability.	Engaging health professionals in environmental sustainability

References

1. World Health Organization. Health. Cambio Climatico 2023. Available online: http://www.who.int/news-room/fact-sheets/detail/climate-change-and-health#:~:text=Climate%20change%20affects%20food%20availability,700%20000%20annually,%20may%20rise (accessed on 24 November 2023).
2. Zikhathile, T.; Atagana, H.; Bwapwa, J.; Sawtell, D. A review of the impact that healthcare risk waste treatment technologies have on the environment. *Int. J. Environ. Res. Public Health* **2022**, *19*, 11967. [CrossRef]
3. Eckelman, M.J.; Sherman, J.D.; MacNeill, A.J. Life cycle environmental emissions and health damages from the Canadian healthcare system: An economic-environmentalepidemiological analysis. *PLoS Med.* **2018**, *15*, e1002623. [CrossRef] [PubMed]
4. Balali, A.; Valipour, A. Prioritization of passive measures for energy optimization designing of sustainable hospitals and health centres. *J. Build. Eng.* **2021**, *35*, 101992. [CrossRef]
5. Alotaibi, D.M.; Akrami, M.; Dibaj, M.; Javadi, A.A. Smart energy solution for an optimized sustainable hospital in the green city of NEOM. *Sustain. Energy Technol. Assess.* **2019**, *35*, 32–40. [CrossRef]
6. Dion, H.; Evans, M. Strategic frameworks for sustainability and corporate governance in healthcare facilities; approaches to energy-efficient hospital management. *Benchmarking* **2023**, *31*, 353–390. [CrossRef]
7. Chomać-Pierzecka, E. Pharmaceutical Companies in the Light of the Idea of Sustainable Development—An Analysis of Selected Aspects of Sustainable Management. *Sustainability* **2023**, *15*, 8889. [CrossRef]
8. Deng, Y.; Cherian, J.; Ahmad, N.; Scholz, M.; Samad, S. Conceptualizing the role of targetspecific environmental transformational leadership between corporate social responsibility and pro-environmental behaviors of hospital employees. *Int. J. Environ. Res. Public Health* **2022**, *19*, 3565. [CrossRef] [PubMed]
9. Peng, J.; Samad, S.; Comite, U.; Ahmad, N.; Han, H.; Ariza-Montes, A.; Vega-Muñoz, A. Environmentally specific servant leadership and employees' energy-specific proenvironmental behavior: Evidence from healthcare sector of a developing economy. *Int. J. Environ. Res. Public Health* **2022**, *19*, 7641. [CrossRef] [PubMed]
10. Luque-Alcaraz, O.M.; Aparicio-Martinez, P.; Gomera, A.; Vaquero-Abellan, M. Nurses as agents for achieving environmentally sustainable health systems: A bibliometric analysis. *J. Nurs. Manag.* **2022**, *30*, 3900–3908. [CrossRef] [PubMed]
11. Ward, A.; Heart, D.; Richards, C.; Bayliss, L.T.; Holmes, M.; Keogh, S.; Best, O. Reimaginando el papel de la educación de enfermería en la reducción de emisiones. *Enseñar. Aprender. Enfermeras.* **2022**, *17*, 410–416. [CrossRef]

12. Holmner, Å.; Ebi, K.L.; Lazuardi, L.; Nilsson, M. Carbon footprint of telemedicine solutions—Unexplored opportunity for reducing carbon emissions in the health sector. *PLoS ONE* **2014**, *9*, e105040. [CrossRef]
13. Cockrell, H.C.; Maine, R.G.; Hansen, E.E.; Mehta, K.; Salazar, D.R.; Stewart, B.T.; Greenberg, S.L.M. Environmental impact of telehealth use for pediatric surgery. *J. Pediatr. Surg.* **2022**, *57*, 865–869. [CrossRef]
14. Sherman, J.D.; Thiel, C.; MacNeill, A.; Eckelman, M.J.; Dubrow, R.; Hopf, H.; Lagasse, R.; Bialowitz, J.; Costello, A.; Forbes, M.; et al. The green print: Advancement of environmental sustainability in healthcare. *Resour. Conserv. Recycl.* **2020**, *161*, 104882. [CrossRef]
15. Sherman, J.D.; MacNeill, A.; Thiel, C. Reducing pollution from the health care industry. *JAMA* **2019**, *322*, 1043–1044. [CrossRef] [PubMed]
16. Page, M.J.; McKenzie, J.E.; Bossuyt, P.M.; Boutron, I.; Hoffmann, T.C.; Mulrow, C.D.; Alonso-Fernández, S. The PRISMA 2020 statement: An updated guideline for reporting systematic reviews. *BMJ* **2021**, *372*, n71, Correction in *Rev. Española Cardiol.* **2021**, *74*, 790–799. [CrossRef]
17. Braun, V.; Clarcke, V. *Thematic Analysis: A Practical Guide*; Sage: London, UK, 2021.
18. Weisz, U.; Pichler, P.-P.; Jaccard, I.S.; Haas, W.; Matej, S.; Bachner, F.; Nowak, P.; Weisz, H. Carbon emission trends and sustainability options in Austrian health care. *Resour. Conserv. Recycl.* **2020**, *160*, 104862. [CrossRef]
19. Hunfeld, N.; Diehl, J.C.; Timmermann, M.; van Exter, P.; Bouwens, J.; Browne-Wilkinson, S.; de Planque, N.; Gommers, D. Circular material flow in the intensive care unit-environmental effects and identification of hotspots. *Intensiv. Care Med.* **2023**, *49*, 65–74. [CrossRef] [PubMed]
20. Geethika, K.; Bhooma Devi, A. A Sustainable Approach on Socio-Ecological and Socio-Economical Impact of Hospitals. *J. Pharm. Negat. Results* **2022**, *13*, 3130–3141.
21. Vaccari, M.; Montasser, W.; Tudor, T.; Leone, L. Environmental audits and process flow mapping to assess management of solid waste and wastewater from a healthcare facility: An Italian case study. *Environ. Monit. Assess.* **2017**, *189*, 239. [CrossRef] [PubMed]
22. Narayanan, H.; Raistrick, C.; Tom Pierce, J.M.; Shelton, C. Carbon footprint of inhalational and total intravenous anaesthesia for paediatric anaesthesia: A modelling study. *Br. J. Anaesth.* **2022**, *129*, 231–243. [CrossRef]
23. Puška, A.; Stević, Ž.; Pamučar, D. Evaluation and selection of healthcare waste incinerators using extended sustainability criteria and multi-criteria analysis methods. *Environ. Dev. Sustain.* **2022**, *24*, 11195–11225. [CrossRef]
24. Power, B.; Brady, R.; Connell, P. Analyzing the carbon footprint of an intravitreal injection. *J. Ophthalmic Vis. Res.* **2021**, *16*, 367–376. [CrossRef] [PubMed]
25. Barbero, S.; Pallaro, A. Systemic design for sustainable healthcare. *Des. J.* **2017**, *20*, S2473–S2485. [CrossRef]
26. Carino, S.; Collins, J.; Malekpour, S.; Porter, J. Environmentally sustainable hospital foodservices: Drawing on staff perspectives to guide change. *Sustain. Prod. Consum.* **2021**, *25*, 152–161. [CrossRef]
27. B oussuge-Roze, J.; Boveda, S.; Mahida, S.; Anic, A.; Conte, G.; Chun, J.K.R.; Marijon, E.; Sacher, F.; Jais, P. Current practices and expectations to reduce environmental impact of electrophysiology catheters: Results from an EHRA/LIRYC European physician survey. *Europace* **2022**, *24*, 1300–1306. [CrossRef]
28. Vishwakarma, A.; Dangayach, G.S.; Meena, M.L.; Gupta, S.; Joshi, D.; Jagtap, S. Can circular healthcare economy be achieved through implementation of sustainable healthcare supply chain practices? Empirical evidence from Indian healthcare sector. *J. Glob. Oper. Strateg. Sourc.* **2022**, *17*, 230–246. [CrossRef]
29. Irianti, S. Hospital waste management in Queensland, Australia, 2010: A case study for sustainable hospital waste management in Indonesia. *Media Penelit. Dan Pengemb. Kesehat.* **2016**, *26*, 109–118. [CrossRef]
30. Scavarda, A.; Daú, G.L.; Scavarda, L.F.; Korzenowski, A.L. A proposed healthcare supply chain management framework in the emerging economies with the sustainable lenses: The theory, the practice, and the policy. *Resour. Conserv. Recycl.* **2019**, *141*, 418–430. [CrossRef]
31. Abhilash; Inamdar, I. Recycling of plastic wastes generated from COVID-19: A comprehensive illustration of type and properties of plastics with remedial options. *Sci. Total Environ.* **2022**, *838 Pt 1*, 155895. [CrossRef] [PubMed]
32. Xu, L.; Cherian, J.; Zaheer, M.; Sial, M.S.; Comite, U.; Cismas, L.M.; Cristia, J.F.E.; Oláh, J. The role of healthcare employees' pro-environmental behavior for DE-carbonization: An energy conservation approach from CSR perspective. *Energies* **2022**, *15*, 3429. [CrossRef]
33. Wei, S.; Sial, M.S.; Zhou, W.; Badulescu, A.; Badulescu, D. Improving the environmental footprint through employees: A case of female leaders from the perspective of CSR. *Int. J. Environ. Res. Public Health* **2021**, *18*, 13082. [CrossRef] [PubMed]
34. Fang, Z.; Kong, X.-Y.; Xiao, Y.-M.; Sun, L.-J.; Cen, J. Factors in waste management of environmentally friendly hospitals. *J. Environ. Prot. Ecol.* **2022**, *23*, 77–83.
35. Simpson, O.; Elliott, M.; Muller, C.; Jones, T.; Hentsch, P.; Rooney, D.; Cowell, N.; Bloss, W.J.; Bartington, S.E. Evaluating actions to improve air quality at University Hospitals Birmingham NHS Foundation Trust. *Sustainability* **2022**, *14*, 11128. [CrossRef]

36. Ryan-Fogarty, Y.; O'Regan, B.; Moles, R. Greening healthcare: Systematic implementation of environmental programmes in a university teaching hospital. *J. Clean. Prod.* **2016**, *126*, 248–259. [CrossRef]
37. Marsden, O.; Clery, P.; Smith, S.D.; Leedham-Green, K. Sustainability in Quality Improvement (SusQI): Challenges and strategies for translating undergraduate learning into clinical practice. *BMC Med. Educ.* **2021**, *21*, 555. [CrossRef] [PubMed]
38. Dagenais, B.; Marquez, A.; Lavoie, J.; Hunter, B.; Mercille, G. RD Adopting sustainable menu practices in healthcare institutions: Perceived barriers and facilitators. *Can. J. Diet. Pr. Res.* **2022**, *83*, 120–127. [CrossRef] [PubMed]
39. Burch, H.; McGain, F. Victorian public healthcare Chief Executive Officers' views on renewable energy supply. *Aust. Health Rev.* **2021**, *45*, 7. [CrossRef]
40. Van Schie, V. Governance related factors influencing the implementation of sustainability in hospitals: A systematic literature review. *Health Policy* **2024**, *146*, 105115. [CrossRef]
41. McCauley, P.R.; Mathur, K.; Miab, R.K.; Cohen, N.; Henriques-Thompson, K.; Gopinath, J. Environmental sustainability, healthcare workers and healthcare students: A literature review of attitudes and learning approaches. *Health Prof. Educ.* **2024**, *10*, 12. [CrossRef]
42. Woods, N.; Melnyk, A.I.; Moalli, P. Waste not want not: The story of surgical trash. *Curr. Opin. Obstet. Gynecol.* **2024**, *36*, 444–449. [CrossRef] [PubMed]
43. Roletto, A.; Zanardo, M.; Bonfitto, G.R.; Catania, D.; Sardanelli, F.; Zanoni, S. The environmental impact of energy consumption and carbon emissions in radiology departments: A systematic review. *Eur. Radiol. Exp.* **2024**, *8*, 35. [CrossRef] [PubMed]
44. Carbery, I.; Bhatnagar, G.; Cooney, R.; Selinger, C. How can we improve the carbon footprint of IBD clinical care? *Front. Gastroenterol.* **2024**, *15*, e55–e61. [CrossRef]
45. Ghotra, S.S.; Champendal, M.; Flaction, L.; Ribeiro, R.T.; Sá dos Reis, C. Approaches to reduce medical imaging departments' environmental impact: A scoping review. *Radiography* **2024**, *30*, 108–116. [CrossRef] [PubMed]
46. Çakmak, B.; Yol, Ş. Medical Device Energy Consumption Analysis. In Proceedings of the 2019 Medical Technologies Congress (TIPTEKNO), Izmir, Turkey, 3–5 October 2019; IEEE: New York, NY, USA, 2019; pp. 1–4.
47. Huo, B.; Eussen, M.M.M.; Marconi, S.; Johnson, S.M.; Francis, N.; Oslock, W.M.; Marfo, N.; Potapov, O.; Bello, R.J.; Lim, R.B.; et al. Scoping review for the SAGES EAES joint collaborative on sustainability in surgical practice. *Surg. Endosc.* **2024**, *38*, 5483–5504. [CrossRef] [PubMed]
48. Davies, J.F.; Ikin, B.; Francis, J.J.; McGain, F. Implementation approaches to improve environmental sustainability in operating theatres: A systematic review. *Br. J. Anaesth.* **2024**, *133*, 1383–1396. [CrossRef] [PubMed]

environments

MDPI

Article

Associations of Exposure to 24 Endocrine-Disrupting Chemicals with Perinatal Depression and Lifestyle Factors: A Prospective Cohort Study in Korea

Nalae Moon, Su Ji Heo and Ju Hee Kim *

College of Nursing Science, Kyung Hee University, Seoul 02447, Republic of Korea; mnl0302@khu.ac.kr (N.M.); tnwl0428@khu.ac.kr (S.J.H.)
* Correspondence: juheekim@khu.ac.kr

Abstract: During pregnancy, reproductive hormonal changes could affect the mental health of women, such as depression and anxiety. Previous studies have shown that exposure to endocrine disrupting chemicals (EDCs) is significantly associated with mental health symptoms; however, the results were inconsistent. We aimed to examine the association between 24 endocrine-disrupting chemicals (EDCs) in maternal urine and perinatal depression and their association with dietary and lifestyle factors. Participants were recruited from the "No Environmental Hazards for Mother–Child" cohort in Korea. Structured questionnaires asking dietary and lifestyle factors and evaluation of depressive symptoms were administered during antepartum (14 weeks of gestation) and postpartum (within four weeks after birth) periods. Urine samples were collected from 242 and 119 women during antepartum and postpartum periods, respectively. To assess perinatal depression, we used the Center for Epidemiological Studies-Depression Scale and the Edinburgh Postnatal Depression Scale. Antepartum depression and mono(2-ethyl-5-carboxypentyl) phthalate (MECPP) (1.50, 1.01–2.23) and 1-hydroxypyrene (1-OHP) (0.05, 0–0.89) showed significant positive association. Additionally, postpartum depression showed significant associations with mono(2-ethyl-5-oxohexyl) phthalate (MEOHP) (2.78, 1.00–7.70), mono(2-ethyl-5-hydroxyhexyl) phthalate (MEHHP) (2.79, 1.04–7.46), 2-hydroxynaphthalene (2-NAP) (7.22, 1.43–36.59), and 2-hydroxyfluorene (2-FLU) (<0.01, 0–0.004). Some dietary factors (consumption of fish, fermented foods, cup noodles, and popcorn) and consumer product factors (use of skin care, makeup, perfume, antibiotics, sunscreen, nail polish, new furniture, plastic tableware, detergent, polish, paint, and pesticide) were associated with the concentration level of chemicals. We found that exposure to several EDCs during pregnancy and the postpartum period was associated with perinatal depression and dietary–lifestyle factors. Women in childbirth need to actively seek out information about exposure to EDCs and make efforts to avoid them for their own and fetal health.

Keywords: perinatal depression; endocrine disrupting chemical; dietary factor; lifestyle factor

1. Introduction

The endocrinology of pregnancy is related to physiological changes during fetal development and growth [1]. During the perinatal period, when a woman is pregnant and gives birth, she undergoes significant hormonal changes. For example, as the placenta develops, the levels of human chorionic gonadotropin (hCG) and placental lactogen, which provide nutrients to the fetus, increase, as do the levels of estrogen and progesterone, which are essential for maintaining pregnancy [2]. However, after birth, the placenta, which secretes reproductive hormones, is expelled, and the levels of these hormones drop rapidly [2]. The concentration of thyroid-stimulating hormone (TSH) in early pregnancy temporarily decreases due to the lowering effect of thyroid function caused by increased hCG levels and then begins to increase again [3]. This thyroid hormonal fluctuation may influence physiological changed that could be associated with mental health, including postpartum depression (PPD) [3]. In addition, pregnancy increases cardiac output and respiratory rate by approximately 30–40%, constituting a physical burden for women [2]. Due to these physical changes and fluctuations in reproductive hormones, women experience mental health symptoms such as anxiety, stress, and depression during the perinatal period [4–6]. Perinatal depression is defined as the occurrence of major depressive episodes, either during pregnancy (antenatal depression, AD) or within the first four weeks of postpartum (PPD). Exposure to EDCs in pregnant women can lead to endocrine disruptions, including immune activation and inflammatory responses [4]. According to a systematic review study, the biological and psychosocial predictors of PPD include hormonal dysregulation of the hypothalamic–pituitary–adrenal (HPA) axis, inflammatory processes, genetic vulnerabilities, severe life events, chronic stress, and social support [7]. Among these, exposure to EDCs has been identified as a biologically significant factor [4,7]. The relationship between EDC concentrations in biological samples reflecting internal exposure in pregnant women and PPD has been the focus of recent research. A study conducted in Korea observed an association between EDC concentrations in breast milk and postpartum depression, underscoring the need for further research [8].

Phthalates, bisphenols, parabens, polycyclic aromatic hydrocarbons (PAHs), and volatile organic compounds (VOCs) are endocrine-disrupting chemicals (EDCs) that people may be ubiquitously exposed to in daily life through oral ingestion, dermal absorption, and inhalation [9,10]. These non-persistent chemicals are characterized by short half-lives ranging from 6 to 24 h, which leads to rapid metabolism and large within-person variability over time [9]. Despite their fast turnover, these chemicals are found consistently in human samples, such as urine or breast milk, indicating that most individuals face regularly daily exposure [4,11]. Although the mechanisms underlying the increased risk of perinatal depression following exposure to non-persistent EDCs are unclear, some possible explanations have been suggested. EDCs have estrogenic effects on the hippocampus and amygdala, regulating the hypothalamic–pituitary–adrenal axis (HPA) or influencing changes in neurotransmitters, causing anxiety and depressive behavioral disorders [12–14]. EDCs may cause depression by interfering with the production, transport, and release of neurotransmitters such as dopamine, causing synaptic plasticity [15,16]. Another mechanism is that EDCs act like fake thyroid hormones, which can induce thyroid dysfunction or hypothyroidism and cause psychopathological effects [4]. In other words, if exposed in early pregnancy, EDCs can interfere with thyroid function, reducing the fetus' neurological development and the mother's metabolic function [17,18]. Other possible mechanisms include elevated proinflammatory cytokine levels, oxidative stress, and epigenetic gene expression [19,20]. Epidemiological studies linking exposure to diverse EDCs and psychosocial disorders, such as depression and anxiety, have been reported in various populations, but the results are inconsistent [9,11,21–28]. Previous epidemiological studies have reported that exposure to phthalates and bisphenols increased the risk of postpartum depression by 1.03 (95% CI: 0.07, 1.99) times with bisphenol A (BPA) and bisphenol F (BPF) [11], 1.22 times (95% CI: 1.00–1.48) with mono(2-ethyl-5-carboxypentyl) phthalate (MECPP), 1.33 times (95% CI: 1.14–1.54) with mono-N-butyl phthalate (MnBP), 1.23 times (95% CI: 0.99–1.51) with mono-isobutyl phthalate (MiBP), and 1.29 times (95% CI: 1.00–1.67) with monobenzyl phthalate (MBzP) [24]; in contrast, several epidemiological studies reported that there was no significant difference between exposure to phthalates, bisphenols, and parabens and postpartum depression [9,11,24]. Although women are vulnerable to depression and anxiety during pregnancy, few studies have reported on perinatal depression. Therefore, the purpose of this study was to determine the level of exposure to EDCs during pregnancy and the postpartum period and to determine the relationship between exposure to EDCs and ante- and postpartum depression. Additionally, we explored the relationship between pregnant women's diet, lifestyle habits, and exposure to 24 selected EDCs.

2. Materials and Methods

2.1. Study Design and Population

The No Environmental Hazards for Mother–Child (NoE-MoC) study is a prospective birth cohort in Korea established from the 1st trimester of pregnancy to three years after childbirth. Pregnant women were recruited from 2022 to 2023 in five hospitals in Korea (three in Seoul, one in Gyeonggi-do, and one in Gangwon-do) if they met the following inclusion criteria: (1) healthy Korean pregnant women at least 18 years of age; (2) 14 weeks of gestation (1st trimester of pregnancy); (3) receiving regular prenatal care from an obstetrician; (4) singleton pregnancy; (5) not taking any medications for mental health symptoms such as depression or anxiety; (6) not having any underlying disease such as hypertension, diabetes mellitus, thyroid, etc. All the participants were Koreans of the same ethnicity, maintained national insurance coverage, and lived with their husbands. They were invited to submit urine samples and answer a structured questionnaire covering sociodemographic and obstetric characteristics, dietary factors, consumer product factors, fetal growth records with ultrasonography, and depression symptoms when they visited the hospital for a medical checkup (1st, 2nd, and 3rd trimesters of pregnancy and within 4 weeks after childbirth). Considering the short half-life of EDCs, we investigated whether the study participant used food and personal care products within one to two days. We simultaneously conducted a structured questionnaire, urine collection, and assessment of depressive symptoms. Structured questionnaires and evaluation of depressive symptoms were conducted during pregnancy (around 14 weeks) and postpartum (within four weeks after birth), and urine samples were collected from 242 and 119 women, respectively, during each period. A total of 242 eligible pregnant women were enrolled in this cohort, and 197 were subsequently followed up, of whom 119 submitted postpartum depression scores. Written consent was obtained after participants received detailed explanations regarding this study from qualified nurses at the first visit. This study was approved by the Ethics and Human Committees of Kyung Hee University (KHSIRB-21-598) and Kangwon National University Hospital (KNUH-2022-02-001-001).

2.2. Perinatal Depression Assessment

Maternal ante- and postpartum depressive symptoms were assessed using a self-administered questionnaire, employing the Korean version of the Center for Epidemiological Studies-Depression Scale (CES-D) [29–31] for antepartum depression and the Korean version of the Edinburgh Postnatal Depression Scale (K-EPDS) [31,32] for postpartum depression. The Korean version of the CES-D consists of 20 items covering depressive mood, guilt, lack of self-valuation, hopelessness, and sleep disturbance. The total score ranges from 0 to 60, with a higher score indicating more depressive symptoms. A four-point Likert scale (0–3) was used, with 0 indicating "not at all" and 3 "severely". A total ≤ 20 was classified as "normal" and $\geq$21 was classified as "at risk, abnormal" based on the validated cut-off point for Korean women [30]. The K-EPDS consists of 10 items covering depressive mood, anxiety, hopelessness, and irritability. The total score ranges from 0 to 22, with a higher score indicating more depressive symptoms. The same four-point Likert scale was used, with a total ≤ 9 being classified as "normal" and $\geq$10 as "at risk, abnormal" based on the validated cut-off point for postnatal Korean women [32]. Standardized z-scores were calculated and used to compare and analyze EPDS and CES-D scores.

2.3. Dietary and Lifestyle Factors Assessment

The questionnaire administered to pregnant women included items on sociodemographic and health information (gestational age, weight, height, marital status, educational level, monthly household income, occupation, residence, medical history, obstetric history, alcohol use, and smoking); dietary factors; and consumer product factors. All items in the dietary and consumer product questions were chosen based on a literature review that showed a significant association with exposure to EDCs. This questionnaire was validated by exposure assessment experts and used in our previous research [12]. Participants were required to indicate the frequency of food consumption and daily life product usage from the past 1 day to 4 weeks. Dietary factors consisted of meat with fat tissue, fish, dairy products, shellfish, fermented food, fried food, fast food, frozen food, cup noodles, ice cream, canned food, vinyl-packed food, and popcorn. Consumer product factors consisted of skincare products, makeup products, hair products, manicures, perfumes, antibiotics, sunscreen, new furniture, plastic bowls, disposable dishware, dishwasher, detergent, polish, water-proofing products, air freshener, glue, insect repellent, and mosquito repellent. Responses were recorded using a nine-point Likert scale interpreted as follows: 1 (none or rarely), 2 (once a month), 3 (2–3 times a month), 4 (once a week), 5 (2–4 times a week), 6 (5–6 times a week), 7 (once a day), 8 (twice a day), and 9 (3 times or more a day). All scores were added to calculate the total score in each domain.

2.4. Analysis of 24 Non-Persistent Chemicals in Urine Samples

We collected 20-mL maternal spot urine samples in polypropylene cups during each follow-up visit, which were directly stored at −80 °C until analysis. We measured the concentrations environmental pollutant chemicals, including nine phthalate metabolites (MnBP, MEP, MCPP, MBzP, MMP, MEOHP, MEHHP, MECPP, and MiBP) [8,10–12,14,21]; five phenols (BPA, BPF, BPS, TCS, and BP-3) [8,10–13,17,18]; four parabens (MP, EP, BP, and PP) [8,11,12,17]; four PAHs (1-OHP, 2-NAP, 1-PHE, and 2-FLU) [23,24,27,28]; and two VOCs (t, t-MA and BMA) [22,26] in the urine samples. The full names of these chemicals and the limit of detection (LOD) are presented in Table 1.

Detailed procedures for sample preparation, quality assurance, and quantification have been previously described [8,33]. Briefly, LC-MS/MS and the Thermo Scientific™ Vanquish™ ultra-high-performance liquid chromatography (UHPLC) system (Thermo Finnigan, San Jose, CA, USA) were used in the chemical analysis employing an ACE Excel 2 C18-AR column (150 mm × 2.1 mm I.D.; Advanced Chromatography Technology, Aberdeen, UK) and a TSQ Altis triple-quadrupole mass spectrometer (Thermo Finnigan) equipped with an electrospray ionization (ESI) source. The mobile phase consisted of water with 0.1% formic acid (solvent A) and acetonitrile with 0.1% formic acid (solvent B), with a gradient elution program optimized for target analytes. The spray voltage was 4500 V in the positive mode and 3500 V in the negative mode. The ion transfer tube temperature was 320 °C, and the vaporizer temperature was 340 °C in both modes. The column temperature was maintained at 35 °C. All experiments were performed in time-dependent reaction monitoring mode for simultaneous analysis. All chemicals used in this study were purchased from Sigma-Aldrich (St. Louis, MO, USA), Merck (Darmstadt, Germany), or Burdick and Jackson (Muskegon, MI, USA). *E. coli* β-glucuronidase (140 U/mg at 37 °C) was purchased from Roche (Mannheim, Germany). Standard reference materials (SRMs) 3672 and 3673 were purchased from the National Institute of Standards and Technology (NIST, Gaithersburg, MD, USA).

Table 1. Creatinine adjusted urinary concentration of chemicals in the ante- and postpartum periods (μg/g creatinine).

Groups	Analytes	Antepartum (14 Weeks of Gestation, n = 242)							Postpartum (One Month after Delivery, n = 119)						t-test *	p-Value
		DF (%)	LOD (μg/L)	GM	25th	50th	75th	Max	DF (%)	GM	25th	50th	75th	Max		
Phthalates	MnBP	100	0.11	14.45	7.72	15.34	26.11	232.82	100	24.95	14.51	22.33	39.44	192.25	−5.430	**<0.001**
	MEP	73.6	0.07	1.23	<LOD	1.80	6.35	684.50	100	3.28	1.11	2.52	8.04	711.64	−2.166	**0.031**
	MCPP	97.1	0.06	0.44	0.30	0.42	0.66	10.31	97.6	0.46	<LOD	0.49	0.63	3.14	−0.461	0.645
	MBzP	90.9	0.04	0.21	0.11	0.22	0.40	7.30	94.4	0.19	0.12	0.16	0.35	8.00	1.120	0.263
	MMP	100	0.01	0.33	0.17	0.33	0.62	11.51	37.3	0.03	<LOD	<LOD	0.21	79.21	2.019	**0.045**
	MEOHP	100	0.03	2.55	1.48	2.61	4.67	34.58	96.0	2.76	1.77	3.02	6.72	84.02	−1.958	0.052
	MEHHP	100	0.03	4.24	2.48	4.40	7.51	55.02	97.6	4.06	2.57	4.27	9.14	125.91	−0.640	0.523
	MECPP	92.1	0.03	3.40	2.48	5.08	10.32	53.47	98.4	8.87	5.63	8.65	18.24	196.18	−6.100	**<0.001**
	MiBP	98.8	0.07	5.35	2.54	5.69	12.00	178.70	82.5	3.34	1.01	5.32	18.30	300.41	0.288	0.774
Bisphenols	BPA	78.5	0.12	0.64	0.36	0.61	1.06	22.7	99.2	0.87	0.50	0.83	1.48	21.34	−5.118	**<0.001**
	BPF	42.1	0.08	0.47	0.09	0.26	2.48	19.9	48.4	0.11	<LOD	<LOD	0.19	2.78	4.100	**<0.001**
	BPS	98.8	0.01	0.30	0.13	0.25	0.63	22.1	100	0.77	0.37	0.64	1.74	86.62	−5.168	**<0.001**
Phenols	TCS	71.5	0.04	0.28	0.13	0.27	0.63	3.11	22.2	0.74	0.48	0.48	0.48	25.12	−6.855	**<0.001**
	BP-3	71.5	0.10	0.43	0.14	0.30	0.93	341	69.8	0.25	<LOD	0.15	0.52	156.64	0.022	0.983
Parabens	MP	100	0.15	6.70	2.77	4.82	9.07	1390	64.3	1.93	<LOD	1.81	13.90	682.09	2.307	**0.022**
	EP	99.6	0.14	32.80	10.2	40.30	126	2900	90.5	29.14	10.50	48.08	168.23	2492.72	−0.431	0.667
	PP	31	0.21	1.99	0.34	0.93	12.7	250	69.8	0.64	<LOD	0.32	1.44	303.40	−2.129	**0.034**
	BP	100	0.07	0.78	0.48	0.70	1.09	23.8	100	1.11	0.73	0.96	1.53	12.52	−3.567	**<0.001**
PAHs	1-OHP	85.5	0.03	0.14	0.07	0.13	0.23	4.08	98.4	0.10	0.07	0.11	0.15	0.97	2.652	**0.008**
	2-NAP	100	0.05	2.39	1.24	2.07	3.96	84.1	99.2	2.06	1.01	1.82	3.67	76.89	0.667	0.505
	1-PHE	77.3	0.02	0.07	0.04	0.06	0.09	37.0	84.9	0.05	0.03	0.05	0.08	0.53	2.077	**0.039**
	2-FLU	95	0.01	0.13	0.08	0.14	0.22	9.10	92.9	0.11	0.07	0.13	0.21	2.43	0.094	0.925
VOCs	t,t-MA	99.6	0.58	45.20	21.40	44.80	92.0	554	100	48.75	28.81	43.56	72.59	395.46	−0.869	0.386
	BMA	99.6	0.04	2.87	1.49	2.49	4.67	10100	99.2	5.57	3.24	5.21	9.43	791.21	−5.2132	**<0.001**

DF, detection frequency; LOD, limit of detection; GM, geometric mean; Min, minimum; Max, maximum; MnBP, mono-N-butyl phthalate; MEP, mono ethyl phthalate; MCPP, Mono(3-carboxypropyl) phthalate; MBzP, monobenzyl phthalate; MMP, mono(2-methylpropyl) phthalate; MEOHP, mono(2-ethyl-5-oxohexyl) phthalate; MEHHP, mono(2-ethyl-5-hydroxyhexyl) phthalate; MECPP, mono(2-ethyl-5-carboxypentyl) phthalate; MiBP, mono-isobutyl phthalate; BPA, Bisphenol A; BPF, Bisphenol F; BPS, Bisphenol S; MP, Methylparaben; EP, Ethylparaben; BP, Butylparaben; PP, Propylparaben; TCS, Triclosan; BP-3, Benzophenon-3; 1-OHP, 1-hydroxypyrene; 2-NAP, 2-hydroxynaphthalene; 1-PHE, 1-hydroxyphenanthrene; 2-FLU, 2-hydroxyfluorene; t,t-MA, trans, trans-muconic acid; BMA, benzylmercapturic acid; * *t*-test after natural log transformation; bold values are statistically significant ($p < 0.05$).

For quality control, a standard calibration curve with a regression coefficient > 0.99 was generated for all curves using 30% methanol in aqueous solution. The standard calibration curve ranged between 0.005 and 20 ng/mL. Urine samples were spiked with isotope-labeled standard material. The signal-to-noise ratio of the matrix used in this analysis was three. The average recovery rate for all targets in the matrix spike sample ranged between 86 and 105%, and the relative standard deviation ranged between 11 and 17%. Matrix spike urine samples with known concentrations (1, 10, and 20 ng/mL) and randomly selected procedural blank samples were used for experimental verification. No target analytes were detected in the blank sample. To evaluate the intra-day precision, the standard solution evaluated six times a day was compared with the target solution, and the inter-day precision was evaluated against the standard solution measured six days in a row. The overall quality and accuracy of the described analysis method were monitored through an interlaboratory comparison program.

2.5. Statistical Analyses

All chemicals were detected in >30% of urine samples. Values below the LOD were substituted with LOD/$\sqrt{2}$ [34]. The urinary creatinine levels were adjusted to reflect changes in the intra- and inter-subject variability in renal filtration dynamics [35]. Demographic characteristics were described as the mean, standard deviation, median, and minimum–maximum for continuous variables and numbers and percentages for categorical variables. A normality test (Kolmogorov–Smirnov test) was conducted for all data; because the level of chemical concentration in urine samples showed a right-skewed distribution, a natural log transformation was performed. The mean differences between the chemicals in both the ante- and postpartum periods were compared using a Student's t-test. Pearson's correlation coefficients were used to identify correlations among chemicals, depression scores, and dietary and lifestyle factors. To examine the association between each analyte (phthalates, phenols, parabens, PAHs, and VOCs) and ante- and postpartum depression, multiple logistic regression with the entry method was used to estimate odds ratios (ORs) and 95% confidence intervals. To confirm the association between each analyte and dietary and consumer product factors, bivariate linear regression was used. To evaluate the mixture effect between urinary chemicals and the perinatal depression score, we used Bayesian Kernel Machine Regression (BKMR). BKMR is a reliable method frequently used in the environmental health research field in which non-linear, non-additive, and mixture interaction effects of all substances are considered [36]. The overall cumulative mixture effects and dose–response effects of each of 24 urinary chemicals were evaluated in relation to the antepartum and postpartum depression scores. Subsequently, we evaluated the mixture effect of each chemical on the depression score by dividing the chemicals into subgroups according to phthalates, bisphenols, parabens, PAHs, and other chemicals. Maternal age, early pregnancy body mass index (BMI), education, income, parity, cotinine level in the urine, and neonatal sex were adjusted for as covariates following the previous studies [8,9,11,12]. Statistical significance was evaluated at $p < 0.05$. All statistical analyses were performed using R 4.1.0 (R Development Core Team, Vienna, Austria) and SPSS 28.0 (IBM SPSS Statistics, Armonk, NY, USA).

3. Results

3.1. Study Participants

The mean maternal age at the first visit was 33.8 years (range 21–42 years), and the mean early pregnancy BMI was 23.2 kg/m^2 (Table 2). Over 81% of the participants had a college or higher educational level, over 51% reported a more than 5000 USD household income monthly, about 65% were employed and lived in metropolitan areas, and over

57% were primipara mothers. The mean maternal urinary cotinine level was 25.4 μg/g creatinine. The mean cotinine level of non-smokers was 0.89 μg/g creatinine, while the mean cotinine level of six possible smokers was 995.76 μg/g creatinine (ranged from 544.88 to 1720 μg/g creatinine). The mean score of antepartum depression was 16.5 (range 1–36), and 23.6% of participants were classified as abnormal, with a score $\geq$ 21. The mean score of postpartum depression was 8.9 (range 0–22), and 45.4% of participants were classified as abnormal, with a score $\geq$ 9.

Table 2. Socioeconomic characteristics and ante- and postpartum depression of participants (n = 242).

Variables	Categories	n/M	%/SD	Median	Min	Max
Age (years)		33.8	4.0	34.0	21.0	42.0
Early-pregnancy BMI (kg/m^2)		23.2	4.2	22.5	14.8	40.2
Education	<college	44	18.2			
	≥college	198	81.8			
Household income ($/month)	≤5000	124	51.2			
	>5000	118	48.8			
Employment status	Yes	157	64.9			
	No	85	35.1			
Residence area	Metropolitan	155	64.0			
	Non-metropolitan	87	36.0			
Parity	Primipara	139	57.4			
	Multipara	103	42.6			
Cotinine level (μg/g creatinine) *		0.31	186.46	0.22	0.04	1720
Antepartum depression score		16.5	6.1	15.5	1	36
	Low (≤20)	185 (76.4)				
	High (≥21)	57 (23.6)				
Postpartum depression score (n = 119)		8.9	3.6	8	0	22
	Low (≤9)	65 (54.6)				
	High (≥10)	54 (45.4)				

M, mean; SD, standard deviation; Min, minimum; Max, maximum; BMI, body mass index; * detection frequency of cotinine was 84.3%.

3.2. Non-Persistent Urinary Chemical Concentrations in the Ante- and Postpartum Periods

Table 2 shows the detailed results for each tested chemical in 242 antepartum and 119 postpartum urine samples. The detection frequency, LOD, geometric mean (GM), median, minimum, and maximum values are shown. The detection frequency ranged from 22.2% for TCS in the postpartum period to 100% for MnBP, MMP, MEOHP, MEHHP, MP, BP, and 2-NAP in the antepartum period and for MnBP, MEP, BPS, BP, and t,t-MA during the postpartum period. Significant mean differences between the ante- and postpartum periods were present in MnBP, MEP, MMP, MECPP, BPA, BPF, BPS, TCS, MP, PP, BP, 1-OHP, 1-PHE, and BMA, with urinary concentrations decreasing from antepartum to postpartum (Figure 1). Each subject's urinary chemical concentration changes between ante the partum and postpartum periods are presented as line graphs (Figure 2). Some chemicals, including MEOHP, MEHHP, MECPP, BPA, BPS, TCS, and BMA, generally showed an increasing tendency, while BPF and 1-PHE showed a decreasing pattern in the postpartum period compared to antepartum period.

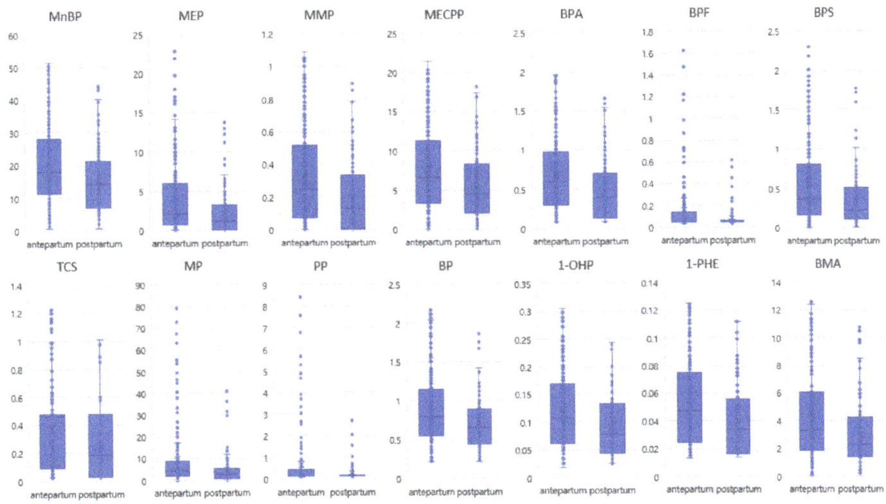

Figure 1. Concentration changes of chemicals in the ante- and postpartum periods. All boxplots show statistically significant higher median, mean, IQR, minimum, maximum, and outliers of chemicals in the antepartum period versus postpartum period. MnBP, mono-N-butyl phthalate; MEP, mono ethyl phthalate; MMP, mono(2-methylpropyl) phthalate; MECPP, mono(2-ethyl-5-carboxypentyl) phthalate; BPA, Bisphenol A; BPF, Bisphenol F; BPS, Bisphenol S; TCS, Triclosan; MP, Methylparaben; PP, Propylparaben; BP, Butylparaben; 1-OHP, 1-hydroxypyrene; 1-PHE, 1-hydroxyphenanthrene; BMA, benzylmercapturic acid. Extreme outliers (<Q1 − 5*IQR, >Q3 + 5*IQR) have been omitted.

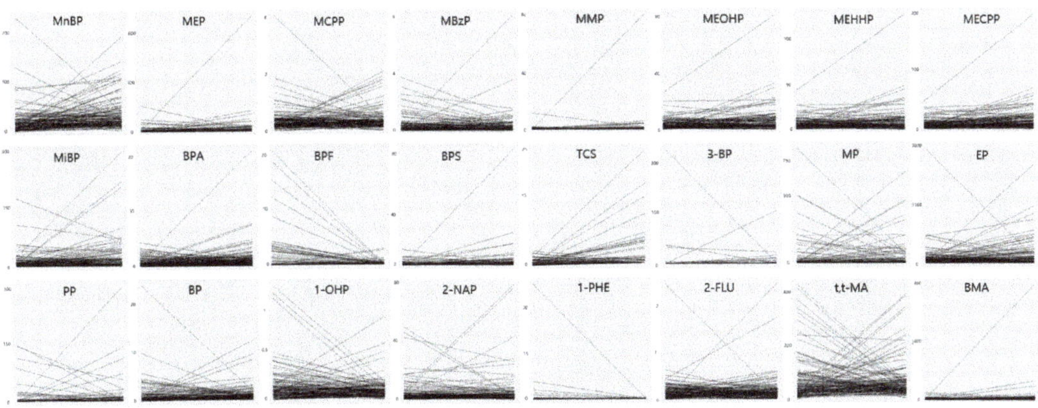

Figure 2. Difference of 24 non-persistent endocrine disrupting chemicals (EDCs) in maternal urine at the points of the 1st trimester and one month after delivery (n = 119). MnBP, mono-N-butyl phthalate; MEP, mono ethyl phthalate; MCPP, Mono(3-carboxypropyl) phthalate; MBzP, monobenzyl phthalate; MMP, mono(2-methylpropyl) phthalate; MEOHP, mono(2-ethyl-5-oxohexyl) phthalate; MEHHP, mono(2-ethyl-5-hydroxyhexyl) phthalate; MECPP, mono(2-ethyl-5-carboxypentyl) phthalate; MiBP, mono-isobutyl phthalate; BPA, Bisphenol A; BPF, Bisphenol F; BPS, Bisphenol S; MP, Methylparaben; EP, Ethylparaben; BP, Butylparaben; PP, Propylparaben; TCS, Triclosan; BP-3, Benzophenon-3; 1-OHP, 1-hydroxypyrene; 2-NAP, 2-hydroxynaphthalene; 1-PHE, 1-hydroxyphenanthrene; 2-FLU, 2-hydroxyfluorene; t,t-MA, trans, trans-muconic acid; BMA, benzylmercapturic acid.

3.3. Association Between Urinary Chemical Concentration and Ante- and Postpartum Depression

In the antepartum period, the depression score of mothers was statistically significantly correlated with MCPP (r = −0.18), MBzP (r = −0.11), MEHP (r = −0.07), and PP (r = −0.06). In the postpartum period, some chemicals showed slight positive correlation with depression score, but there was no statistical significance at the significance level $p < 0.05$. The distribution of each depression score at the antepartum and postpartum periods is presented as scatter plots (Supplementary Figure S1).

In the adjusted multiple logistic regression model with covariates of maternal age, early pregnancy BMI, education, income, parity, gestational age, urine cotinine level, and neonatal sex, we observed a significant association with antepartum depression scores in MECPP (aOR = 1.50, 95% CI = 1.010–2.227) and 1-OHP (aOR = 0.05, 95% CI = 0.003–0.888) (Table 3). In the postpartum period, the antepartum depression score was adjusted with other covariates. Several phthalates and PAHs were significantly associated with maternal postpartum depression scores. In the phthalate group, this consisted of MEOHP (aOR = 2.78, 95% CI = 1.004–7.700) and MEHHP (aOR = 2.79, 95% CI = 1.040–7.459) and, in the PAH group, of 2-NAP (aOR = 7.22, 95% CI = 1.426–36.593) and 2-FLU (aOR <0.01, 95% CI = 0–0.004).

Table 3. Multiple logistic regression of the association between 24 chemicals and antepartum and postpartum depression.

		Antepartum Depression (n = 242)			Postpartum Depression (n = 119)		
Groups	Chemical	aOR	*p*-Value	95% CI	aOR	*p*-Value	95% CI
Phthalates	MnBP	0.97	0.863	0.682–1.379	0.46	0.185	0.144–1.455
	MEP	0.79	0.081	0.603–1.030	1.03	0.936	0.536–1.970
	MCPP	0.27	0.065	0.064–1.088	0.30	0.562	0.005–17.788
	MBzP	0.38	0.130	0.113–1.325	9.92	0.307	0.121–NA
	MMP	0.67	0.473	0.217–2.031	<0.01	0.180	0–NA
	MEOHP	1.04	0.874	0.645–1.675	**2.78**	**0.049**	**1.004–7.700**
	MEHHP	1.09	0.710	0.697–1.700	**2.79**	**0.042**	**1.040–7.459**
	MECPP	**1.50**	**0.045**	**1.010–2.227**	2.73	0.056	0.973–7.641
	MiBP	1.09	0.604	0.797–1.477	1.08	0.749	0.668–1.751
Bisphenols	BPA	0.87	0.731	0.400–1.901	1.00	1.000	0.106–9.446
	BPF	0.82	0.467	0.475–1.407	0.02	0.326	0–49.044
	BPS	0.99	0.984	0.523–1.886	0.41	0.296	0.078–2.174
Phenols	TCS	0.96	0.944	0.320–2.890	0.77	0.805	0.100–5.983
	BP-3	0.90	0.642	0.589–1.386	0.94	0.947	0.168–5.314
Parabens	MP	0.85	0.222	0.660–1.102	0.77	0.335	0.448–1.315
	EP	1.03	0.725	0.865–1.232	0.89	0.506	0.622–1.264
	PP	0.91	0.562	0.671–1.242	0.64	0.399	0.228–1.801
	BP	1.00	0.993	0.439–2.294	0.06	0.087	0.002–1.511
PAHs	1-OHP	**0.05**	**0.041**	**0.003–0.888**	0.01	0.511	0–NA
	2-NAP	1.10	0.660	0.727–1.654	**7.22**	**0.017**	**1.426–36.593**
	1-PHE	0.27	0.355	0.016–4.364	<0.01	0.144	0–NA
	2-FLU	0.37	0.423	0.032–4.217	**<0.01**	**0.017**	**0–0.004**
VOCs	t,t-MA	1.08	0.621	0.796–1.466	0.68	0.442	0.250–1.832
	BMA	0.97	0.852	0.691–1.356	0.67	0.603	0.148–3.027

Multiple logistic regression results adjusted for maternal age, early-pregnancy body mass index, education, income, parity, gestational age, and maternal urine cotinine level. Postpartum pregnancy depression score was adjusted for antepartum depression score and neonatal sex; bold characters indicate statistical significance ($p < 0.05$). MnBP, mono-N-butyl phthalate; MEP, mono ethyl phthalate; MCPP, Mono(3-carboxypropyl) phthalate; MBzP, monobenzyl phthalate; MMP, mono(2-methylpropyl) phthalate; MEOHP, mono(2-ethyl-5-oxohexyl) phthalate; MEHHP, mono(2-ethyl-5-hydroxyhexyl) phthalate; MECPP, mono(2-ethyl-5-carboxypentyl) phthalate; MiBP, mono-isobutyl phthalate; BPA, Bisphenol A; BPF, Bisphenol F; BPS, Bisphenol S; MP, Methylparaben; EP, Ethylparaben; BP, Butylparaben; PP, Propylparaben; TCS, Triclosan; BP-3, Benzophenon-3; 1-OHP, 1-hydroxypyrene; 2-NAP, 2-hydroxynaphthalene; 1-PHE, 1-hydroxyphenanthrene; 2-FLU, 2-hydroxyfluorene; t,t-MA, trans, trans-muconic acid; BMA, benzylmercapturic acid; aOR, adjusted odds ratio; CI, confidence interval.

We used the BKMR method to assess the mixture effects of 24 non-persistent EDCs on antepartum (Figure 3a) and postpartum (Figure 3d) depression. The overall effect regression models were adjusted for maternal age, early-pregnancy BMI, education, income, parity, gestational age, maternal urine cotinine level, and neonatal sex. Both antepartum and postpartum depression scores showed no statistically significant association between urinary chemicals in terms of overall mixture effect when other chemical levels were fixed at similar percentiles from the 10th to 90th. Figure 3b,e show the dose–response relationship for the association between each non-persistent chemical level and antepartum and postpartum depression scores, with other chemical levels fixed at their median. Each chemical showed different dose–response results, including positive, negative, and non-linear patterns. Figure 3c,f show the estimated effect and 95% confidence intervals of interquartile change of each chemical and antepartum and postpartum depression scores after fixing the other chemical levels at their 25th (red), 50th (green), and 75th (blue) percentiles. No individual chemical showed a statistically significant interquartile change effect in this analysis.

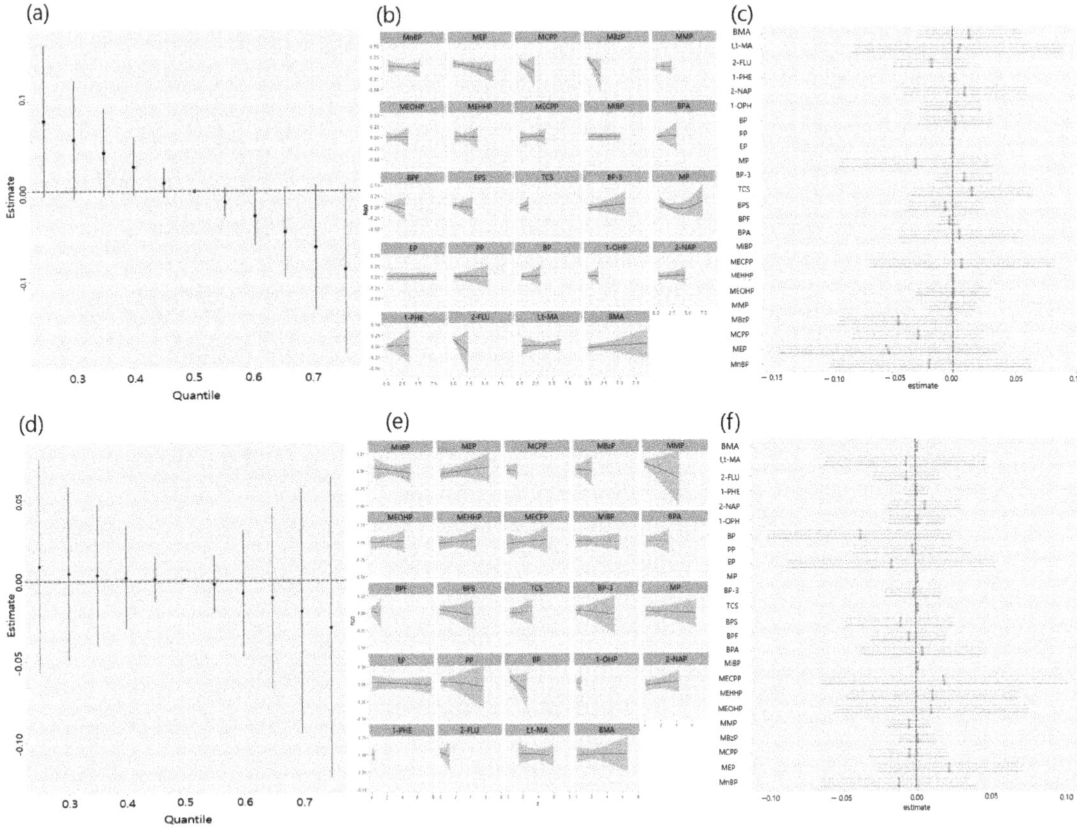

Figure 3. Bayesian Kernel Machine Regression between phthalates, bisphenols, parabens, PAHs, and other chemicals and antepartum and postpartum depression scores. (**a**) The overall effects of bisphenols; parabens; polycyclic aromatic hydrocarbons (PAHs); and other chemicals (TCS, BP-3, and VOCs) on the antepartum depression score were estimated using the Bayesian Kernel Machine Regression (BKMR) adjusted for maternal age, early-pregnancy body mass index, education, income, parity, gestational weeks, maternal urine cotinine level, and neonatal sex; ln: natural log. (**b**) Exposure–response relationship for the association between each chemical and antepartum depression score, fixing other chemical levels at their median. (**c**) The red, green, and blue bars and dots shows the estimated effect and 95% confidence intervals of an interquartile range change of each urinary chemical and antepartum depression score when the level of each of the other chemicals was held at

their corresponding 25th, 50th, and 75th percentiles, respectively. (**d**) The overall effects of bisphenols; parabens; polycyclic aromatic hydrocarbons (PAHs); and other chemicals (TCS, BP-3, and VOCs) on the postpartum depression score were estimated using the Bayesian Kernel Machine Regression (BKMR) adjusted for early pregnancy depression score, maternal age, early-pregnancy body mass index, education, income, parity, gestational weeks, maternal urine cotinine level, and neonatal sex; ln: natural log. (**e**) Exposure–response relationship for the association between each chemicals and postpartum depression score, fixing other chemical levels at their median. (**f**) The red, green, and blue bars and dots shows the estimated effect and 95% confidence intervals of an interquartile range change of each urinary chemical and postpartum depression score when the level of each of the other chemicals was held at their corresponding 25th, 50th, and 75th percentiles, respectively.

3.4. Association Between Dietary/Lifestyle Factors and Depression

In this study, the consumption of fish (MiBP), fermented food (MMP), cup noodle (MBzP), and popcorn (MEP) and use of manicure (MBzP), perfume (MiBP), plastic tableware (MMP), paint (MEHHP), and pesticides (MCPPs) were significantly associated with an increase in urinary phthalate concentration in pregnant women during the antepartum and postpartum periods. The increase in bisphenol levels was correlated with the consumption of fish (BPF) and popcorn (BPF) and the use of paint (BPA and BPF). TCS was significantly associated with the consumption of frozen food and use of new furniture. Increased paraben concentrations were significantly correlated with fermented foods (BP), consumption of cup noodles (MP and PP), skincare, makeup, sunscreen (EP), perfumes (PP), pesticides (MP), and the use of polishes (BP). Increased levels of PAHs in urine were significantly associated with the consumption of fermented and frozen foods; use of skin care, perfume, hand washer, and sunscreen products; and use of detergent, polish, air fresheners, and paint. There was a significant increase in VOCs in urine with the use of skincare products and polish (Tables 4 and 5).

Table 4. Associations between chemicals in maternal urine and dietary factors and consumer products in the antepartum period (n = 242).

Chemical	Dietary Factors						Consumer Products Factor											
	Fish	Dairy Products	Fermented Foods	Frozen Foods	Cup Noodle	Popcorn	Skincare Products	Makeup Products	Perfume	Antimicrobial Products	Sunscreen	New Furniture	Plastic Bowl	Detergent	Polish	Air Freshener	Paint	Pesticides
			B									B						
MnBP	beta 0.03	0.01	0.00	−0.06	−0.06	−0.05	−0.01	−0.03	−0.04	−0.02	−0.01	−0.10 *	−0.01	−0.02	−0.09	−0.02	0.00	0.00
MEP	beta 0.03	−0.07	0.04	−0.07	−0.11	−0.19	0.06	0.01	0.09	0.00	−0.01	−0.04	−0.02	−0.02	−0.10	0.00	−0.17	0.05
MCPP	beta 0.02	0.00	0.01	−0.01	0.00	−0.01	0.00	−0.01	0.00	0.00	−0.01	−0.02	−0.01	0.00	−0.03	0.00	−0.01	0.00
MBzP	beta 0.02	0.02	0.01	−0.01	−0.01	−0.03	0.01	0.00	−0.01	0.01	0.01	0.00	0.00	0.01	0.01	0.00	0.06	0.02
MMP	beta 0.00	0.00	**0.03** *	−0.01	−0.01	0.00	0.01	−0.01	0.00	0.00	0.00	0.00	**0.02** *	0.01	−0.01	0.01	0.02	0.00
MEOHP	beta 0.05	0.03	0.01	0.02	−0.01	−0.02	0.01	−0.01	−0.04	0.01	−0.01	−0.01	0.00	0.02	0.00	−0.02	0.14	−0.01
MEHHP	beta 0.05	0.04	0.00	0.02	−0.01	0.01	0.01	−0.01	−0.04	0.01	−0.02	−0.01	0.00	0.01	0.04	−0.03	**0.23** *	0.01
MECPP	beta 0.05	0.05	0.00	0.02	−0.01	0.00	0.03	−0.01	−0.05	0.01	−0.02	−0.04	0.00	0.02	−0.01	−0.03	0.18	0.01
MiBP	beta **0.15** *	0.02	−0.05	0.02	0.06	0.06	−0.01	−0.01	−0.07	0.00	0.02	−0.08	−0.01	−0.04	−0.12	−0.05	−0.09	0.02
BPA	beta 0.03	0.01	0.03	0.01	−0.01	0.04	0.02	0.00	0.01	0.00	0.02	0.00	0.01	0.00	0.04	0.00	**0.12** *	0.00
BPF	beta **0.07** *	0.04	−0.02	0.00	−0.01	0.05	0.02	−0.02	−0.01	−0.01	−0.02	−0.04	−0.03	−0.01	0.06	−0.02	**0.18** *	0.01
BPS	beta 0.00	0.01	−0.02	0.03	−0.04	0.03	0.00	−0.01	0.01	0.01	−0.01	**0.05** *	0.01	0.01	0.00	0.00	0.10	−0.01
TCS	beta −0.01	0.00	0.00	**0.03** *	0.02	−0.02	0.00	0.01	0.01	0.00	0.00	**0.02** *	0.02	0.00	−0.02	0.00	0.04	0.01
BP-3	beta 0.03	−0.04	0.02	0.00	−0.04	−0.03	0.01	−0.02	0.06	0.00	0.02	0.03	0.02	−0.01	0.05	0.00	0.20	0.07
MP	beta 0.05	0.03	0.00	0.08	−0.17 *	0.10	0.06	0.02	0.00	−0.02	0.00	0.05	0.02	−0.01	−0.01	0.01	−0.13	**0.21** *
EP	beta 0.08	0.03	0.04	0.02	−0.07	−0.01	**0.14** *	**0.10** *	0.08	0.03	**0.09** *	0.04	−0.04	0.04	−0.11	0.00	−0.46	0.04
PP	beta −0.02	0.06	−0.01	0.01	−0.10 *	−0.03	0.04	0.00	0.00	0.00	−0.01	0.04	0.01	0.03	−0.12	0.01	−0.05	0.10
BP	beta −0.01	0.00	**0.04** *	0.00	0.00	0.03	−0.01	0.00	0.00	0.01	0.01	**0.03** *	0.01	0.01	0.04	0.01	−0.06	0.01
1-OHP	beta 0.01	0.00	**0.02** *	0.01	0.00	0.00	**0.02** *	0.00	**0.02** *	**0.01** *	**0.01** *	0.00	0.00	0.01	**0.04** *	**0.01** *	**0.10** *	−0.01
2-NAP	beta 0.00	−0.01	0.04	**0.07** *	0.00	0.07	0.02	0.00	0.02	0.02	0.03	−0.01	−0.01	**0.06** *	−0.04	**0.05** *	0.01	−0.02
1-PHE	beta 0.03	−0.01	0.02	−0.01	0.00	−0.03	0.00	−0.01	−0.01	−0.01	0.00	−0.01	0.01	0.00	−0.02	−0.01	−0.01	0.00
2-FLU	beta 0.00	0.00	**0.02** *	0.01	−0.01	0.01	0.00	0.01	0.00	0.00	0.00	0.00	0.00	0.00	−0.01	0.01	0.00	0.00
t,tMA	beta 0.01	0.00	0.05	0.04	0.05	0.09	**0.07** *	0.03	0.05	0.04	0.01	0.01	0.00	−0.03	−0.05	0.00	0.20	−0.02
BMA	beta −0.03	−0.04	0.05	−0.02	0.04	0.08	−0.04	0.00	0.02	−0.02m	0.00	−0.05	−0.03	−0.02	−0.02	0.02	0.02	0.05

Multiple linear regression results adjusted for maternal age, early-pregnancy body mass index, education, income, parity, gestational age, and maternal urine cotinine level after natural log transformation for chemical concentrations; *p*, *p*-value; bold and asterisk (*) characters indicate a statistically significant positive association ($p < 0.05$). MnBP, mono-N-butyl phthalate; MEP, mono ethyl phthalate; MCPP, mono(3-carboxypropyl) phthalate; MBzP, monobenzyl phthalate; MMP, mono(2-methylpropyl) phthalate; MEOHP, mono(2-ethyl-5-oxohexyl) phthalate; MEHHP, mono(2-ethyl-5-hydroxyhexyl) phthalate; MECPP, Mono(2-ethyl-5-carboxypentyl) phthalate; MiBP, mono-isobutyl phthalate; BPA, Bisphenol A; BPF, Bisphenol F; BPS, Bisphenol S; MP, Methylparaben; EP, Ethylparaben; BP, Butylparaben; PP, Propylparaben; TCS, Triclosan; BP-3, Benzophenon-3; 1-OHP, 1-hydroxypyrene; 2-NAP, 2-hydroxynaphthalene; 1-PHE, 1-hydroxyphenanthrene; 2-FLU, 2-hydroxyfluorene; t,t-MA, trans, trans-muconic acid; BMA, benzylmercapturic acid.

Table 5. Associations between chemicals in maternal urine and dietary factors and consumer products in the postpartum period (n = 119).

Chemical		Dietary Factors						Consumer Products											
		Fish	Dairy Products	Fermented Foods	Frozen Foods	Cup Noodle	Popcorn	Skincare Products	Makeup Products	Manicure	Perfume	Antimicrobial Products	Sunscreen	New Furniture	Plastic Bowl	Detergent	Polish	Air Freshener	Pesticide
		B						B											
MnBP	beta	0.020	−0.009	0.023	−0.023	−0.016	0.097	−0.056	−0.007	−0.204	0.114	0.004	−0.043	−0.008	−0.033	−0.037	0.031	−0.027	0.058
MEP	beta	0.067	−0.003	−0.011	0.027	0.063	**0.258 ***	0.051	0.150	0.780	0.016	0.024	0.087	0.138	−0.037	0.009	−0.048	0.000	0.212
MCPP	beta	−0.001	0.016	0.002	−0.004	−0.005	0.011	−0.004	0.007	0.051	0.024	−0.006	−0.011	−0.022	0.003	0.003	−0.034	−0.009	**0.068 ***
MBzP	beta	−0.011	0.016	0.011	−0.004	**0.053 ***	0.053	0.018	0.030	**0.227 ***	−0.003	0.004	0.006	−0.022	−0.004	0.012	−0.040	0.007	−0.016
MMP	beta	0.014	−0.021	0.021	−0.012	−0.051	0.038	−0.020	−0.023	−0.164	0.045	−0.003	−0.032	0.024	0.012	−0.014	−0.075	−0.044	0.004
MEOHP	beta	0.01	−0.01	0.01	−0.01	0.02	−0.04	−0.01	0.04	−0.40	0.25	0.03	−0.04	−0.08	0.00	−0.01	−0.20	0.00	0.02
MEHHP	beta	0.02	−0.01	0.01	0.00	0.05	−0.04	−0.01	0.03	−0.38	0.21	0.03	−0.05	−0.08	0.01	0.00	−0.27 *	−0.01	0.01
MECPP	beta	0.02	0.02	0.04	0.02	0.06	0.04	−0.02	0.05	−0.11	0.23	0.05	−0.06	−0.10	0.01	−0.02	−0.23 *	0.00	0.04
MiBP	beta	0.03	−0.02	0.06	0.07	0.03	0.19	0.00	0.03	−0.68	**0.47 ***	−0.01	0.00	−0.03	0.05	0.00	−0.16	−0.07	0.12
BPA	beta	−0.04	0.02	−0.02	−0.05	−0.06	0.07	0.02	−0.01	−0.02	0.07	−0.02	−0.01	−0.02	0.00	0.02	0.04	−0.03	−0.05
BPF	beta	−0.01	0.00	−0.01	−0.01	−0.01	**0.09 ***	−0.01	−0.02	−0.04	−0.01	0.00	0.00	0.01	−0.01	−0.01	−0.03	0.00	−0.02
BPS	beta	0.01	−0.07	−0.03	−0.01	0.05	−0.02	−0.01	0.06	0.05	0.07	0.02	0.03	−0.02	−0.01	−0.02	−0.03	0.00	−0.03
TCS	beta	−0.08 *	−0.03	−0.08 *	−0.06	−0.11 *	−0.04	0.03	0.02	−0.18	0.15	0.02	−0.01	−0.01	−0.02	0.02	0.02	−0.04	−0.07
BP-3	beta	−0.08 *	−0.03	−0.08 *	−0.06	−0.11 *	−0.04	0.03	0.02	−0.18	0.15	0.02	−0.01	−0.01	−0.02	0.02	0.02	−0.04	−0.07
MP	beta	−0.13	0.00	−0.06	−0.04	−0.07	0.11	0.13	0.08	−0.21	0.57	0.04	0.05	0.06	−0.10	−0.03	−0.05	−0.01	0.18
EP	beta	0.01	0.03	−0.24 *	−0.27 *	−0.26	−0.34	0.06	−0.09	0.06	0.20	−0.08	0.00	−0.01	−0.11	−0.05	0.18	0.03	−0.01
PP	beta	−0.07	0.01	−0.02	−0.01	−0.09	0.00	0.07	0.14	0.00	**0.37 ***	0.02	0.06	0.01	−0.07	−0.04	−0.02	−0.06	0.10
BP	beta	0.00	0.01	0.01	−0.01	0.01	0.05	0.01	0.01	0.16	−0.01	0.01	0.00	0.01	0.00	0.00	**0.14 ***	0.01	0.00
1-OHP	beta	0.00	0.01	0.01	−0.01	0.01	0.05	0.01	0.01	0.16	−0.01	0.01	0.00	0.01	0.00	0.00	**0.14 ***	0.01	0.00
2-NAP	beta	0.00	0.01	0.01	−0.01	0.01	0.05	0.01	0.01	0.16	−0.01	0.01	0.00	0.01	0.00	0.00	**0.14 ***	0.01	0.00
1-PHE	beta	0.00	0.01	0.01	−0.01	0.01	0.05	0.01	0.01	0.16	−0.01	0.01	0.00	0.01	0.00	0.00	**0.14 ***	0.01	0.00
2-FLU	beta	0.00	0.01	0.01	−0.01	0.01	0.05	0.01	0.01	0.16	−0.01	0.01	0.00	0.01	0.00	0.00	**0.14 ***	0.01	0.00
t,tMA	beta	0.00	0.01	0.01	−0.01	0.01	0.05	0.01	0.01	0.16	−0.01	0.01	0.00	0.01	0.00	0.00	**0.14 ***	0.01	0.00
BMA	beta	0.05	0.02	0.04	−0.06	−0.06	0.07	−0.01	−0.08	0.04	0.15	−0.02	−0.07	−0.02	−0.02	−0.05	0.00	−0.05	0.18

Multiple linear regression results adjusted for maternal age, early-pregnancy body mass index, education, income, parity, maternal urine cotinine level, and neonatal sex after natural log transformation for chemical concentrations; *p*, *p*-value; bold and asterisk (*) characters indicate statistically significant positive association ($p < 0.05$). MnBP, mono-N-butyl phthalate; MEP, mono ethyl phthalate; MCPP, mono(3-carboxypropyl) phthalate; MBzP, monobenzyl phthalate; MMP, mono(2-methylpropyl) phthalate; MEOHP, mono(2-ethyl-5-oxohexyl) phthalate; MEHHP, mono(2-ethyl-5-hydroxyhexyl) phthalate; MECPP, mono(2-ethyl-5-carboxypentyl) phthalate; MiBP, mono-isobutyl phthalate; BPA, Bisphenol A; BPF, Bisphenol F; BPS, Bisphenol S; MP, Methylparaben; EP, Ethylparaben; BP, Butylparaben; PP, Propylparaben; TCS, Triclosan; BP-3, Benzophenon-3; 1-OHP, 1-hydroxypyrene; 2-NAP, 2-hydroxynaphthalene; 1-PHE, 1-hydroxyphenanthrene; 2-FLU, 2-hydroxyfluorene; t,t-MA, trans, trans-muconic acid; BMA, benzylmercapturic acid.

4. Discussion

We found that some phthalates and PAHs in maternal urine were significantly associated with ante- and postpartum depression and confirmed the relationship between dietary and lifestyle factors and depression. However, it is difficult to discuss the relationship between EDC exposure and perinatal depression, because few studies have compared them. Therefore, we compared our results with those of previous studies in other population groups, such as children, adults in general, and the elderly.

In the present study, we found that the secondary metabolites of MEHP (MECPP, MEOHP, and MEHHP) in the maternal urine were significantly associated with ante- and postpartum depression, which is supported by several previous studies [9,11,21,24,25]. A Chinese epidemiological study involving 278 pregnant women reported that exposure to a mixture of phthalates, bisphenols, and parabens resulted in a 1.03-fold increase in postpartum depression [11]. Another Chinese study demonstrated an association (OR = 1.490, 95% CI = 1.051–2.112) and a mediating effect (β = 0.1027, 95% CI = 0.0288–0.1971) between MEHP levels in urine samples from the general elderly population and depressive symptoms [21]. Another study found that MECPP was significantly related to depressive symptoms in American adults [24], and concentrations of DEHP metabolites, including MEOHP, MEHHP, and MECPP, were positively associated with an increased risk of depressive symptoms in a Korean elderly population (OR = 1.92, 95% CI = 1.17–3.13) [25]. In toxicological animal studies, female rats exposed to multiple EDCs showed a multigenerational reduction in maternal behaviors such as nursing, grooming, and licking their babies, which is similar to human postpartum depression symptoms [37]. In another animal study, mice exposed to dibutyl phthalate in the peri-gestational period showed impaired maternal behavior, regarded as typical symptoms in maternal postpartum depression [38].

With respect to the link between PAHs and depression, we found that some PAHs (1-OHP, 2-NAP, and 2-FLU) were significantly associated with ante- and postpartum depression, similar to the results of previous studies [23,27,28]. A recent meta-analysis concluded that prenatal exposure to PAHs can be associated with an increased risk of social behavior (OR = 1.60), attention deficits (OR = 2.99), motor skill deficits (OR = 1.91), and other neurodevelopmental problems (OR = 2.10) in children [27]. In addition, exposure to 2-hydroxyfluorene in the general adult population could increase the risk of depression (OR = 1.43). A study in the US that assessed the association between PAH metabolites and the risk of depression using the National Health and Nutrition Examination Survey (NHANES) [23] revealed positive associations between the urinary 1-NAP (OR = 2.78) and 2-NAP level (OR = 3.17) and depressive symptoms in women within the highest quantile of exposure [28].

However, in our study, there was no significant relationship with perinatal depression for bisphenols, parabens, phenols, and VOCs, with the exception of some phthalates and PAHs. A Chinese birth cohort study found that maternal exposure to BPA and BPF during pregnancy was associated with higher postpartum depression scores, suggesting that pregnancy constituted an important window of vulnerability [11]. Another longitudinal study determined the association between exposure to total volatile organic compounds (TVOCs) by air freshener use and maternal postpartum depression symptoms at 6–8 months after delivery (OR = 1.19) [22]. Environmental tobacco smoke, a complex mixture of nicotine, tar, carbon monoxide, carbon dioxide, and PAHs, represents one of the main pollutants influencing maternal depression [4]. A recent meta-analysis found that perinatal exposure to secondhand smoke in non-smoking women significantly increased the risk of maternal depression symptoms at any time during pregnancy or the postpartum period (OR = 1.77) and increased antenatal suicidal ideation (OR = 1.75) [26]. The range of outcomes in these studies can be understood as differences in populations, sample sizes, mixture effects, time when depression was measured, and research design. While our study measured depression in the first trimester of pregnancy (before the 14 week), a previous study measured depression in the second trimester (14–28 weeks) and focused on twin pregnancies [11]. Differences in the composition of reproductive hormones between these trimesters [2] may also feature here.

To the best of our knowledge, limited studies have reported mixture effects of non-persistent EDC exposure on perinatal depression to date [11]. This implies that the present univariate models may underestimate or overestimate the health effects compared to the more advanced mixture model approach like BKMR. In this study, we evaluated the mixture effect of 24 non-persistent EDCs on antepartum and postpartum depression scores after adjusting covariates. Although no chemicals showed a statistically significant association with the depression score at the significance level of $p < 0.05$ in both periods, a distinct trend difference between two periods was observed. Our result aligns with those of a previous study, which reported weak mixture effects of non-persistent EDCs on anxiety and depression during pregnancy and the postpartum period using BKMR and quantile-based g-computation methodologies [11].

In the present study, the consumption of fish, fermented foods, cup noodles, and popcorn and use of nail polish and perfume, plastic tableware, paint, and pesticides were significantly associated with an increased phthalate urinary concentration in pregnant women. This was consistent with the results of previous studies [12,39–46]. Phthalates are classified into low-molecular-weight types (dimethyl, diethyl, dibutyl, and diisobutyl phthalate) and high-molecular-weight types (di(2-ethylhexyl), diisononyl, and diphenyl phthalate). The former are used as solvents in personal hygiene products, cosmetics, and pharmaceuticals, while the latter are used as plasticizers in PVC products, including medical devices and children's toys [47]. Most environmental phenols are also significantly associated with the consumption of fermented foods; frozen foods; cup noodles; and the use of skin care products, makeup products, sunscreen products, perfumes, and pesticides, as reported in previous studies [12,13,48–52]. Increased PAH levels in urine are significantly associated with the use of detergents, polishes, air fresheners, and paints, as well as the use of personal hygiene products such as skin care, perfume, hand wash, and sunscreen products [53–55]. These are compounds of interest in human biomonitoring because of their potential to bioaccumulate and exert carcinogenic, mutagenic, and teratogenic effects [53]. The most common sources of exposure to PAHs are factory and traffic exhaust derived from gasoline and diesel fuels, residential fossil fuel heating, wood-burning ovens and fireplaces, cigarette smoke, fires, and charcoal-based food smoke [55,56]. The present study confirmed that most exposure to EDCs occurs in everyday life, such as from food commonly consumed by pregnant women, personal hygiene, household products, and automobile exhaust. Therefore, pregnant women who are environmentally vulnerable and sensitive should avoid these products and exposures as much as possible.

This study was subject to some limitations. First, we measured depression levels during the first trimester of pregnancy. However, as pregnancy is a time when reproductive hormones change dramatically depending on the trimester, depression scores from that trimester are not representative for the entire pregnancy period. Secondly, the successful follow-up rate of pregnant women was low at approximately 50%. Third, discrepancies in time point between urine sample collection and food and lifestyle factors were observed. Thirdly, we did not have information on family interactions or social support, such as intimacy with the husband, receiving aid from the mother's family, and relationships with friends, which are known to influence perinatal depression. Fourth, compared to other countries, South Korea exhibits greater homogeneity in factors such as ethnicity, marital status, cohabitation with a spouse, and insurance coverage. This introduces limitations in generalizing or extrapolating the findings from the cohort of pregnant women in this study to populations of pregnant women in other countries or regions. Additionally, it should be noted that many participants in this study were residents of metropolitan areas with relatively higher levels of education and income, which should be considered when interpreting and comparing the results. Despite these limitations, our study targeted hard-to-reach pregnant women and was able to obtain information on EDC exposure and depressive symptoms from the same study participants, both during pregnancy and postpartum. Additionally, we attempted to measure the effects of a mixture of 24 EDCs that can be obtained in everyday life.

5. Conclusions

We observed an association between exposure to non-persistent chemicals and an increased risk of ante- or postpartum depression and its association with dietary and lifestyle factors. Our findings provide meaningful information about the identification of toxic chemicals potentially linked to perinatal depression. It is imperative that clinical obstetricians, psychologists, public health organizations, and harmful chemical regulatory governance provide practical guidelines and counseling to mitigate exposure to toxic chemicals. Pregnant women and their families should also pay attention to reducing their exposure to multiple EDCs that are commonly absorbed through various pathways to help prevent antenatal and postnatal depression.

Supplementary Materials: The following supporting information can be downloaded at: https://www.mdpi.com/article/10.3390/environments12010015/s1, Figure S1: Distribution of antepartum and postpartum depression score.

Author Contributions: Conceptualization, J.H.K.; methodology, J.H.K.; software, N.M.; validation, N.M.; formal analysis, N.M., S.J.H. and J.H.K.; investigation, N.M., S.J.H. and J.H.K.; resources, N.M. and J.H.K.; data curation, N.M., S.J.H. and J.H.K.; writing—original draft preparation, N.M., S.J.H. and J.H.K.; writing—review and editing, N.M., S.J.H. and J.H.K.; visualization, N.M.; supervision, J.H.K.; project administration, J.H.K.; funding acquisition, J.H.K. All authors have read and agreed to the published version of the manuscript.

Funding: This study was supported by the National Research Foundation of Korea (NRF) and funded by the Korean Government (Ministry of Science, ICT) [grant number NRF-2021R1A2C4001788].

Data Availability Statement: Data is available on request due to privacy restrictions. The data used in this study contains sensitive pregnancy-related information about the participants and can only be made available upon reasonable request to the corresponding author.

Conflicts of Interest: The authors declare no conflicts of interest.

References

1. Kumar, P.; Magon, N. Hormones in pregnancy. *Niger. Med. J.* **2012**, *53*, 179–183. [CrossRef]
2. Cunningham, F.G.; Leveno, K.J.; Dashe, J.S.; Hoffman, B.L.; Spong, C.Y.; Casey, B.M. Maternal Physiology. In *Williams Obstetrics, 26e*; McGraw Hill: New York, NY, USA, 2022. Available online: https://accessmedicine.mhmedical.com/content.aspx?bookid=2977&sectionid=254987027 (accessed on 1 December 2024).
3. Soma-Pillay, P.; Nelson-Piercy, C.; Tolppanen, H.; Mebazaa, A. Physiological changes in pregnancy. *Cardiovasc. J. Afr.* **2016**, *27*, 89–94. [CrossRef]
4. Jacobson, M.H.; Ghassabian, A.; Gore, A.C.; Trasande, L. Exposure to environmental chemicals and perinatal psychopathology. *Biochem. Pharmacol.* **2022**, *195*, 114835. [CrossRef]
5. Li, S.H.; Graham, B.M. Why are women so vulnerable to anxiety, trauma-related and stress-related disorders? The potential role of sex hormones. *Lancet Psychiatry* **2017**, *4*, 73–82. [CrossRef]
6. Schiller, C.E.; Meltzer-Brody, S.; Rubinow, D.R. The role of reproductive hormones in postpartum depression. *CNS Spectr.* **2015**, *20*, 48–59. [CrossRef] [PubMed]

7. Yim, I.S.; Stapleton, L.R.T.; Guardino, C.M.; Hahn-Holbrook, J.; Schetter, C.D. Biological and psychosocial predictors of postpartum depression: Systematic review and call for integration. *Annu. Rev. Clin. Psychol.* **2015**, *11*, 99–137. [CrossRef]
8. Kim, J.H.; Moon, N.; Ji, E.; Moon, H.B. Effects of postnatal exposure to phthalate, bisphenol a, triclosan, parabens, and per- and poly-fluoroalkyl substances on maternal postpartum depression and infant neurodevelopment: A korean mother-infant pair cohort study. *Environ. Sci. Pollut. Res. Int.* **2023**, *30*, 96384–96399. [CrossRef] [PubMed]
9. Kim, J.H.; Shin, H.S.; Lee, W.H. Impact of endocrine-disrupting chemicals in breast milk on postpartum depression in Korean mothers. *Int. J. Environ. Res. Public. Health* **2021**, *18*, 4444. [CrossRef]
10. Townsend, M.K.; Franke, A.A.; Li, X.; Hu, F.B.; Eliassen, A.H. Within-person reproducibility of urinary bisphenol A and phthalate metabolites over a 1 to 3 year period among women in the Nurses' Health Studies: A prospective cohort study. *Environ. Health* **2013**, *12*, 80. [CrossRef] [PubMed]
11. Hu, L.; Mei, H.; Feng, H.; Huang, Y.; Cai, X.; Xiang, F.; Chen, L.; Xiao, H. Exposure to bisphenols, parabens and phthalates during pregnancy and postpartum anxiety and depression symptoms: Evidence from women with twin pregnancies. *Environ. Res.* **2023**, *221*, 115248. [CrossRef]
12. Kim, J.H.; Kim, D.; Moon, S.M.; Yang, E.J. Associations of lifestyle factors with phthalate metabolites, bisphenol A, parabens, and triclosan concentrations in breast milk of Korean mothers. *Chemosphere* **2020**, *249*, 126149. [CrossRef]
13. Xu, X.; Hong, X.; Xie, L.; Li, T.; Yang, Y.; Zhang, Q.; Zhang, G.; Liu, X. Gestational and lactational exposure to bisphenol-A affects anxiety- and depression-like behaviors in mice. *Horm. Behav.* **2012**, *62*, 480–490. [CrossRef]
14. Xu, X.; Yang, Y.; Wang, R.; Wang, Y.; Ruan, Q.; Lu, Y. Perinatal exposure to di-(2-ethylhexyl) phthalate affects anxiety- and depression-like behaviors in mice. *Chemosphere* **2015**, *124*, 22–31. [CrossRef]
15. Gaum, P.M.; Gube, M.; Esser, A.; Schettgen, T.; Quinete, N.; Bertram, J.; Putschögl, F.M.; Kraus, T.; Lang, J. Depressive symptoms after PCB exposure: Hypotheses for underlying pathomechanisms via the thyroid and dopamine system. *Int. J. Environ. Res. Public Health* **2019**, *16*, 950. [CrossRef] [PubMed]
16. Putschögl, F.M.; Gaum, P.M.; Schettgen, T.; Kraus, T.; Gube, M.; Lang, J. Effects of occupational exposure to polychlorinated biphenyls on urinary metabolites of neurotransmitters: A cross-sectional and longitudinal perspective. *Int. J. Hyg. Environ. Health* **2015**, *218*, 452–460. [CrossRef]
17. Aker, A.M.; Johns, L.; McElrath, T.F.; Cantonwine, D.E.; Mukherjee, B.; Meeker, J.D. Associations between maternal phenol and paraben urinary biomarkers and maternal hormones during pregnancy: A repeated measures study. *Environ. Int.* **2018**, *113*, 341–349. [CrossRef]
18. Huang, H.; Liang, J.; Tang, P.; Yu, C.; Fan, H.; Liao, Q.; Long, J.; Pan, D.; Zeng, X.; Liu, S.; et al. Associations of bisphenol exposure with thyroid hormones in pregnant women: A prospective birth cohort study in China. *Environ. Sci. Pollut. Res.* **2022**, *29*, 87170–87183. [CrossRef]
19. Del Río, J.P.; Alliende, M.I.; Molina, N.; Serrano, F.G.; Molina, S.; Vigil, P. Steroid Hormones and Their Action in Women's Brains: The Importance of Hormonal Balance. *Front. Public. Health* **2018**, *6*, 141. [CrossRef]
20. Eleiwa, N.Z.H.; Elsayed, A.S.F.; Said, E.N.; Metwally, M.M.M.; Abd-Elhakim, Y.M. Di (2-ethylhexyl) phthalate alters neurobehavioral responses and oxidative status, architecture, and GFAP and BDNF signaling in juvenile rat's brain: Protective role of Coenzyme10. *Food Chem. Toxicol.* **2024**, *184*, 114372. [CrossRef] [PubMed]
21. Bao, C.; Lv, J.; Chen, J.R.; Wei, G.Z.; Liu, N.; Wang, Y.T.; Ding, Z.; Liu, W.B.; Cao, H.J.; Sheng, J.; et al. Chronic inflammation as a potential mediator between phthalate exposure and depressive symptoms. *Ecotoxicol. Environ. Saf.* **2022**, *233*, 113313. [CrossRef]
22. Farrow, A.; Taylor, H.; Northstone, K.; Golding, J. Symptoms of Mothers and Infants Related to Total Volatile Organic Compounds in Household Products. *Arch. Environ. Health: Int. J.* **2003**, *58*, 633–641. [CrossRef]
23. Farhan, J.A.; Iwaniuk, P.; Kaczyński, P.; Łozowicka, B.; Mroczko, B.; Orywal, K.; Perkowski, M.; Socha, K.; Zoń, W. Urinary polycyclic aromatic hydrocarbon metabolites and depression: A cross-sectional study of the National Health and Nutrition Examination Survey 2005-2016. *Env. Sci Pollut Res Int.* **2022**, *29*, 39067–39076. [CrossRef]
24. Shiue, I. Urinary heavy metals, phthalates and polyaromatic hydrocarbons independent of health events are associated with adult depression: USA NHANES, 2011–2012. *Environ. Sci. Pollut. Res.* **2015**, *22*, 17095–17103. [CrossRef] [PubMed]
25. Lee, K.S.; Lim, Y.H.; Kim, K.N.; Choi, Y.H.; Hong, Y.C.; Lee, N. Urinary phthalate metabolites concentrations and symptoms of depression in an elderly population. *Sci. Total Environ.* **2018**, *625*, 1191–1197. [CrossRef] [PubMed]
26. Suzuki, D.; Wariki, W.M.; Suto, M.; Yamaji, N.; Takemoto, Y.; Rahman, M.M.; Ota, E. Association of secondhand smoke and depressive symptoms in nonsmoking pregnant Women: A systematic review and meta-analysis. *J. Affect. Disord.* **2019**, *245*, 918–927. [CrossRef] [PubMed]
27. Zhen, H.; Zhang, F.; Cheng, H.; Hu, F.; Jia, Y.; Hou, Y.; Shang, M.; Yu, H.; Jiang, M. Association of polycyclic aromatic hydrocarbons exposure with child neurodevelopment and adult emotional disorders: A meta-analysis study. *Ecotoxicol. Environ. Saf.* **2023**, *255*, 114770. [CrossRef]
28. Zhang, L.; Sun, J.; Zhang, D. The relationship between urine polycyclic aromatic hydrocarbons and depressive symptoms in American adults. *J. Affect. Disord.* **2021**, *292*, 227–233. [CrossRef]

29. Radloff, L.S. The CES-D Scale:A Self-Report Depression Scale for Research in the General Population. *Appl. Psychol. Meas.* **1977**, *1*, 385–401. [CrossRef]
30. Jeon, G.; Choi, S.; Yang, B. Integrated Korean version of CES-D development. *J. Korean Psychol. Assoc. Health* **2001**, *6*, 59–76.
31. Cox, J.L.; Holden, J.M.; Sagovsky, R. Detection of Postnatal Depression: Development of the 10-item Edinburgh Postnatal Depression Scale. *Br. J. Psychiatry* **1987**, *150*, 782–786. [CrossRef]
32. Kim, Y.K.; Hur, J.W.; Kim, K.H.; Oh, K.S.; Shin, Y.C. Clinical Application of Korean Version of Edinburgh Postnatal Depression Scale. *J. Korean Neuropsychiatr. Assoc.* **2008**, *47*, 36–44.
33. Kim, J.H.; Moon, N.; Heo, S.J.; Jeong, Y.W.; Kang, D.R. Repeated measurements and mixture effects of urinary bisphenols, parabens, polycyclic aromatic hydrocarbons, and other chemicals on biomarkers of oxidative stress in pre- and postpartum women. *Environ. Pollut.* **2024**, *342*, 123057. [CrossRef]
34. Hornung, R.W.; Reed, L.D. Estimation of average concentration in the presence of nondetectable values. *Appl. Occup. Environ. Hyg.* **1990**, *5*, 46–51. [CrossRef]
35. Barr, D.B.; Wilder, L.C.; Caudill, S.P.; Gonzalez, A.J.; Needham, L.L.; Pirkle, J.L. Urinary creatinine concentrations in the US population: Implications for urinary biologic monitoring measurements. *Environ. Health Perspect.* **2005**, *113*, 192–200. [CrossRef] [PubMed]
36. Bobb, J.F.; Valeri, L.; Claus Henn, B.; Christiani, D.C.; Wright, R.O.; Mazumdar, M.; Godleski, J.J.; Coull, B.A. Bayesian kernel machine regression for estimating the health effects of multi-pollutant mixtures. *Biostatistics* **2015**, *16*, 493–508. [CrossRef]
37. López-Rodríguez, D.; Aylwin, C.F.; Delli, V.; Sevrin, E.; Campanile, M.; Martin, M.; Franssen, D.; Gérard, A.; Blacher, S.; Tirelli, E.; et al. Multi- and Transgenerational Outcomes of an Exposure to a Mixture of Endocrine-Disrupting Chemicals (EDCs) on Puberty and Maternal Behavior in the Female Rat. *Environ. Health Perspect.* **2021**, *129*, 87003. [CrossRef] [PubMed]
38. Lee, S.M.; Jeon, S.; Jeong, H.J.; Kim, B.N.; Kim, Y. Dibutyl phthalate exposure during gestation and lactation in C57BL/6 mice: Maternal behavior and neurodevelopment in pups. *Environ. Res.* **2020**, *182*, 109025. [CrossRef] [PubMed]
39. Ding, S.; Zhang, Z.; Chen, Y.; Qi, W.; Zhang, Y.; Xu, Q.; Liu, H.; Zhang, T.; Zhao, Y.; Han, X.; et al. Urinary levels of phthalate metabolites and their association with lifestyle behaviors in Chinese adolescents and young adults. *Ecotoxicol. Environ. Saf.* **2019**, *183*, 109541. [CrossRef] [PubMed]
40. Liao, C.; Liu, W.; Zhang, J.; Shi, W.; Wang, X.; Cai, J.; Zou, Z.; Lu, R.; Sun, C.; Wang, H.; et al. Associations of urinary phthalate metabolites with residential characteristics, lifestyles, and dietary habits among young children in Shanghai, China. *Sci. Total Environment.* **2018**, *616*, 1288–1297. [CrossRef]
41. Luo, C.; Deng, J.; Chen, L.; Wang, Q.; Xu, Y.; Ping, L.Y.; Zhou, L.; Shi, Y.; Mao, W.; Yang, X.; et al. Phthalate acid esters and polycyclic aromatic hydrocarbons concentrations with their determining factors among Chinese pregnant women: A focus on dietary patterns. *Sci. Total Environ.* **2022**, *852*, 158344. [CrossRef]
42. Di Napoli, I.; Tagliaferri, S.; Sommella, E.; Salviati, E.; Porri, D.; Raspini, B.; Cena, H.; Campiglia, P.; La Rocca, C.; Cerbo, R.M.; et al. Lifestyle Habits and Exposure to BPA and Phthalates in Women of Childbearing Age from Northern Italy: A Pilot Study. *Int. J. Environ. Res. Public. Health* **2021**, *18*, 9710. [CrossRef] [PubMed]
43. Zheng, Y.; Cheng, B.; You, W.; Yu, J.; Ho, W. 3D hierarchical graphene oxide-NiFe LDH composite with enhanced adsorption affinity to Congo red, methyl orange and Cr (VI) ions. *J. Hazard. Mater.* **2019**, *369*, 214–225. [CrossRef]
44. Fišerová, P.S.; Melymuk, L.; Komprdová, K.; Domínguez-Romero, E.; Scheringer, M.; Kohoutek, J.; Přibylová, P.; Andrýsková, L.; Piler, P.; Koch, H.M.; et al. Personal care product use and lifestyle affect phthalate and DINCH metabolite levels in teenagers and young adults. *Environ. Res.* **2022**, *213*, 113675. [CrossRef] [PubMed]
45. Fréry, N.; Santonen, T.; Porras, S.P.; Fucic, A.; Leso, V.; Bousoumah, R.; Duca, R.C.; El Yamani, M.; Kolossa-Gehring, M.; Ndaw, S.; et al. Biomonitoring of occupational exposure to phthalates: A systematic review. *Int. J. Hyg. Environ. Health* **2020**, *229*, 113548. [CrossRef]
46. EFSA Panel on Food Contact Materials; Enzymes and Processing Aids (CEP); Silano, V.; Barat Baviera, J.M.; Bolognesi, C.; Chesson, A.; Cocconcelli, P.S.; Crebelli, R.; Gott, D.M.; Grob, K.; et al. Update of the risk assessment of di-butylphthalate (DBP), butyl-benzyl-phthalate (BBP), bis(2-ethylhexyl)phthalate (DEHP), di-isononylphthalate (DINP) and di-isodecylphthalate (DIDP) for use in food contact materials. *EFSA J.* **2019**, *17*, e05838. [CrossRef]
47. Bethea, T.N.; Wesselink, A.K.; Weuve, J.; McClean, M.D.; Hauser, R.; Williams, P.L.; Ye, X.; Calafat, A.M.; Baird, D.D.; Wise, L.A. Correlates of exposure to phenols, parabens, and triclocarban in the Study of Environment, Lifestyle and Fibroids. *J. Expo. Sci. Environ. Epidemiol.* **2020**, *30*, 117–136. [CrossRef] [PubMed]
48. Husøy, T.; Andreassen, M.; Hjertholm, H.; Carlsen, M.H.; Norberg, N.; Sprong, C.; Papadopoulou, E.; Sakhi, A.K.; Sabaredzovic, A.; Dirven, H.A. The Norwegian biomonitoring study from the EU project EuroMix: Levels of phenols and phthalates in 24-h urine samples and exposure sources from food and personal care products. *Environ. Int.* **2019**, *132*, 105103. [CrossRef] [PubMed]
49. Kang, H.S.; Ko, A.; Kwon, J.E.; Kyung, M.S.; Im Moon, G.; Park, J.H.; Lee, H.S.; Suh, J.H.; Lee, J.M.; Hwang, M.S.; et al. Urinary benzophenone concentrations and their association with demographic factors in a South Korean population. *Environ. Res.* **2016**, *149*, 1–7. [CrossRef] [PubMed]

50. Machtinger, R.; Berman, T.; Adir, M.; Mansur, A.; Baccarelli, A.A.; Racowsky, C.; Calafat, A.M.; Hauser, R.; Nahum, R. Urinary concentrations of phthalate metabolites, bisphenols and personal care product chemical biomarkers in pregnant women in Israel. *Environ. Int.* **2018**, *116*, 319–325. [CrossRef] [PubMed]
51. Peinado, F.M.; Ocón-Hernández, O.; Iribarne-Durán, L.M.; Vela-Soria, F.; Ubiña, A.; Padilla, C.; Mora, J.C.; Cardona, J.; León, J.; Fernández, M.F.; et al. Cosmetic and personal care product use, urinary levels of parabens and benzophenones, and risk of endometriosis: Results from the EndEA study. *Environ. Res.* **2021**, *196*, 110342. [CrossRef]
52. Arfaeinia, H.; Dobaradaran, S.; Mahmoodi, M.; Farjadfard, S.; Tahmasbizadeh, M.; Fazlzadeh, M. Urinary profile of PAHs and related compounds in women working in beauty salons. *Sci. Total Environ.* **2022**, *851 Pt 2*, 158281. [CrossRef] [PubMed]
53. Cao, L.; Wang, D.; Wen, Y.; He, H.; Chen, A.; Hu, D.; Tan, A.; Shi, T.; Zhu, K.; Ma, J.; et al. Effects of environmental and lifestyle exposures on urinary levels of polycyclic aromatic hydrocarbon metabolites: A cross-sectional study of urban adults in China. *Chemosphere* **2020**, *240*, 124898. [CrossRef] [PubMed]
54. Hoseini, M.; Nabizadeh, R.; Delgado-Saborit, J.M.; Rafiee, A.; Yaghmaeian, K.; Parmy, S.; Faridi, S.; Hassanvand, M.S.; Yunesian, M.; Naddafi, K. Environmental and lifestyle factors affecting exposure to polycyclic aromatic hydrocarbons in the general population in a Middle Eastern area. *Environ. Pollut.* **2018**, *240*, 781–792. [CrossRef]
55. Evci, Y.M.; Esen, F.; Taşdemir, Y. Monitoring of Long-Term Outdoor Concentrations of PAHs with Passive Air Samplers and Comparison with Meteorological Data. *Arch. Environ. Contam. Toxicol.* **2016**, *71*, 246–256. [CrossRef] [PubMed]
56. Gurung, G.; Bradley, J.; Delgado-Saborit, J.M. Effects of shisha smoking on carbon monoxide and PM2.5 concentrations in the indoor and outdoor microenvironment of shisha premises. *Sci. Total Environ.* **2016**, *548*, 340–346. [CrossRef] [PubMed]

environments MDPI

Article

Evidence About the Possible Role of Phthalates and Bisphenol A in Recurrent Pregnancy Loss and Endocrine Dysfunctions: A Case–Control Study

Lidia Caporossi [1,*], Paola Viganò [2], Enrico Paci [1], Silvia Capanna [1], Alessandra Alteri [3], Mariangela De Rosa [1], Daniela Pigini [1], Elisa Partenzi [1] and Bruno Papaleo [1]

[1] Department of Occupational and Environmental Medicine, Epidemiology and Hygiene, National Institute of Insurance Against Accidents at Work, 00078 Monte Porzio Catone, Italy; e.paci@inail.it (E.P.); s.capanna@inail.it (S.C.); m.derosa@inail.it (M.D.R.); d.pigini@inail.it (D.P.); e.partenzi@inail.it (E.P.); b.papaleo@inail.it (B.P.)

[2] Infertility Center, Fondazione IRCCS Ca'Granda, Ospedale Maggiore Policlinico, 20122 Milan, Italy; paola.vigano@policlinico.mi.it

[3] Unit of Obstetrics and Gynecology, IRCCS San Raffaele Scientific Institute, 20132 Milan, Italy; alteri.alessandra@hsr.it

* Correspondence: l.caporossi@inail.it

Abstract: Objectives. A case–control study was conducted to investigate the exposure levels to some specific chemicals, in women with infertility issues, compared with fertile women. Methods. A total of 186 cases and 196 controls were recruited. Each participant provided a urine sample for the determination of six phthalate metabolites (mono-ethyl phthalate, MEP; mono-n-butyl phthalate, MnBP; mono-n-ottyl phthalate, MnOP; monobenzyl phthalate, MBzP; and two metabolites of the diethyl-hexyl phthalate (DEHP): mono(2-ethyl-5-hydroxyhexyl) phthalate, MEHHP and mono(2-ethylhexyl) phthalate, MEHP) in addition to bisphenol A, BPA. Each woman also completed a questionnaire. The urine samples were analyzed using HPLC/MS/MS methods. Results. The analysis revealed significantly higher metabolite concentrations in cases than in controls for all metabolites, except MnOP. Stratification based on infertility factors, showed a significant association of MnBP, MBzP, BPA and DEHP with ovulatory and endocrine dysfunctions. Furthermore, higher mean concentrations of MEP and DEHP were observed in women with recurrent pregnancy loss (RPL) and idiopathic infertility, respectively. Conclusion. These findings suggest that some of the analyzed chemicals may play a role in female infertility. Exposure to DEP (diethyl phthalate) and DEHP appears to be associated with RPL and idiopathic infertility. Further investigation is required to explore potential sources of these risks.

Keywords: phthalates; reproduction; women; BPA; endocrine disrupters

1. Introduction

Infertility is defined as the inability to conceive after 12 months, or more, of unprotected sexual intercourse [1]. It has a multifactorial etiology, influenced by a range of risk factors that may affect female reproductive capacity. This risk factor can arise from both personal and occupational exposures [2]. In recent years, increasing attention has been focused on xenobiotics classified as endocrine disruptors, which interact with estrogen and androgen receptors [3–5]. Historically, these chemicals have been widely used [6], notably as additives in plastic materials, solvents and stabilizing agents in cosmetics. They were also present in thermal papers and as coating agents in food cans. Currently, numerous legal restrictions exist, particularly in Europe, to reduce this type of risk.

Phthalates represent a class of structurally similar molecules that have been used industrially since the early 20th century. Their reprotoxicity is well documented in the literature [7]. In vivo studies have demonstrated embryotoxicity and fetotoxicity [8,9] in chronically exposed female mice. In human studies, long-term exposure to phthalates has yielded conflicting results regarding their role in pregnancy loss [10–12]. Moreover, other studies have identified associations between phthalate exposure and reduced follicle numbers [13], as well as a decreased number of retrieved, mature and fertilized oocytes [14,15]. Further investigations have highlighted the potential reproductive toxicity of di-(2-ethylhexyl) phthalate (DEHP), diethyl phthalate (DEP), dibenzyl phthalate (DBzP), di-n-butyl phthalate (DnBP), butylbenzyl phthalate (BBzP), and more recently di-n-octyl phthalate (DnOP) and di-iso-nonyl phthalate (DiNP) [16].

Bisphenol A (BPA), structurally similar to 17-β-estradiol, can bind to estrogen receptors (α and β) [17–19]. Both in vivo and in vitro experimental studies have emphasized the reprotoxic effects of BPA, which result in oocyte aneuploidy [20], chromosome segregation [21] and effects on meiotic segregation [22]. However, results from human studies remain inconclusive. While some studies found BPA levels to be negatively correlated with estradiol levels [23,24] and reduced useful oocyte numbers in assisted reproductive technology (ART) cycles [25], other studies have yielded contradictory findings [26]. Furthermore, BPA has also been shown to exhibit antiandrogenic activity [27]. In vitro and in silico assays have demonstrated that BPA significantly antagonizes the androgen receptor (AR) by 5α-dihydrotestosterone (DHT)-induced AR transcriptional activity [27].

Exposure to these chemicals occurs primarily through inhalation, dermal absorption and ingestion [28,29], particularly via food contamination [30,31]. Phthalates are rapidly metabolized into monoesters and oxidative metabolites [32], which are excreted predominantly in urine. For this reason, measuring urinary metabolites of phthalates and BPA is considered the most reliable method to assess environmental exposure, and such molecules are useful as biomarkers. Complete urinary excretion occurs within 24 h, with a peak in urinary levels approximately 4 h after exposure [33,34].

Given the potential reproductive toxicity of these substances, studying infertile women may provide insights into their heightened vulnerability [35]. Therefore, identifying circumstances under which exposure occurs, whether in the workplace or daily life, could help to clarify the real routes of exposure and promote reproductive health.

The present study was conducted to assess if exposure to phthalates and BPA could be linked with reproductive problems in a population of women with diagnosis of infertility, and to explore possible ways of exposure. The aim of this study is to understand whether the infertile population actually shows, as suggested in the literature, higher exposure values for these substances and whether these exposure levels can be correlated with specific infertility factors.

2. Materials and Methods

2.1. Study Population

This epidemiological study enrolled female users of a fertility center as cases. Inclusion criteria were as follows: age under 43 years, no history of chemotherapy related to genital problems, and no infertility issues related to surgery or anatomical alterations. The minimum age of the sample of infertile women was 34 years, as younger women were not present at the assisted reproduction center during the sampling period. It should be noted that the average age of the first pregnancy in Italy is estimated at 32 years, which may contribute to the likelihood of noticing reproductive issues at an older age.

Urine samples were taken from non-pregnant women diagnosed with infertility at the clinic. In this survey, women were explicitly selected from couples where infertility was exclusively attributed to the female partner, while the semen quality of their partners was analyzed.

Confounding factors considered in the statistical elaboration, prioritized in relation to the studied situation, included body mass index (BMI), smoking habits, alcohol consumption, age between 35 and 43 years, prior chemotherapy treatments (excluding genital treatment), insulin-dependent diabetes [36] and thyroid disorders [37]. A final exclusion criterion was an abnormal urinary creatinine level, based on World Health Organization (WHO) guidelines [38].

The calculation of the sample size useful for the significance of the data was carried out starting from the prevalence of the considered pathology: the prevalence data of female infertility in Italy is equal to 15% [39], and a margin of maximum error of 5% and a confidence level of 95% was set.

After applying all criteria, a total sample of 186 eligible women with infertility issues was identified.

The control group consisted of women who had recently given birth in the same hospital's obstetrics unit, without undergoing hormonal or fertility treatment, and who achieved pregnancy within 12 months. Control samples were collected at least 4 days postpartum, resulting in an overall control sample of 196 female subjects.

The Institutional Review Board of the IRCCS San Raffaele Scientific Institute in Milan approved the investigation protocol, assigning it the identification code 73/INT/2017. All procedures involving human participants were conducted in accordance with the Declaration of Helsinki.

All participants signed an informed consent form and subsequently completed a structured questionnaire to collect data on clinical status, with a focus on endocrine conditions, lifestyles and occupational habits. The questionnaire adopted involved a multidisciplinary team in its drafting, made up of gynecologists expert in assisted reproduction, embryologists, statisticians and experts in chemical risk in living and working environments.

A well-trained researcher assisted in the completion of the clinical anamnesis. The questionnaire's life habits section collected information on smoking, alcohol consumption, the use of plastic containers, the use of cosmetics such as scents, hair sprays and nail polish, and dietary habits.

Every participant provided a random spot urine sample during her morning clinical visit. These urine samples were analyzed for chemicals of interest.

The sampling period extended from October 2017 to June 2019, covering the geographic area of Northen Italy.

2.2. *Analytical Procedure*

The analytical phase employed previously published HPLC tandem mass spectrometry methods [40,41]. Briefly, for phthalates analysis, urine samples underwent a pretreatment involving enzymatic digestion with β-glucuronidase-from E. Coli, followed by solid-phase extraction (SPE OASIS HBL, 6 cm^3, 200 mg cartridges) before the chromatographic column injection. For BPA analysis, the samples were first incubated at 38 °C for 2 h with β-glucuronidase-arylsulfatase enzyme from Elix Pomatia, followed by acidification with acetic acid 2% (*v*/*v*). The analyte was then extracted using SPE extraction with SPE OASIS HBL (6 cm^3, 200 mg) cartridges, before the HPLC-MS/MS analysis.

The main metabolites of phthalates of interest were analyzed: in detail, mono-ethyl phthalate (MEP) from DEP; mono-n-butyl phthalate (MnBP) from DnBP and BBzP; mono-n-ottyl phthalate (MnOP) from DnOP; monobenzyl phthalate (MBzP) from BBzP and DBzP; two metabolites of the DEHP: mono(2-ethyl-5-hydroxyhexyl) phthalate (MEHHP) and mono(2-ethylhexyl) phthalate (MEHP); and total BPA.

Urinary levels were normalized by dividing by urinary creatinine, obtained using the Jaffè's method [42].

Samples with creatinine levels exceeding 3 g/L or below 0.3 g/L were rejected, following the WHO guidelines [38] and the American Conference of Governmental Industrial Hygienists (ACGIH) recommendation [43]. Values outside this range could indicate kidney issues or other diseases, leading to erroneous results.

2.3. Statistical Elaboration

The SPSS® 25.0 (IBM, Armonk, NY, USA SPSS) software was used for statistical analysis. A preliminary descriptive analysis was conducted to assess the characteristics of the sample population and the distribution of urinary metabolite concentrations. For results below the limit of detection (LOD), values were established to LOD divided by two [44]. Non-parametric methods were employed to analyze the phthalate metabolite concentrations, to discriminate the differences between different groups, including occupational activities, personal habits and demographic categories.

To highlight the differences between cases and controls, the odds ratio was calculated, considering working activities and the daily life habits. Associations between urinary metabolites and infertility factors were assessed using the Kruskal–Wallis test and Dunn post hoc test. The statistical elaboration considered the confounding factors using multivariate logistic regressions.

3. Results

Table 1 shows information about the populations studied, highlighting possible significant differences in specific parameters. The two groups of women display similar characteristics, although infertile women had a higher mean older age and a greater tendency to smoke. Regarding the body mass index, the women controls were asked to indicate their weight before the beginning of the pregnancy.

Table 1. Characteristics of population under study.

	Cases (n = 186)	**Controls (n = 196)**	**p Value**
Age (range)	37.6 (29–43)	33.4 (21–44)	0.000 *
BMI [a] (% of subjects in the class)			
Normal	73.3	59.2	0.101
Overweight	11.3	14.8	
Obese	4.3	8.7	
Underweight	9.1	8.7	
Unknown	1.6	8.7	
Present smokers (%)	16.1	6.1	0.010 *
Previously smokers (%)	23.1	20.4	
Alcohol consumption (%)			
Daily	5.9	7.7	0.000 *
Weekly	44.6	26.0	
Monthly	23.7	28.1	
Never	21.0	37.2	
Missing	4.8	1.0	
Residence area (%)			
Urban	79.0	85.7	0.469
Rural	11.8	9.2	
Coast	2.2	1.0	
Industrial	1.1	0.0	
Urban and industrial	1.1	0.0	

Table 1. *Cont.*

	Cases (n = 186)	Controls (n = 196)	p Value
Other	3.7	0.5	
Missing	1.1	1.5	
Use of plastic containers for fat food storage (%)			
Never	17.2	14.3	0.244
Daily	23.1	21.4	
Weekly	38.2	46.9	
Monthly	18.8	16.8	
Missing	2.7	0.5	
Eating canned food at least weekly (%)	43.5	40.3	0.290
Eating soya products at least weekly (%)	17.8	11.8	0.070
Use of scents at least weekly (%)	80.1	80.7	0.560
Use of nail polishes at least weekly (%)	40.9	32.6	0.148
Use of hair sprays at least weekly (%)	16.6	14.3	0.399
Working activity (%)			
Armed forces	0.5	0.0	0.110
Industrial workers	1.1	2.6	
Education/learning area/ professionals/PC operators	60.7	58.2	
Health workers	8.6	11.7	
Cleaning activity/catering	7.5	6.6	
Trade	8.1	5.6	
Unemployed	2.2	4.1	
Others	11.3	11.2	

[a] BMI: body mass index. * Significant difference; Mann–Whitney test for continuous variables; χ^2 test for qualitative variables.

Table 2 presents the results of the urine sample analysis, detailing the number of samples with metabolites exceeding the limit of detection (LOD) of the methods, and the potential differences highlighted using the Mann–Whitney test. Overall, the results showed significantly higher values in infertile women for all the metabolites, with the only exception being for MnOP. Higher exposure was confirmed by the elevated urinary analyte levels in the cases group.

Table 2. Results (μg/g creatinine) of urinary metabolites of phthalates and BPA.

Parameters	MnBP [1]		MEP [2]		MBzP [3]		MnOP [4]		DEHP [5]		BPA [6]	
	Cases	Controls	Cases	Controls	Cases	Controls	Cases	Controls	Cases	Controls	Cases	Controls
N subjects	186	196	186	196	186	196	186	196	186	196	125	112
Arithmetic mean	25.69	21.76	191.82	101.06	5.53	2.75	2.14	1.86	16.52	11.08	1.73	0.90
Median	16.29	11.55	13.26	28.59	2.62	1.33	1.25	1.03	8.57	5.65	0.57	0.24
Standard deviation	38.39	53.24	762.55	292.23	11.47	3.83	2.69	1.86	24.30	11.08	3.82	4.16
5° percentile	1.25	1.25	0.77	1.50	0.27	0.38	0.08	0.29	1.15	0.92	0.05	0.07
95° percentile	108.39	58.02	635.08	421.62	23.72	9.71	8.44	6.18	58.26	28.52	8.49	2.88
p value (Mann–Whitney test)	0.011 *		0.036 *		0.000 *		0.526		0.000 *		0.000 *	
LOD [7] (μg/L)	0.8		3.0		1.2		0.1		0.15 MEHP [8] 0.05 MEHHP [9]		0.02	
% > LOD	97.3	97.4	62.9	79.1	69.4	51.5	91.4	100.0	99.5	100.0	99.2	100.0

[1] MnBP—mono-n-butyl phthalate; [2] MEP—mono ethyl phthalate; [3] MBzP—monobenzyl phthalate; [4] MnOP—mono-n-octyl phthalate; [5] DEHP—di-(2-ethylhexyl) phthalate, molar sum of two metabolites; [6] BPA—bisphenol A; [7] LOD—limit of detection; [8] MEHP—mono(2-ethylhexyl) phthalate; [9] MEHHP—mono(2-ethyl-5-hydroxyhexyl) phthalate. * Significant value.

MEP levels, despite showing considerable variability, were consistently higher than the concentrations of other phthalates. This may be because DEP is the only compound considered here that is not subject to legal restrictions in Europe [45]. The exposure values were also one or two orders of magnitude higher, with peaks reaching up to 7000 μg/L.

Instead, Table 3 stratifies the data according to the infertility factors reported by the infertile women. Differences among the groups were evaluated using the Kruskal–Wallis test, followed by Dunn's post hoc test for a more detailed analysis of the differences between each infertility factor and the controls. Statistically significant differences, between cases and controls, in urinary levels of MEP MnBP, BPA and DEHP were observed in women with infertility related to ovulatory factors or endocrine dysfunction. MEP levels also differed significantly from controls in women with recurrent pregnancy loss and reduced ovarian reserve. Additionally, DEHP levels were significantly elevated in women with ovulatory, endocrine and idiopathic infertility compared to controls.

DEHP showed higher mean concentration levels, compared with mean value in controls, in all groups of the different infertility factors, except for reduced ovarian reserve, with statistical significance in ovulatory and endocrine dysfunction and idiopathic infertility groups (sine causa infertility). MnBP levels were twice as high in women with ovulatory and endocrine dysfunction, and the same trend was observed for MBzP.

MEP levels were notably higher in women with RPL, with the geometric mean concentration being twice that of the controls. Finally, BPA levels were statistically significantly elevated in women with ovulatory and endocrine dysfunction, and an increasing trend was observed in women with endometriosis (mean value: 0.94 ± 3.93 μg/g creatinine), tubal factors (1.07 ± 5.43 μg/g creatinine) and reduced ovarian reserve (0.61 ± 2.58 μg/g creatinine) compared with controls (0.28 ± 3.06 μg/g creatinine), although these differences were not statistically significant.

Table 3. Phthalates levels with stratification for infertility factors vs. controls.

		μg/g Creatinine (Geometric Mean ± SD [a])					
Infertility Factors	N	**MnBP**	**MEP**	**MBzP**	**MnOP**	**DEHP**	**BPA**
Controls	196	9.32 ± 3.76	22.86 ± 6.45	1.49 ± 2.94	1.11 ± 2.48	5.46 ± 2.76	0.28 ± 3.06
Ovulatory and endocrine dysfunctions	30	21.95 ± 3.84 *	10.71 ± 9.08	3.97 ± 3.80 *	0.81 ± 4.27	12.64 ± 3.06 *	0.64 ± 2.31 *
Endometriosis	20	15.07 ± 2.94	29.04 ± 6.02	2.02 ± 3.33	1.14 ± 3.21	8.78 ± 2.43	0.94 ± 3.93
Idiopathic	52	13.44 ± 2.74	19.49 ± 10.81	2.26 ± 3.48	1.38 ± 4.35	9.69 ± 2.99 *	0.44 ± 4.56
Recurrent Pregnancy Losses (RPL)	18	14.52 ± 4.50	40.07 ± 21.03 *	2.38 ± 2.54	0.56 ± 3.25	10.61 ± 2.56	0.41 ± 3.68
Reduced ovarian reserve	50	8.72 ± 3.66	7.67 ± 7.07 *	1.74 ± 3.48	1.02 ± 3.11	5.39 ± 3.50	0.61 ± 2.58
Reduced ovarian reserve + endometriosis	3	14.70 ± 1.08	10.88 ± 7.19	0.57 ± 1.54	1.30 ± 1.51	6.03 ± 1.81	-
Tubal factors	13	13.82 ± 2.73	12.86 ± 8.87	3.31 ± 5.28	1.64 ± 3.50	11.77 ± 3.84	1.07 ± 5.43
p value Kruskal-Wallis		0.027 *	0.021 *	0.001 *	0.135	0.000 *	0.000 *
p value Dunn post hoc test		0.029 *	0.029 * 0.025 *	0.004 *	0.135	0.019 * 0.007 *	0.016 *

[a] SD—geometric standard deviation; * statistically significant ($p < 0.05$).

Tables 4 and 5 show the calculated odds ratio between cases and controls, considering the different occupational activities and daily life habits, respectively.

No specific occupation or habit seems to be of higher concern in our sample, with the only exception being the use of canned food (OR = 2.021, 95% CI 1.022–3.996).

Table 4. Odds ratio for working activity, adjusted for age, BMI, smoke, alcohol and pathologies.

Working Activity	Cases	Controls	OR	95% CI	*p* Value
Soldiers/policewomen	1	0	-	-	-
Industrial workers	2	5	2.307	0.348–15.293	0.386
Teachers/professionals	112	114	0.699	0.412–1.187	0.185
Nurses/doctors/health professionals	16	23	0.759	0.330–1.747	0.517
Cleaning women/caterer	14	13	2.060	0.721–5.887	0.177
Cashier/traders	15	11	2.580	0.870–7.646	0.087
Other	4	8	0.559	0.107–2.919	0.490

Table 5. Odds ratio for life habits, adjusted for age, BMI, smoke, alcohol and pathologies.

Habits	Cases	Controls	OR	95% CI	*p* Value
Use of plastic containers for storage of fat food	147	167	0.930	0.480–1.804	0.830
Use of canned food	155	154	2.021	1.022–3.996	0.043 *
Use of soya products	90	86	1.111	0.669–1.844	0.685
Use of scents	162	180	0.607	0.265–1.387	0.236
Use of nail polish	150	160	0.634	0.327–1.228	0.176
Use of hair spray	51	49	1.357	0.749–2.459	0.313

* Significant value.

4. Discussion

The results of this study suggest a possible association between exposure to phthalates and BPA and certain female infertility factors. Overall, there was a statistically significant difference between cases and controls, with higher levels of all metabolites in the infertile women, except for MnOP.

Data stratified by infertility factors indicated significantly higher concentrations of MnBP, MBzP, DEHP and BPA in women with ovulatory problems and endocrine dysfunctions. Otherwise, MEP levels were particularly elevated in women with RPL and reduced ovarian reserve, while DEHP levels were higher in women with idiopathic infertility.

The interaction between these chemicals and the endocrine system may directly interfere with endocrine function, potentially leading to ovulatory problems, as shown in experimental studies. These chemicals can affect the quality of the oocyte [46], and recently, some authors [47] have demonstrated a direct interference action of phthalates on the key pathways involved in oocyte maturation.

Experimental data support our findings with the group of women with endocrine and ovulatory problems. Many of the chemicals examined interact with estrogenic or androgen receptors, often involving the aryl hydrocarbon receptor in biochemical mechanisms [48]. BPA can interfere, at different stages, with the feedback control system of the hypothalamic–pituitary–gonadal (HPG) axis, contributing to reproductive toxicity by altering the gonadotropin-releasing hormone levels, which affect follicle-stimulating hormone (FSH) and luteinizing hormone (LH) release [49]. Similar mechanisms are supposed to be involved for phthalates through the HPG axis alteration. Although the involved mechanism remains uncertain, phthalates have been shown to either trigger or inhibit receptor activity, inducing both positive or negative responses on androgen and estrogenic receptors [50]. In vivo studies have demonstrated that phthalate exposure can impair oogenesis [51–53] and folliculogenesis [54], causing damage to deoxyribonucleic acid in oocytes and altering steroidogenesis and the expression of gonadotropin and hormone receptor signaling [55]. Some studies [16] have suggested that phthalates may contribute to the onset of endometriosis through the action of phthalates on inflammation, cytokine production, oxidative stress increase and proliferation of endometrial cells, though our results did not confirm this hypothesis.

BPA exposure has been associated with a reduced likelihood of embryo implantation and oocyte counts [56,57], as well as other gynecological disorders [58]. BPA tends to bioaccumulate, promoting nongenomic signaling pathways, altering women's metabolism and reproductive function leading to conditions such as hyperandrogenism, insulin resistance, obesity, dyslipidemia, chronic inflammation, anovulation and polycystic ovary syndrome (PCOS) [59]. A case–control study [60] on 321 women with PCOS and 412 controls revealed an increased odds ratio for bisphenol exposure (OR 1.26, 95%, CI 1.12–1.45). Other authors have confirmed the positive association between blood BPA concentrations and PCOS [61]. The current evidence [60,61] suggests a role for BPA, similar to other plasticizers, in female reproductive health, with mean concentrations ranging from 1.00 to 2.70 μg/g of creatinine. This warrants further investigations into the mechanism of action.

Otherwise, epidemiological studies have also highlighted an association between phthalate exposure and infertility, particularly focused on possible effects on oocyte yield [62]; some authors suggested effects like ovarian failure, anovulation and a decrease in steroidogenesis [53]. Though these results are controversial [24].

Regarding the possible association between phthalate exposure and RPL, different studies have focused mainly on DEP, DEHP and DnBP, either individually or in mixtures. However, the evidence remains inconclusive or conflicting [11,63].

Some authors [52] conducted a case–control study focused on RPL (260 patients and 203 controls), finding significantly higher levels of phthalates in cases, especially DEHP (the highest quartile of concentration was strongly related to RPL). The geometric mean of that group of women was 0.27 μg/L (unfortunately, results were presented without creatinine correction), which is markedly lower than the value found in our population (DEHP 10.61 μg/g of creatinine). Messerlian et al. [64] found a similar correlation between DEHP and RPL. Elevated MEP and DEHP levels have been associated with an increased risk of miscarriage [10] in 3220 pregnant women (OR = 1.99 and OR = 2.19, respectively), particularly during early gestation (6-10 weeks of gestation). In later gestation, an association was found only with MEHHP levels (OR = 2.41). However, other authors [12] have not confirmed these findings.

The present study does not highlight a particular risk for DnBP exposure in women with RPL, though previous studies have suggested such an effect [65], observing a solid significance for DnBP exposure and an elevated risk for RPL, with a less consistent correlation with DEHP and DEP metabolite levels [65]. Comparisons with these studies reveal higher DEHP and DEP exposure levels in our sample, up to two orders of magnitude higher, with similar results for DnBP. Conflicting results could be attributed to the differences in study design, exclusion criteria, or the sample size. A meta-analysis considering data on 4713 women (651 cases and 4062 controls) identified an elevated risk of pregnancy loss for MnBP and DEHP (OR = 1.34 and 1.79, respectively), though the authors advised caution due to limited study numbers (only eight) [66]. These data suggest the need to compare findings coming from similar geographic areas to avoid differences due to lifestyle habits and different laws for consumer protection.

Considerations about exposure to mixtures of compounds are mandatory, because even at low doses, different chemicals could determine the same effect. Precisely, in light of these considerations, in a cohort study on 132 women, MEP, MnBP and MiBP levels were associated with a higher risk of RPL [67]. Comparing these results with the data herein presented a significantly higher geometric mean for MEP (40.07 vs. 13.26 μg/g creatinine).

Epidemiological studies about women undergoing ART are of particular interest for our debate. DEHP confirmed its reprotoxicity, with lower probability of implantation (−22%) and lower possibility of clinical pregnancy (−24%) or the birth of an alive child (−38%) in case of higher concentrations [66]. Higher exposure (to DnBP and DEHP) and exposure to multiple phthalates (DEHP, DiNP, BBzP) led to a significant association with a lower chance of pregnancy [68]. With a female population of 663 subjects, urinary MnBP was negatively correlated with the odds of normal fertilization [15]. Finally, a risk of preterm birth was highlighted in the case of preconception exposure, studying a sample of 386 women, considering DEHP exposure [69].

Our findings strongly suggest a role of DEP exposure in the RPL, endorsing what other authors suggested. Instead, epidemiological investigations carried out to understand the role of phthalates in idiopathic infertility have not been conducted to date, to our knowledge, even though our results showed a possible role of DEHP exposure.

The higher urinary levels of the examined metabolites call for considerations regarding the sources of exposure. The stratification of data in relation to occupational activities was not significant, not allowing us to identify specific workplaces with a higher potential exposure. The difference between cases and controls, however, requires further investigation in daily life habits, as certainly some sources of exposure in the context of life led to higher exposures in the studied infertile women.

Furthermore, data related to DEP exposure are quite interesting, particularly as the DEP is currently not subject to any regulatory restriction in Europe. The mean values of DEP metabolite in cases are twice as high as those of controls, in particular, for women affected by RPL, and at least one order of magnitude higher than the other metabolites.

Limitations

A limitation of this study is the use of random spot urine samples, as these reflect exposure over the 12–24 h preceding sampling. However, as some researchers have observed [70], multiple urinary samples tend to fall within the same quartile of concentrations, possibly due to low variability in the underlined exposure in daily life. In particular, intra-subject variability studies [71–73] have shown that the use of a spot urine sample can be considered moderately representative of exposure to phthalates, with some differences from phthalate to phthalate.

Another potential bias is the possibility that women who had given birth a few days before, a major part of our controls, could have a faster toxicokinetic than other women, and this could, to a certain extent, underestimate the level of exposure. While no specific data exist for phthalates and alkylphenols, pharmacokinetic studies [73] support this possibility. On the other hand, some authors [74–76] indicate that for pregnant women there may be higher values of some phthalates, particularly DEHP, linked to hospitalization and the possible use of drips or catheters. Furthermore, it is documented in the literature how renal clearance is modified during pregnancy [77], and therefore, creatinuria levels generally decrease. It must be said however that in the postpartum days, the levels tend to return to the prepartum ones; therefore, in our case, this specific aspect should not have a significant impact.

There is also the possibility that women during pregnancy have adopted healthier lifestyles which may affect levels of phthalates, even if the questionnaire asked for elements related to possible sources of exposure and many of these do not fall into a bad lifestyle such as makeup or storing fatty foods in plastic containers.

Finally, there are numerous reprotoxic chemicals, and there are further substances that could act on the endocrine system producing adverse effects on reproduction. For this reason, there is an inevitable limitation of the obtained results, even considering the main confounding factors, and there could be exposures due to particular lifestyle habits that could affect the results.

5. Conclusions

The results of this epidemiological study suggest that exposure to DEP and DEHP, among other substances, may play a role in the RPL and idiopathic infertility. Other substances like BPA or DnBP have shown, with different magnitudes, a higher level in women with specific infertility factors, and this calls for further research to better clarify their role.

These findings highlight the urgent need for more epidemiological investigations focused on idiopathic infertility, because of a lack of information in this field and the possible cumulative effects of chemical mixtures on female reproductive health. In fact, the real exposure is hardly to one substance, but usually to a mixture of substances, and these must be taken into consideration for probable cumulative adverse health effects.

Regarding DEP, there is still no sufficient evidence in the scientific literature to support the hypothesis of its role in infertility problems. However, it should be taken in mind that "it is the dose that makes a substance a poison", and since the MEP concentrations found in our samples are very high, more accurate studies should be carried out to exclude or confirm the possible risk due to DEP exposure in women.

Author Contributions: Conceptualization, L.C.; data curation, L.C., S.C. and M.D.R.; formal analysis, L.C. and S.C.; investigation, L.C., E.P. (Elisa Partenzi), P.V. and A.A.; methodology, L.C., E.P. (Elisa Partenzi), E.P. (Enrico Paci) and D.P.; project administration, B.P.; software, S.C.; writing—original draft, L.C.; validation, E.P. (Enrico Paci) and D.P. writing—review and editing, L.C., P.V., A.A., B.P. and E.P. (Enrico Paci). All authors have read and agreed to the published version of the manuscript.

Funding: This research received no external funding.

Institutional Review Board Statement: The study was conducted according to the guidelines of the Declaration of Helsinki and approved by the Institutional Review Board of the IRCCS San Raffaele Scientific Institute in Milan (identification code 73/INT/2017).

Informed Consent Statement: Informed consent was obtained from all subjects involved in the study.

Data Availability Statement: The data presented in this study are available on request from the corresponding author. The data are not publicly available due to privacy and ethical reasons.

Conflicts of Interest: The authors declare no conflicts of interest.

References

1. WHO. *Infertility Prevalence Estimates, 1990–2021*; World Health Organization Geneva: Geneva, Switzerland, 2023.
2. Ribeiro, E.; Ladeira, C.; Viegas, S. Occupational Exposure to Bisphenol A (BPA): A Reality That Still Needs to Be Unveiled. *Toxics* **2017**, *5*, 22. [CrossRef] [PubMed]
3. Meeker, J.D.; Calafat, A.M.; Hauser, R. Urinary metabolites of di(2-ethylhexyl) phthalate are associated with decreased steroid hormone levels in adult men. *J. Androl.* **2009**, *30*, 287–297. [CrossRef]
4. Pan, G.; Hanaoka, T.; Yoshimura, M.; Zhang, S.; Wang, P.; Tsukino, H.; Inoue, K.; Nakazawa, H.; Tsugane, S.; Takahashi, K. Decreased serum free testosterone in workers exposed to high levels of di-n-butyl phthalates (DBP) and di-2-ethylhexyl phthalate (DEHP): A cross sectional study in China. *Environ. Health Perspect.* **2006**, *114*, 1643–1648. [CrossRef] [PubMed]
5. Konieczna, A.; Rutkowska, A.; Rachon, D. Health risk of exposure to bisphenol A (BPA). *Rocz. Panstw. Zakl. Hig.* **2015**, *66*, 5–11.
6. Wang, Y.; Qian, H. Phthalates and their impacts on human health. *Healthcare* **2021**, *9*, 603. [CrossRef]
7. Hauser, R.; Calafat, A. Phthalates and human health. *Occup. Environ. Med.* **2005**, *62*, 806–818. [CrossRef] [PubMed]
8. Chiang, C.; Lewis, L.R.; Borkowski, G.; Flaws, J.A. Late-life consequences of short-term exposure to di(2-ethylhexyl) phthalate and diisononyl phthalate during adulthood in female mice. *Reprod. Toxicol.* **2020**, *93*, 28–42. [CrossRef] [PubMed]
9. Zong, T.; Lai, I.; Hu, J.; Guo, M.; Li, M.; Zhang, L.; Zhong, C.; Yang, B.; Wu, L.; Zhang, D.; et al. Maternal exposure to di-(2-ethylhexyl) phthalate disrupts placental growth and development in pregnant mice. *J. Hazard. Mater.* **2015**, *297*, 25–33. [CrossRef] [PubMed]

10. Gao, H.; Zhang, Y.W.; Huang, K.; Yan, S.Q.; Mao, L.J.; Ge, X.; Xu, Y.Q.; Xu, Y.Y.; Sheng, J.; Jin, Z.X.; et al. Urinary concentrations of phthalate metabolites in early pregnancy associated with clinical pregnancy loss in Chinese women. *Sci. Rep.* **2017**, *7*, 6800. [CrossRef] [PubMed]
11. Liao, K.W.; Kuo, P.L.; Huang, H.B.; Chang, J.W.; Chiang, H.C.; Huang, P.C. Increased risk of phthalates exposure for recurrent pregnancy loss in reproductive aged women. *Environ. Pollut.* **2018**, *241*, 969–977. [CrossRef] [PubMed]
12. Jukic, A.M.; Calafat, A.M.; McConnaughey, D.R.; Longnecker, M.P.; Hoppin, J.A.; Weinberg, C.R.; Wilcox, A.J.; Baird, D.D. Urinary concentrations of phthalate metabolites and bisphenol A and associations with follicular-phase length, luteal phase length, fecundability and early pregnancy loss. *Environ. Health Perspect.* **2016**, *124*, 321–328. [CrossRef] [PubMed]
13. Messerlian, C.; Souter, I.; Gaskins, A.J.; Williams, P.I.; Ford, J.B.; Chiu, Y.H.; Calafat, A.M.; Hauser, R. Urinary phthalate metabolites and ovarian reserve among women seeking infertility care. *Hum. Reprod.* **2016**, *31*, 75–83. [CrossRef] [PubMed]
14. Machtinger, R.; Gaskins, A.J.; Racowsky, C.; Mansur, A.; Adir, M.; Baccarelli, A.A.; Calafat, A.M.; Hauser, R. Urinary concentrations of biomarkers of phthalates and phthalate alternatives and IVF outcomes. *Environ. Int.* **2018**, *111*, 23–31. [CrossRef]
15. Deng, T.; Du, Y.; Wang, Y.; Teng, X.; Hua, X.; Yuan, X.; Yao, Y.; Guo, N.; Li, Y. The associations of urinary phthalate metabolites with the intermediate and pregnancy outcomes of women receiving IVF/ICSI treatments: A prospective single-center study. *Ecotoxicol. Environ. Saf.* **2020**, *188*, 109884. [CrossRef] [PubMed]
16. Hlisníková, H.; Petrovičová, I.; Kolena, B.; Šidlovská, M.; Sirotkin, A. Effects and mechanisms of phthalates' action on reproductive processes and reproductive health: A literature review. *Int. J. Environ. Res. Public Health* **2020**, *17*, 6811. [CrossRef]
17. Miao, M.; Yuan, W.; Yang, F.; Liang, H.; Zhou, Z.; Li, R.; Gao, E.; Li, D.K. Associations between bisphenol A exposure and re-productive hormones among female workers. *Int. J. Environ. Res. Public Health* **2015**, *12*, 13240–13250. [CrossRef] [PubMed]
18. Kuiper, G.G.J.M.; Lemmen, J.G.; Carlsson, B.; Christopher Corton, J.; Safe, S.H.; van der Saag, P.T.; van der Burg, B.; Gustafsson, J.A. Interaction of estrogenic chemicals and phytoestrogens with estrogen receptor β. *Endocrinology* **1998**, *139*, 4252–4263. [CrossRef] [PubMed]
19. Gould, J.C.; Leonard, L.S.; Maness, S.C.; Wagner, S.B.L.; Conner, K.; Zacharewski, T.; Safe, S.; McDonnell, D.P.; Gaido, K.W. Bisphenol A interacts with the estrogen receptor alpha in a distinct manner from estradiol. *Mol. Cell. Endocrinol.* **1998**, *142*, 203–214. [CrossRef] [PubMed]
20. Hunt, P.A.; Koehler, K.E.; Susiarjo, M.; Hodges, C.A.; Ilagan, A.; Voigt, R.C.; Thomas, S.; Thomas, B.F.; Hassold, T.J. Bisphenol A exposure causes meiotic aneuploidy in the female mouse. *Curr. Biol.* **2003**, *13*, 546–553. [CrossRef] [PubMed]
21. Machtinger, R.; Combelles, C.M.; Missmer, S.A.; Correira, K.F.; Fox, J.H.; Racowsky, C. The association between severe obesity and characteristics of failed fertilized oocytes. *Hum. Reprod.* **2012**, *27*, 3198–3207. [CrossRef]
22. Can, A.; Semiz, O.; Cinar, O. Bisphenol A induces cell cycle delay and alters centrosome and spindle microtubular organization in oocytes during meiosis. *Mol. Hum. Reprod.* **2005**, *11*, 389–396. [CrossRef] [PubMed]
23. Bloom, M.S.; Kim, D.; vom Saal, F.S.; Taylor, J.A.; Cheng, T.G.; Lamb, J.D.; Fujimoto, V.J. Bisphenol A exposure reduces the estradiol response to gonadotropin stimulation during in vitro fertilization. *Fertil. Steril.* **2011**, *96*, 672–677.e2. [CrossRef] [PubMed]
24. Mok-Lin, E.; Ehrlich, S.; Williams, P.L.; Petrozza, J.; Wright, D.L.; Calafat, A.M.; Ye, X.; Hauser, R. Urinary bisphenol A concentrations and ovarian response among women undergoing IVF. *Int. J. Androl.* **2010**, *33*, 385–393. [CrossRef] [PubMed]
25. Ehrlich, S.; Williams, P.L.; Missmer, S.A.; Flaws, J.A.; Ye, X.; Calafat, A.M.; Petrozza, J.C.; Wright, D.; Hauser, R. Urinary bisphenol A concentrations and early reproductive health outcomes among women undergoing IVF. *Hum. Reprod.* **2021**, *27*, 3583–3592. [CrossRef]
26. Minguez-Alarcón, L.; Gaskins, A.J.; Chiu, Y.H.; Williams, P.I.; Ehrlich, S.; Chavarro, J.E.; Petrozza, J.C.; Ford, J.B.; Calafat, A.M.; Hauser, R. Urinary bisphenol A concentrations and association with in vitro fertilization outcomes among women from a fertility clinic. *Hum. Reprod.* **2015**, *30*, 2120–2128. [CrossRef] [PubMed]
27. Huang, X.; Cang, X.; Liu, J. Molecular mechanism of bisphenol A on androgen receptor antagonism. *Toxicol. Vitr.* **2019**, *61*, 104621. [CrossRef]
28. Koch, H.M.; Lorber, M.; Christensen, K.L.; Palmke, C.; Koslitz, S.; Brüning, T. Identifying sources of phthalate exposure with human biomonitoring: Results of a 48 h fasting study with urine collection and personal activity patterns. *Int. J. Hyg. Environ. Health* **2013**, *216*, 672–681. [CrossRef] [PubMed]
29. Huo, X.; Chen, D.; He, Y.; Zhu, W.; Zhou, W.; Zhang, J. Bisphenol-A and female infertility: A possible role of gene-environment interactions. *Int. J. Environ. Res. Public Health* **2015**, *12*, 11101–11116. [CrossRef] [PubMed]
30. Rudel, R.A.; Gray, J.M.; Engel, C.L.; Rawsthorne, T.W.; Dodson, R.E.; Ackerman, J.M.; Rizzo, J.; Nudelman, J.L.; Brody, J.G. Food packaging and bisphenol A and bis(2-ethyhexyl) phthalate exposure: Findings from a dietary intervention. *Environ. Health Perspect.* **2011**, *119*, 914–920. [CrossRef]
31. Sajiki, J.; Miyamoto, F.; Fukata, H.; Mori, C.; Yonekubo, J.; Hayakawa, K. Bisphenol A (BPA) and its source in foods in Japanese markets. *Food Addit. Contam.* **2007**, *24*, 103–112. [CrossRef] [PubMed]

32. Frederiksen, H.; Skakkebaek, N.E.; Andersson, A.M. Metabolism of phthalates in humans. *Mol. Nutr. Food Res.* **2007**, *51*, 899–911. [CrossRef]
33. Krais, A.M.; Andersen, C.; Eriksson, A.C.; Johnsson, E.; Nielsen, J.; Pagels, J.; Gudmundsson, A.; Lindh, C.H.; Wierzbicka, A. Excretion of urinary metabolites of the phthalate esters DEP and DEHP in 16 volunteers after inhalation and dermal exposure. *Int. J. Environ. Res. Public Health* **2018**, *15*, 2514. [CrossRef] [PubMed]
34. Völkel, W.; Bittner, N.; Dekant, W. Quantitation of bisphenol A and bisphenol A glucuronide in biological samples by high performance liquid chromatography tandem mass spectrometry. *Drug Metab. Dispos.* **2005**, *33*, 1748–1757. [CrossRef] [PubMed]
35. Pizzorno, J. Environmental toxins and infertility. *Integr. Med.* **2018**, *17*, 8–11.
36. Thong, E.P.; Codner, E.; Laven, J.S.E.; Teede, H. Diabetes: A metabolic and reproductive disorder in women. *Lancet Diabetes Endocrinol.* **2020**, *8*, 134–149. [CrossRef] [PubMed]
37. Concepción-Zavaleta, M.J.C.; Coronado-Arroyo, J.C.; Quiroz-Aldave, J.E.; Concepción-Urteaga, L.A.; Paz-Ibarra, J. Thyroid dysfunction and female infertility. A comprehensive review. *Diabetes Metab. Syndr.* **2023**, *17*, 102876. [CrossRef]
38. WHO. *Biological Monitoring of Chemical Exposure in the Workplace*; World Health Organization: Geneva, Switzerland, 1996; Volume 1.
39. Scaravelli, G.; De Luca, R.; Spoletini, R.; Speziale, L.; Fedele, F.; Bolli, S.; Mazzola, M.; Bertini, A.; Di Monte, C.; Vigiliano, V. Medically assisted reproduction in Italy, 2020 data from the Italian MAR register. *Minerva Obstet Gynecol* **2024**, *76*, 118–126. [CrossRef] [PubMed]
40. Tranfo, G.; Caporossi, L.; Paci, E.; Aragona, C.; Romanzi, D.; De Carolis, C.; De Rosa, M.; Capanna, S.; Papaleo, B.; Pera, A. Urinary phthalate monoesters concentration in couples with infertility problems. *Toxicol. Lett.* **2012**, *213*, 15–20. [CrossRef]
41. Caporossi, L.; Alteri, A.; Campo, G.; Paci, E.; Tranfo, G.; Capanna, S.; Papaleo, E.; Pigini, D.; Viganò, P.; Papaleo, B. Cross sectional study on exposure to BPA and phthalates and semen parameters in men attending a fertility center. *Int. J. Environ. Res. Public Health* **2020**, *17*, 489. [CrossRef] [PubMed]
42. Kroll, M.H.; Chesler, R.; Hagengruber, C.; Blank, D.W.; Kestner, J.; Rawe, M. Automated determination of urinary creatinine without sample dilution: Theory and practice. *Clin. Chem.* **1986**, *32*, 446–452. [CrossRef] [PubMed]
43. ACGIH—American Conference of Governmental Industrial Hygienists. *Recommendation, TLVs and BEIs*; Signature Publications: Salt Lake City, UT, USA, 2014.
44. Giskeødegård, G.F.; Lydersen, S. Many methods for measuring levels of a substance in a sample have a lower detection limit. Data from these measurements must be handled in a way that avoids systematic errors. *Tidsskr. Nor. Legeforen* **2022**, *142*. [CrossRef]
45. European Chemical Agency. Substance Information. Available online: https://echa.europa.eu/it/substance-information/-/substanceinfo/100.001.409 (accessed on 22 January 2025).
46. Land, K.L.; Miller, F.G.; Fugate, A.C.; Hannon, P.R. The effects of endocrine disrupting chemicals on ovarian and ovulation related fertility outcomes. *Mol. Reprod. Dev.* **2022**, *89*, 608–631. [CrossRef] [PubMed]
47. Hannon, P.R.; Akin, J.W.; Curry, T.E. Exposure to a phthalate mixture disrupts ovulatory progesterone receptor signaling in human granulosa cells in vitro. *Biol. Reprod.* **2023**, *109*, 552–565. [CrossRef] [PubMed]
48. Koch, H.M.; Rossbach, B.; Drexler, H.; Angerer, J. Internal exposure of the general population to DEHP and other phthalate—Determination of secondary and primary phthalate monoester metabolites in urine. *Environ. Res.* **2003**, *93*, 177–185. [CrossRef] [PubMed]
49. Marques-Pinto, A.; Carvalho, D. Human infertility: Are endocrine disruptors to blame? *Endocr. Connect.* **2013**, *2*, R15–R29. [CrossRef]
50. Ma, Y.; Liu, H.; Wu, J.; Yuan, L.; Wang, Y.; Du, X.; Wang, R.; Marwa, P.W.; Petlulu, P.; Chen, X.; et al. The adverse health effects of bisphenol A and related toxicity mechanisms. *Environ. Res.* **2019**, *176*, 108575. [CrossRef]
51. Mariana, M.; Feiteiro, J.; Verde, I.; Cairrao, E. The effects of phthalates in the cardiovascular and reproductive systems: A review. *Environ. Int.* **2016**, *94*, 758–776. [CrossRef] [PubMed]
52. Chang, W.H.; Chou, W.C.; Waits, A.; Liao, K.W.; Kuo, P.L.; Huang, C. Cumulative risk assessment of phthalates exposure for recurrent pregnancy loss in reproductive-aged women population using multiple hazard indices approaches. *Environ. Int.* **2021**, *154*, 106657. [CrossRef]
53. Patel, S.; Zhou, C.; Rattan, S.; Flaws, J.A. Effects of Endocrine-Disrupting Chemicals on the Ovary. *Biol. Reprod.* **2015**, *93*, 20. [CrossRef] [PubMed]
54. Hannon, P.R.; Flawes, J.A. The effects of phthalates on the ovary. *Front. Endocrinol.* **2015**, *6*, 8. [CrossRef]
55. Zhang, T.; Shen, W.; De Felici, M.; Zhang, X.F. Di(2-ethylhexyl)phthalate: Adverse effects on folliculogenesis that cannot be neglected. *Environ. Mol. Mutagen.* **2016**, *57*, 579–588. [CrossRef]
56. Radwan, P.; Wielgomas, B.; Radwan, M.; Krasinski, R.; Klimowska, A.; Kaleta, D.; Jurewicz, J. Urinary bisphenol A concentrations and in vitro fertilization outcomes among women from a fertility clinic. *Reprod. Toxicol.* **2020**, *96*, 216–220. [CrossRef]
57. Shen, J.; Kang, Q.; Mao, Y.; Yuan, M.; Le, F.; Yang, X.; Xu, X.; Jinet, F. Urinary bisphenol A concentration is correlated with poorer oocyte retrieval and embryo implantation outcomes in patients with tubal factor infertility undergoing in vitro fertilization. *Ecotoxicol. Environ. Saf.* **2020**, *187*, 109816. [CrossRef]

58. Park, S.Y.; Jeon, J.H.; Jeong, K.; Chung, H.W.; Lee, H.; Sung, Y.A.; Ye, S.; Ha, S.H. The association of ovarian reserve with exposure to bisphenol A and phthalate in reproductive-aged women. *J. Korean Med. Sci.* **2021**, *36*, e1. [CrossRef]
59. Lara Urbanetz, L.A.M.; Soares, M.S.J.; Rosa Maciel, G.A.; dos Santos Simões, R.; Pinheiro Baracat, M.C.; Baracat, E.C. Does bisphenol A (BPA) participate in the pathogenesis of Polycystic Ovary Syndrome (PCOS)? *Clinics* **2023**, *78*, 100310. [CrossRef]
60. Zhan, W.; Tang, W.; Shen, X.; Xu, H.; Zhang, J. Exposure to bisphenol A and its analogs and polycystic ovarian syndrome in women of childbearing age: A multicenter case-control study. *Chemosphere* **2023**, *313*, 137463. [CrossRef]
61. Ghanati, K.; Jahanbakhsh, M.; Shakoori, A.; Aghebat-Bekheir, S.; Khalili-Rikabadi, A.; Sadighara, P. The association between polycystic ovary syndrome and environmental pollutants based on animal and human study—A systematic review. *Rev. Environ. Health* **2023**, *39*, 651–657. [CrossRef] [PubMed]
62. Chou, Y.C.; Tzeng, C.R. The impact of phthalate on reproductive function in women with endometriosis. *Reprod. Med. Biol.* **2021**, *20*, 159–168. [CrossRef] [PubMed]
63. Hauser, R.; Gaskins, A.J.; Souter, I.; Smith, K.W.; Dodge, L.E.; Ehrlich, S.; Meeker, J.D.; Calafat, A.M.; Williams, P.L. Urinary Phthalate Metabolite Concentrations and Reproductive Outcomes among Women Undergoing in Vitro Fertilization: Results from the EARTH Study. *Environ. Health Perspect.* **2016**, *124*, 831–839. [CrossRef] [PubMed]
64. Messerlian, C.; Wylie, B.J.; Mínguez-Alarcón, L.; Williams, P.L.; Ford, J.B.; Souter, I.C.; Calafat, A.M.; Hauser, R. Urinary concentrations of phthalate metabolites and pregnancy loss among women conceiving with medically assisted reproduction. *Epidemiology* **2016**, *27*, 879–888. [CrossRef]
65. Minguez-Alarcon, L.; Messerlian, C.; Bellavia, A.; Gaskins, A.J.; Chiu, Y.H.; Ford, J.B.; Azevedo, A.R.; Petrozza, J.C.; Calafa, A.M.; Hauser, R.; et al. Urinary concentrations of bisphenol A, parabens and phthalate metabolite mixtures in relation to reproductive success among women undergoing in vitro fertilization. *Environ. Int.* **2019**, *126*, 355–362. [CrossRef] [PubMed]
66. Zhang, H.; Gao, F.; Ben, Y.; Su, Y. Association between phthalate exposure and risk of spontaneous pregnancy loss: A systematic review and meta-analysis. *Environ. Pollut.* **2020**, *267*, 115446. [CrossRef]
67. Mu, D.; Gao, F.; Fan, Z.; Shen, H.; Peng, H.; Hu, J. Levels of phthalate metabolites in urine of pregnant women and risk of clinical pregnancy loss. *Environ. Sci. Technol.* **2015**, *49*, 10651–10657. [CrossRef] [PubMed]
68. Begum, T.F.; Fujimoto, V.Y.; Gerona, R.; McGough, A.; Lenhart, N.; Wong, R.; Mok-Lin, E.; Melamed, J.; Butts, C.D.; Bloom, M.S. A pilot investigation of couple-level phthalates exposure and in vitro fertilization (IVF) outcomes. *Reprod. Toxicol.* **2021**, *99*, 56–64. [CrossRef]
69. Yland, J.J.; Zhang, Y.; Williams, P.L.; Mustieles, V.; Vagios, S.; Souter, I.; Calafat, A.M.; Hauser, R.; Messerlian, C. Phthalate and DINCH urinary concentrations across pregnancy and risk of preterm birth. *Environ. Pollut.* **2022**, *292*, 118476. [CrossRef] [PubMed]
70. Pariente, G.; Leibson, T.; Carls, A.; Adams-Webber, T.; Ito, S.; Koren, G. Pregnancy-Associated Changes in Pharmacokinetics: A Systematic Review. *PLoS Med.* **2016**, *13*, e1002160. [CrossRef] [PubMed]
71. Frommea, H.; Boltea, G.; Koch, H.M.; Angererb, J.; Boehmera, S.; Drexlerb, H.; Mayerc, R.; Lieblc, B. Occurrence and daily variation of phthalate metabolites in the urine of an adult population. *Int. J. Hyg. Environ. Health* **2007**, *210*, 21–33. [CrossRef] [PubMed]
72. Hoppin, J.A.; Brock, J.W.; Davis, B.J.; Baird, D.D. Reproducibility of urinary phthalate metabolites in first morning urine samples. *Environ. Health Perspect.* **2002**, *110*, 515–518. [CrossRef] [PubMed]
73. Hauser, R.; Meeker, J.D.; Park, S.; Silva, M.J.; Calafat, A.M. Temporal variability of urinary phthalate metabolite levels in men of reproductive age. *Environ. Health Perspect.* **2004**, *112*, 1734–1740. [CrossRef]
74. Yan, X.; Calafat, A.; Lashley, S.; Smulian, J.; Ananth, C.; Barr, D.; Silva, M.; Ledoux, T.; Hore, P.; Robson, M.G. Phthalates biomarker identification and exposure estimates in a population of pregnant women. *Hum. Ecol. Risk Assess.* **2009**, *15*, 565–578. [CrossRef] [PubMed]
75. Vandentorren, S.; Zeman, F.; Morin, L.; Sarter, H.; Bidondo, M.L.; Oleko, A.; Leridon, H. Bisphenol-A and phthalates contamination of urine samples by catheters in the Elfe pilot study: Implications for large-scale biomonitoring studies. *Environ. Res.* **2011**, *111*, 761–764. [CrossRef] [PubMed]
76. Zeman, F.A.; Boudet, C.; Tack, K.; Floch Barneaud, A.; Brochot, C.; Péry, A.R.R.; Oleko, A.; Vandentorren, S. Exposure assessment of phthalates in French pregnant women: Results of the ELFE pilot study. *Int. J. Hyg. Environ. Health* **2013**, *216*, 271–279. [CrossRef]
77. Kuromoto, K.; Watanabe, M.; Adachi, K.; Ohashi, K.; Iwatani, Y. Increases in urinary creatinine and blood pressure during early pregnancy in pre-eclampsia. *Ann. Clin. Biochem.* **2010**, *47*, 336–342. [CrossRef] [PubMed]

environments

MDPI

Article

Unveiling Stress Vulnerability and Occupational Noise Perception as Burnout Predictors: Results of an Exploratory Study in Industrial Environments

Carlos Carvalhais [1,2,*], Luísa Antunes Ribeiro [3] and Cristiana C. Pereira [2,4,5]

1 RISE-Health, Center for Translational Health and Medical Biotechnology Research (TBIO), ESS, Polytechnic of Porto, Rua Dr. António Bernardino de Almeida, no. 400, 4200-072 Porto, Portugal
2 ITR/EPIUnit—Instituto de Saúde Pública, Universidade do Porto, Rua das Taipas, no. 135, 4050-600 Porto, Portugal; cristiana.costapereira@lns.etat.lu
3 Research Centre for Human Development, Faculty of Education and Psychology, Universidade Católica Portuguesa, Rua de Diogo Botelho, no. 1327, 4169-005 Porto, Portugal; laribeiro@ucp.pt
4 Environmental Hygiene and Human Biological Monitoring Unit, Department of Health Protection, Laboratoire National de Santé, 1, rue Louis Rech, L-3555 Dudelange, Luxembourg
5 Environmental Health Department, National Institute of Health, Rua Alexandre Herculano, no. 321, 4000-055 Porto, Portugal
* Correspondence: caa@ess.ipp.pt

Abstract: Burnout is a complex phenomenon influenced by both environmental and individual factors. This pilot study explores the predictive role of occupational noise perception and stress vulnerability on burnout symptoms among industrial workers. A cross-sectional survey was conducted with 119 Portuguese workers exposed to occupational noise. Participants completed validated self-report measures assessing noise perception, stress vulnerability, and burnout. Path analysis revealed that both higher stress vulnerability and greater perceived occupational noise were significant predictors of elevated burnout levels. Furthermore, gender emerged as a relevant predictor, with women reporting significantly higher burnout symptoms than men. Age was inversely related to stress vulnerability, indicating greater resilience among older workers. These findings suggest that individual differences in stress vulnerability and noise perception contribute meaningfully to burnout risk, beyond traditional occupational hazard assessments. The study underscores the need for holistic occupational health strategies, integrating both environmental modifications and psychosocial interventions aimed at enhancing workers' coping capacities. This study contributes novel insights into the interplay between perceived noise and psychological vulnerability in industrial settings, supporting broader preventive measures for work-related mental health outcomes.

Keywords: burnout; occupational noise; stress; industrial workers; psychosocial risks

1. Introduction

Occupational noise exposure is a well-established risk factor for hearing loss and other auditory impairments. However, emerging evidence suggests that its effects may extend beyond auditory damage, potentially contributing to psychological stress and burnout symptoms [1]. While most studies on workplace noise have focused on its impact on hearing, less attention has been given to its influence on other health outcomes such as mental health disorders [2]. Moreover, the experience of noise-related stress may be modulated by individual differences in stress vulnerability [1]. Some evidence indicates that noise contributes to psychological strain among workers exposed to multiple occupational hazards, including both physical (e.g., noise) and chemical agents [3].

1.1. Noise and Noise Perception

Noise can be defined as an unwanted sound that acts as a psychosocial stressor adversely affecting the health and well-being of individuals through the activation of the sympathetic and endocrine systems [4–7]. Evidence shows that noise exposure increases systolic and diastolic blood pressure, changes heart rate, and causes the release of stress hormones (including catecholamines and glucocorticoids) [4,8]. The General Stress Model proposed by Babisch [5] explains the rationale behind these reactions (Figure 1). Potential mechanisms are emotional stress reactions due to perceived discomfort (indirect pathway) and non-conscious physiological stress from interactions between the central auditory system and other regions of the CNS (direct pathway) [5,6].

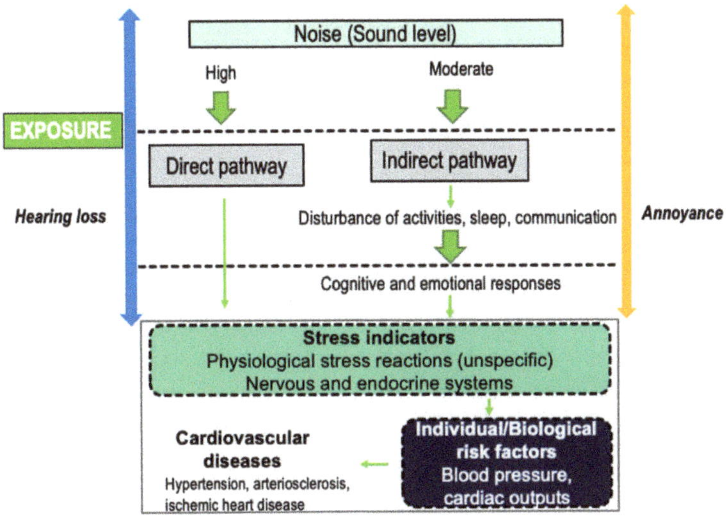

Figure 1. Noise reaction scheme (adapted from Babisch [5]).

High noise perception may contribute to increased stress levels [9]. Noise perception refers to how an individual interprets and responds to auditory stimuli in their environment. In fact, workers' noise perceptions have been studied in several occupational contexts, namely in relation to creating health and safety legislation, so that workers are not exposed to noise that they consider excessive (e.g., patient areas in hospital environments) [10,11].

Noise pollution has emerged as a significant, yet often underestimated, contributor to chronic stress [12]. The incessant exposure to noise—whether from urban traffic, construction, industrial machinery, or the omnipresence of electronic devices—not only affects the auditory system but also impacts cognitive and emotional functioning [13]. Research has increasingly highlighted the adverse effects of noise on human health, with prolonged exposure linked to heightened stress responses, disrupted sleep patterns, and reduced cognitive performance [9]. These effects are particularly relevant in occupational settings, where noise exposure during cognitive tasks can lead to elevated physiological and psychological stress, as well as other non-auditory disorders [3,6,13–17]. Additionally, chronic exposure to psychosocial stressors in the workplace—including noise—has been associated with an increased risk of cardiovascular disease, reinforcing the broader health implications of persistent stressors in the work environment [14].

1.2. Vulnerability to Stress

Vulnerability to stress refers to an individual's susceptibility or predisposition to experience negative effects in response to stressors [18]. Stressors are events, situations, or conditions that can elicit a stress response, which involves the body and mind's efforts to cope with challenges. It can be influenced by various factors, including biological, psychological, and environmental elements [19,20]. An individual's vulnerability to stress significantly shapes their response to environmental stressors. Factors such as sociocultural environment, personal resilience, coping mechanisms, and overall mental health are contributing factors to an individual's profile of stress response [21]. Those already pushing their stress tolerance limit due to work pressures, personal responsibilities, or existing mental health conditions are particularly susceptible to the detrimental effects of noise [21–24]. Recent research has also shown that noise exposure, when combined with high stress from other sources, can lead to severe outcomes such as cardiovascular strain, sleep disturbances, and increased anxiety [22,25,26]. When stress tolerance is already near its limit, the added burden of noise can significantly amplify its harmful effects [8,27].

1.3. Burnout

Burnout is a state of chronic physical and emotional exhaustion, often accompanied by feelings of cynicism and detachment from work [28]. Burnout syndrome is transversal across occupations, since the stressors that can instigate it may be present at any workplace [29]. Consequently, it is expected that burnout has a negative effect on workers' performance, inhibiting creativity and innovation and causing more work-related accidents and absenteeism [30,31]. Both noise perception and vulnerability to stress can be hypothesized as potential predictors of burnout, since, theoretically, individuals with prolonged exposure to noise stressors and higher vulnerability to stress may struggle to cope with yet another work-related challenge [20]. Over time, these heightened stress levels can contribute to burnout [32].

1.4. Rationale and Aim of the Study

Understanding the interaction between environmental stressors and individual psychological traits is essential for developing comprehensive frameworks to address occupational burnout. In particular, the theoretical link between perceived occupational noise (PON) and stress vulnerability (SV) offers valuable insight into the multifaceted nature of burnout. Despite increasing evidence of the impact of occupational stressors on mental health, few studies have integrated both environmental and dispositional variables into explanatory models of burnout.

Perceived occupational noise, a subjective and often underestimated stressor, may play a critical role in the development of burnout, particularly among individuals with high vulnerability to stress. Recognizing the interplay between environmental stimuli and psychological susceptibility underscores the need for holistic approaches to preventing and mitigating burnout. Such approaches should address not only environmental factors, such as noise exposure but also individual factors. This dual perspective may inform the design of more targeted interventions that combine environmental modifications with psychological strategies aimed at enhancing coping mechanisms and reducing vulnerability.

The main aim of this pilot study is to investigate whether noise perception and vulnerability to stress predict burnout symptoms among industrial workers. We also examine the moderating effects of demographic variables, specifically gender and age.

2. Materials and Methods

2.1. Participants

A total of 119 industrial manual workers exposed to occupational noise were recruited through a convenience sampling method from five different industrial settings (metalworking and chemical sectors). This non-probabilistic approach was chosen due to the exploratory nature of the study and the practical accessibility of participants within the selected workplaces. The sample comprised 64 men (54%) and 53 women (45%), while two participants (1%) did not report their gender. The overall response rate was 61.0%. Individuals were aged between 19 and 66 years (M = 34.9, SD = 12.8). Most participants were single (52.1%) or married/living with a partner (37.8%). Only 8 participants (6.7%) were separated/divorced and 4 widowed (3.4%). Regarding education, 59 (49.6%) participants completed 10 to 12 years of education, and 34 (28.6%) completed 9 years or less. Nearly all participants (96.7%) were Portuguese citizens, with the remaining workers originating from Brazil. Seventy-eight (78%) workers reported the need to raise their voice to be able to communicate with their colleagues at the workplace, but just 35 (29.4%) reported using hearing protection devices, at least sometimes. Permission was not obtained to access the noise exposure levels expressed in dB (A).

2.2. Measures

Perception of Occupational Noise (PON): In line with Abbasi et al. [33], who included two standardized items from ISO/TS 15666 [34] to assess noise annoyance in occupational settings, we used the equivalent adapted items from the Portuguese Standard NP 4476 [35], which is based on the first edition of ISO/TS 15666. The questions are as follows: PN1—"Considering the last 12 months, to what extent has the noise at your workplace bothered and disturbed you?", with a 10-point response scale. Higher numbers on the 0–10 scale indicate greater agreement with the statement. PN2—"Considering the last 12 months, indicate from 0 to 10 the extent to which you feel harmed or disturbed by the noise at your workplace". Higer numbers on the scale of 0–10 represent greater reported disturbance.

Stress Vulnerability Scale (23QVS [36]): The Stress Vulnerability Scale is a self-report questionnaire composed of 23 questions used to measure individual vulnerability to stress as a trait. Based on a sample of 368 individuals of the general Portuguese population, the original version had a good internal consistency (Cronbach's $\alpha = 0.83$ for all items). The questionnaire assessed the following seven factors characterizing vulnerability to stress: (i) Perfectionism and Intolerance to Frustration; (ii) Inhibition and Functional Dependence; (iii) Lack of Social Support; (iv) Adverse Life Conditions; (v) Dramatization of Existence; (vi) Subjugation; and (vii) Deprivation of Affection and Rejection. A value of 43 is the cut-off point above which a person is considered to be vulnerable to stress. Appendix A presents an informative English translation of the items included in the 23-item Stress Vulnerability Scale (23QVS), originally validated in Portuguese. This translation is provided for illustrative purposes only.

Shirom-Melamed Burnout Measure (SMBM) [37]: We used the Portuguese version of the SMBM adapted and translated by Gomes [38] to measure Burnout (B). The scale is composed of 14 items assessing feelings of burnout, such as the following: "When I wake up, I feel no energy to go to work"; "I have trouble concentrating at work"; etc. The 14 items are divided into three subscales as follows: (a) Physical Fatigue (6 items), (b) Cognitive Fatigue (5 items), and (c) Emotional Exhaustion (3 items). Respondents rate each item from "never" (1) to "always" (7), with higher scores corresponding to higher levels of burnout. The instrument has shown good psychometric properties in Portuguese samples [38,39].

2.3. Procedure

Questionnaires were distributed at industry sites, mostly in paper format, to facilitate the participation of workers without computer access. Participation was voluntary, and workers were asked to give informed consent with regard to the use of their data for research purposes. All data were confidential and anonymized. The study was approved by the Institutional Ethical Board Committee and was conducted in accordance with the ethical principles of the Declaration of Helsinki. The questionnaire started with a demographic section, followed by the three measures described above. The workers took approximately 10 min to complete the questionnaire. Data were entered into an Excel spreadsheet and further analyzed using R software (version 4.2.3), R Studio Desktop (version 3.6.1), and the R packages "Lavaan" [40] and "semPlot" [41].

3. Results

3.1. Missing Data

There were, in total, five missing values in our data (only two of which were in the same case). The missing pattern was as follows: one missing value each on the variables Age, Stress Vulnerability, and Burnout; two missing values for the variable Sex. Missingness was therefore quite low. Nevertheless, we used both the default ML estimator and listwise deletion for handling missing data. The results of our prediction models were identical, so we present here the ML model only.

3.2. Descriptive Statistics

The means and standard deviations of the variables (by gender) used in the analysis can be seen in Table 1. There were no significant differences between men and women for the variables PN1 (Portuguese Standard item #1), PN2 (Portuguese Standard item #2), and Stress Vulnerability (SV). Men were significantly older than women (t (114) = 3.18, $p < 0.001$), and women had significantly higher levels of Burnout (B) (t (114) = −4.42, $p < 0.001$). Figure 2 shows the separate histograms for the dependent variable Burnout by gender.

Table 1. Means and standard deviations of the variables age, PN1, PN2, Stress Vulnerability (SV), and Burnout (B).

	Female (n = 53)	Male (n = 64)	Total (n = 119)
	M (SD)	M (SD)	M (SD)
Age	30.6 (11.12)	37.75 (12.78)	34.92 (12.76)
PN1	5.74 (2.31)	5.86 (2.65)	5.76 (2.53)
PN2	5.55 (2.44)	5.53 (2.57)	5.50 (2.53)
SV	2.42 (0.39)	2.35 (0.51)	2.38 (0.45)
B	3.73 (1.19)	2.68 (1.36)	3.18 (1.39)

Note: There were two individuals who did not indicate their gender.

By analyzing Figure 2, the histogram suggests a tendency for lower burnout levels among men, with a higher concentration of scores in the lower range of the scale. In contrast, women's scores appear more evenly distributed, with a noticeable peak around the mid-range values and a greater proportion reporting moderate to high levels of burnout. This visual pattern may indicate gender-related differences in the experience or perception of occupational burnout within the sample.

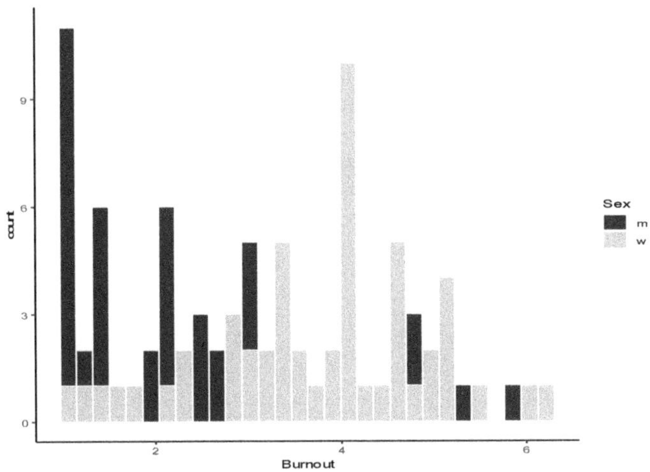

Figure 2. Distribution of burnout scores among male (dark bars) and female (light bars) participants ($n = 116$). Separate histograms are shown by sex to illustrate differences in the frequency of burnout levels.

3.3. Simple Correlation Analyses

Being male was significantly associated with older age and lower levels of Burnout. There was a significant negative correlation between age and Stress Vulnerability, with older individuals being less vulnerable. The same happened for the relation between age and Burnout: the older the individuals, the lower the burnout levels they reported. As expected, the variables PN1 (Portuguese Standard item #1) and PN2 (Portuguese Standard item #2) referring to the perception of occupational noise in the workplace showed significant positive correlations between them, and both were positively and significantly correlated with reported Burnout. Finally Stress Vulnerability was significantly associated with Burnout levels, with more vulnerable individuals reporting higher levels of Burnout. Table 2 shows the correlation matrix between all variables.

Table 2. Correlation matrix for the variable sex, age, PN1, PN2, Stress Vulnerability (SV), and Burnout (B).

	Sex	Age	PN1	PN2	SV	B
Sex	1					
Age	−0.29 **	1				
PN1	−0.03	0.12	1			
PN2	0.003	0.14	0.87 **	1		
SV	0.08	−0.21 *	0.14	0.16	1	
B	0.38 **	−0.18 *	0.24 **	0.29 **	0.40 **	1

* $p < 0.05$, ** $p < 0.01$ Sex: 0 = male; 1 = female.

3.4. Prediction Models

The main estimation models (displayed as path diagrams) are shown in Figure 3. A latent variable PON (Perception of Occupational Noise) was created with the indicators PN1 and PN2, which consider the two questions included in the Portuguese standard for noise perception, as described in the methods section. The variables SV (Stress Vulnerability) and B (Burnout) are manifest variables and correspond to the total scores obtained from the questionnaire measures 23QVS and SMBM, respectively.

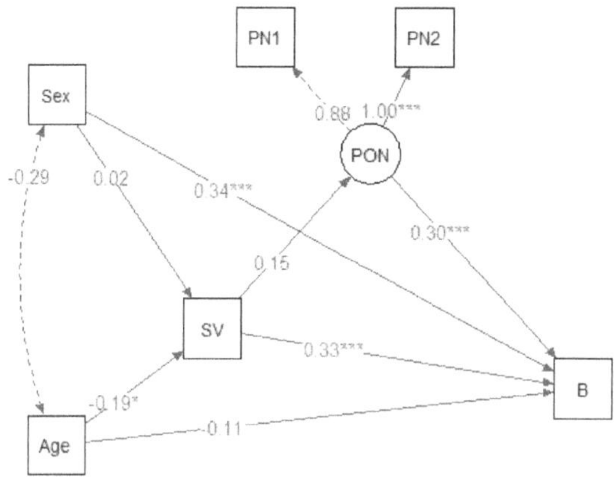

Figure 3. Path model illustrating regressions predicting B (Burnout) from PON (Perception of Occupational Noise) and SV (Stress Vulnerability). Standardized coefficients are depicted (n = 119). Men = 0; Women = 1. * $p < 0.05$; ** $p < 0.01$; *** $p < 0.001$.

Burnout was significantly and directly predicted by gender, Stress Vulnerability, and Perception of Occupational Noise. Being female (B = 0.91, SE = 0.21, $p < 0.001$) and having higher levels of both Stress Vulnerability (B = 1.01, SE = 0.23, $p < 0.001$) and Perception of Occupational Noise (B = 0.19, SE = 0.05, $p < 0.001$) were associated with higher Burnout scores. In addition, age significantly predicted Stress Vulnerability (B = −0.007, SE = 0.003, $p < 0.05$), with older workers showing lower levels on that scale.

4. Discussion

This exploratory study investigated the predicting role of the perception of occupational noise and stress vulnerability on burnout levels in a sample of Portuguese industrial workers. We have also investigated the moderating role of the variables age and gender. The results of the path analysis model revealed that being female, having higher levels of stress vulnerability, and greater levels of perceived occupational noise were significantly associated with increased burnout symptoms. The positive association between perceived occupational noise and burnout is consistent with previous research showing that noisy environments can impair concentration, disrupt communication, and lead to both physiological arousal and psychological strain [42]. These stress responses, if sustained over time, can contribute to emotional exhaustion and other components of burnout. While noise exposure has been more commonly studied in relation to auditory outcomes, our findings emphasize its broader psychosocial impact. The results align with studies in both educational [16] and industrial settings [43], where subjective noise perception was linked to irritation, fatigue, and stress-related outcomes. Stress vulnerability also emerged as a robust predictor of burnout, reinforcing the hypothesis that dispositional factors significantly influence how individuals respond to occupational stressors. As previously suggested [44], individuals with higher vulnerability may lack adequate coping strategies, making them more susceptible to emotional exhaustion and reduced psychological resilience in demanding work environments. This finding supports models of stress–burnout relationships that integrate both environmental and personal dimensions [22]. An interesting and theoretically grounded result concerns the inverse relationship between age and stress vulnerability. Older workers reported significantly lower vulnerability, which is consistent with the Strength and Vulnerability Integration (SAVI) model [45]. According to this framework, aging is associated with improved emotion regulation and more adaptive coping, which may buffer against the effects of chronic stressors in the workplace.

Gender differences in burnout were also observed, with women reporting significantly higher levels of burnout than men. This finding echoes the previous literature attributing higher burnout risk in women to increased emotional labor demands [46], work–family role conflict [47], and systemic gender-based inequities in the workplace [48]. It is also plausible that task assignment, support structures, and reporting patterns differ by gender, especially in male-dominated industrial contexts. Further studies should consider a more granular analysis of job roles, psychosocial hazards, and coping resources by gender. Taken together, these findings support a biopsychosocial model of occupational burnout, where both external stressors (e.g., noise exposure) and individual traits (e.g., stress vulnerability) interact to shape mental health outcomes. Importantly, this study highlights the relevance of subjective perception—how workers interpret and internalize environmental demands—as a key factor in understanding burnout.

5. Conclusions

To our knowledge, this is the first study on the role of noise perception and vulnerability to stress as predictors of burnout in an industrial environment. In these environments, occupational health and safety professionals are typically more focused on preventing professional hearing loss than on non-auditory effects, such as burnout. The assessment and prevention of non-auditory disorders, which can occur at exposure levels much lower than the recommended maximum levels for hearing loss prevention, represent a step forward in relation to the classic assessment of noise exposure at the workplace, typically focused on preventing hearing damage. The integration of occupational health psychologists in multidisciplinary teams could provide a valuable contribution to designing interventions against the detrimental psychological effects of noise exposure, namely, by focusing on coping mechanisms and stress management skills. While our exploratory study provides valuable insights that can guide future studies, it is essential to acknowledge some limitations. First, the cross-sectional design limits causal inferences. Future research should employ longitudinal designs to examine the temporal relations among these variables. Second, this study employed the self-report method, which is vulnerable to participants' reporting style, motivation, and social desirability. Third, our study focused on a specific population of industrial workers and a relatively small sample. Replicating these findings in other occupational settings would strengthen the generalizability of our results. Future studies on noise exposure (including objective measurements or eventually scales validated to quantify noise exposure) and other environmental factors, such as lightening, thermal environment, indoor air quality, and other variables, such as job demands, job control, and social support, could provide a more comprehensive understanding of burnout. In summary, this study highlights the importance of considering both environmental perceptions and psychological traits in understanding burnout among industrial workers. Perceived occupational noise and stress vulnerability emerged as significant predictors of burnout, reinforcing the need for integrated workplace interventions. These should include not only physical noise control measures, but also psychosocial support strategies tailored to individual profiles.

Author Contributions: Formal analysis, L.A.R., C.C. and C.C.P.; investigation, L.A.R. and C.C.P.; resources, L.A.R. and C.C.P.; data curation, L.A.R.; writing—original draft preparation, C.C.; writing—review and editing, C.C., L.A.R. and C.C.P. All authors have read and agreed to the published version of the manuscript.

Funding: This research received no external funding.

Institutional Review Board Statement: The study was conducted in accordance with the Declaration of Helsinki, authorized by the National Data Protection Commission (CNPD) (protocol no.7087/2028,

24 May 2018) and approved by the Ethics Committee for Health of National Institute of Health (CES-INSA) (18 June 2019).

Informed Consent Statement: Informed consent was obtained from all subjects involved in the study.

Data Availability Statement: The original contributions presented in this study are included in the article. Further inquiries can be directed to the corresponding author.

Acknowledgments: We would like to thank Adélia Monarca for her support in establishing contact with the industrial settings where the study took place and the students Joana Batista and Sara Reis for their collaboration in data collection.

Conflicts of Interest: The authors declare no conflicts of interest.

Appendix A

English translation of the Stress Vulnerability Scale (23QVS).

1. I am a determined person when it comes to solving my problems
2. I have difficulty relating to unfamiliar people
3. When I have problems that bother me, I can count on one or more friends who serve as confidents
4. I usually have enough money to meet my personal needs
5. I worry easily about everyday setbacks
6. When I have a problem to solve, I usually find someone who can help me
7. I regularly give and receive affection
8. It is rare for me to be overwhelmed by unpleasant events that happen to me
9. When faced with daily difficulties, I tend to complain more than make an effort to solve them
10. I am the kind of person who gets easily upset
11. In most cases, the solutions to the important problems in my life do not depend on me
12. When I am criticized, I tend to feel guilty
13. People only pay attention to me when they need something for their own benefit
14. I spend more time responding to other people's demands than attending to my own needs
15. I prefer to stay quiet rather than contradict someone, even when they are wrong
16. I get nervous and annoyed when I do not perform as well as I expected
17. There are unpleasant aspects of myself that cause others to distance themselves
18. At the right moments, I find it difficult to express what I truly feel
19. I get nervous and upset if I don't get what I want immediately
20. I am the kind of person who, due to my sense of humor, can laugh about unpleasant events that happen to me
21. The money I have barely covers my essential expenses
22. When faced with life's problems, I am more likely to run away than to fight
23. I feel bad when I am not perfect in what I do

References

1. Chaharaghran, F.; Tabatabaei, S.; Rostamzadeh, S. The impact of noise exposure and work posture on job stress in a food company. *Work* **2022**, *73*, 1227–1234. [CrossRef] [PubMed]
2. Heinonen-Guzejev, M.; Whipp, A.M.; Wang, Z.; Ranjit, A.; Palviainen, T.; van Kamp, I.; Kaprio, J. Perceived Occupational Noise Exposure and Depression in Young Finnish Adults. *Int. J. Environ. Res. Public Health* **2023**, *20*, 4850. [CrossRef] [PubMed]
3. Lu, Y.; Zhang, Z.; Yan, H.; Rui, B.; Liu, J. Effects of Occupational Hazards on Job Stress and Mental Health of Factory Workers and Miners: A Propensity Score Analysis. *BioMed Res. Int.* **2020**, *2020*, 1754897. [CrossRef] [PubMed]
4. Aminian, O.; Saraie, M.; Ahadi, M.; Eftekhari, S. Association of the working environment noise with occupational stress in industrial workers. *J. Public Health* **2023**, *31*, 979–984. [CrossRef]

5. Babisch, W. The noise/stress concept, risk assessment and research needs. *Noise Health* **2002**, *4*, 1–11. Available online: http://www.noiseandhealth.org/article.asp?issn=1463-1741;year=2002;volume=4;issue=16;spage=1;epage=11;aulast=Babisch (accessed on 29 June 2023).
6. Basner, M.; Babisch, W.; Davis, A.; Brink, M.; Clark, C.; Janssen, S.; Stansfeld, S. Auditory and non-auditory effects of noise on health. *Lancet* **2014**, *383*, 1325–1332. [CrossRef]
7. Münzel, T.; Sørensen, M.; Schmidt, F.; Schmidt, E.; Steven, S.; Kröller-Schön, S.; Daiber, A. The Adverse Effects of Environmental Noise Exposure on Oxidative Stress and Cardiovascular Risk. *Antioxid. Redox Signal.* **2018**, *28*, 873–908. [CrossRef]
8. Babisch, W. Cardiovascular effects of noise. *Noise Health* **2011**, *13*, 201–204. [CrossRef]
9. Luzzi, S.; Vasilyev, A.V. Auditory and non-auditory effects, monitoring and mapping of occupational exposure to noise. *Noise Mapp.* **2022**, *9*, 146–156. [CrossRef]
10. Carvalhais, C.; Rodrigues, C.; Xavier, A.; Silva, M.V.; Santos, J. The impact of structural changes on sound pressure levels in a neonatal intensive care unit. *Arch. Acoust.* **2021**, *46*, 435–442. [CrossRef]
11. Santos, J.; Carvalhais, C.; Xavier, A.; Silva, M.V. Assessment and characterization of sound pressure levels in Portuguese neonatal intensive care units. *Arch. Environ. Occup. Health* **2018**, *73*, 121–127. [CrossRef] [PubMed]
12. Behzad Fouladi, D.; Nassiri, P.; Mohammadreza Monazzam, E.; Farahani, S.; Hassanzadeh, G.; Hoseini, M. Industrial noise exposure and salivary cortisol in blue collar industrial workers. *Noise Health* **2012**, *14*, 184–189. [CrossRef]
13. Dzhambov, A.; Tilov, B.; Makakova-Tilova, D.; DImitrova, D. Pathways and contingencies linking road traffic noise to annoyance, noise sensitivity, and mental ill-health. *Noise Health* **2019**, *21*, 248–257. [CrossRef] [PubMed]
14. Kivimäki, M.; Kawachi, I. Work Stress as a Risk Factor for Cardiovascular Disease. *Curr. Cardiol. Rep.* **2015**, *17*, 74. [CrossRef]
15. Oenning, N.S.X.; Ziegelmann, P.K.; Goulart, B.N.G.; Niedhammer, I. Occupational factors associated with major depressive disorder: A Brazilian population-based study. *J. Affect. Disord.* **2018**, *240*, 48–56. [CrossRef]
16. Sjödin, F.; Kjellberg, A.; Knutsson, A.; Landström, U.; Lindberg, L. Noise and stress effects on preschool personnel. *Noise Health* **2012**, *14*, 166–178. [CrossRef]
17. Tennant, C. Work-related stress and depressive disorders. *J. Psychosom. Res.* **2001**, *51*, 697–704. [CrossRef]
18. Monteiro, A.A.; Vaz-Serra, A. 2661—Psychometric properties of the Russian version of the stress vulnerability questionnaire—23QVS (Serra, 2000), in a sample of 556 Russian-speaking immigrants in Portugal. *Eur. Psychiatry* **2013**, *28*, 1. [CrossRef]
19. Ingram, R.E.; Luxton, D.D. Vulnerability-stress models. In *Development of Psychopathology: A Vulnerability-Stress Perspective*; Sage Publications, Inc.: Thousand Oaks, CA, USA, 2018. [CrossRef]
20. Orgambídez-Ramos, A.; Borrego-Alés, Y.; Ruiz-Frutos, C. Empowerment, vulnerabilidad al estrés y burnout en enfermeros portugueses. *Cienc. Saude Colet.* **2018**, *23*, 259–266. [CrossRef]
21. James, K.A.; Stromin, J.I.; Steenkamp, N.; Combrinck, M.I. Understanding the relationships between physiological and psychosocial stress, cortisol and cognition. *Front. Endocrinol.* **2023**, *14*, 1085950. [CrossRef]
22. Hahad, O.; Prochaska, J.H.; Daiber, A.; Muenzel, T. Environmental Noise-Induced Effects on Stress Hormones, Oxidative Stress, and Vascular Dysfunction: Key Factors in the Relationship between Cerebrocardiovascular and Psychological Disorders. *Oxid. Med. Cell. Longev.* **2019**, *2019*, 4623109. [CrossRef] [PubMed]
23. Goines, L.; Hagler, L. Noise pollution and public health: A critical review. *Environ. Health Perspect.* **2019**, *127*, 950–956. [CrossRef]
24. Kirkbride, J.B.; Anglin, D.M.; Colman, I.; Dykxhoorn, J.; Jones, P.B.; Patalay, P.; Pitman, A.; Soneson, E.; Steare, T.; Wright, T.; et al. The social determinants of mental health and disorder: Evidence, prevention and recommendations. *World Psychiatry* **2024**, *23*, 58–90. [CrossRef] [PubMed]
25. Basner, M.; McGuire, S. WHO Environmental Noise Guidelines for the European Region: A systematic review on environmental noise and effects on sleep. *Int. J. Environ. Res. Public Health* **2018**, *15*, 519. [CrossRef]
26. Ising, H.; Kruppa, B. Health effects caused by noise: Evidence in the literature from the past 25 years. *Noise Health* **2003**, *6*, 5–13. Available online: https://journals.lww.com/nohe/fulltext/2004/06220/health_effects_caused_by_noise__evidence_in_the.3.aspx (accessed on 29 June 2023).
27. Jafari, M.J.; Khosrowabadi, R.; Khodakarim, S.; Mohammadian, F. The Effect of Noise Exposure on Cognitive Performance and Brain Activity Patterns. *Open Access Maced J. Med. Sci.* **2019**, *7*, 2924–2931. [CrossRef]
28. Hespanhol, A. Burnout e Stress ocupacional. *Rev. Port. Picossomática* **2005**, *7*, 153–162.
29. Maslach, C.; Leiter, M.P. Understanding the burnout experience: Recent research and its implications for psychiatry. *World Psychiatry* **2016**, *15*, 103–111. [CrossRef]
30. Bakker, A.B.; Demerouti, E.; Sanz-Vergel, A.I. Burnout and Work Engagement: The JDR Approach. *Annu. Rev. Organ. Psychol. Organ. Behav.* **2014**, *1*, 389–411. [CrossRef]
31. Gabriel, K.P.; Aguinis, H. How to prevent and combat employee burnout and create healthier workplaces during crises and beyond. *Bus. Horiz.* **2022**, *65*, 183–192. [CrossRef]
32. Li, X.; Jiang, T.; Sun, J.; Shi, L.; Liu, J. The relationship between occupational stress, job burnout and quality of life among surgical nurses in Xinjiang, China. *BMC Nurs.* **2021**, *20*, 181. [CrossRef] [PubMed]

33. Abbasi, M.; Yazdanirad, S.; Habibi, P.; Arabi, S.; Fallah Madvari, R.; Mehri, A.; Poursadeghiyan, M.; Ebrahimi, M.H.; Ghaljahi, M. Relationship among noise exposure, sensitivity, and noise annoyance with job satisfaction and job stress in a textile industry. *Noise Vib. Worldw.* **2019**, *50*, 195–201. [CrossRef]
34. *ISO/TS 15666:2021*; Acoustics—Assessment of Noise Annoyance by Means of Social and Socio-Acoustic Surveys. International Organization for Standardization: Geneva, Switzerland, 2021.
35. *NP 4476 2008*; Avaliação da Incomodidade Devida ao Ruído por Meio de Inquéritos Sociais e Sócio-Acústicos. Instituto Português da Qualidade: Lisboa, Portugal, 2008.
36. Vaz Serra, A. Construção de uma escala para avaliar a vulnerabilidade ao stress: A 23 QVS. *Psiquiatr. Clín.* **2000**, *21*, 279–308.
37. Shirom, A.; Melamed, S. A comparison of the construct validity of two burnout measures in two groups of professionals. *Int. J. Stress Manag.* **2006**, *13*, 176–200. [CrossRef]
38. Gomes, A.R. *Medida de "Burnout" de Shirom-Melamed (MBSM)*; Relatório técnico não publicado; Escola de Psicologia, Universidade do Minho: Braga, Portugal, 2006. Available online: http://repositorium.sdum.uminho.pt/bitstream/1822/87555/4/2-MBSM-SMBM-Medida%20Burnout-Burnout%20Measure-Shirom-Melamed.pdf (accessed on 14 January 2023).
39. Reisa, S.B.; Gomes, A.R.; Simães, C. Stress e burnout em professores: Importância dos processos de avaliação cognitiva. *Psicol. Saúde Doenças* **2018**, *19*, 208–221.
40. Rosseel, Y. Lavaan: An R package for structural equation modeling. *J. Stat. Softw.* **2012**, *48*, 1–36. [CrossRef]
41. Epskamp, S. SemPlot: Path Diagrams and Visual Analysis of Various SEM Packages' Output, Version 1.1.6. 2022. Available online: https://CRAN.R-project.org/package=semPlot (accessed on 19 June 2023).
42. Stansfeld, S.A.; Matheson, M.P. Noise pollution: Non-auditory effects on health. *Br. Med. Bull.* **2003**, *68*, 243–257. [CrossRef]
43. Madvari, R.F.; Bidel, H.; Mehri, A.; Babaee, F.; Laal, F. Analysis of the relationships between noise exposure and stress/arousal mood at different levels of workload. *Sound Vib.* **2024**, *58*, 119–131. [CrossRef]
44. Maslach, C.; Schaufeli, W.B.; Leiter, M.P. Job burnout. *Annu. Rev. Psychol.* **2001**, *52*, 397–422. [CrossRef]
45. Charles, S.T.; Carstensen, L.L. Social and emotional aging. *Annu. Rev. Psychol.* **2010**, *61*, 383–409. [CrossRef]
46. Grzywacz, J.G.; Marks, N.F. Reconceptualizing the work-family interface: An ecological perspective on the correlates of positive and negative spillover between work and family. *J. Occup. Health Psychol.* **2000**, *5*, 111–126. [CrossRef] [PubMed]
47. Wharton, A.S. The sociology of emotional labor. *Annu. Rev. Sociol.* **2009**, *35*, 147–165. [CrossRef]
48. Berdahl, J.L.; Moore, C. Workplace harassment: Double jeopardy for minority women. *J. Appl. Psychol.* **2006**, *91*, 426–436. [CrossRef]

environments

MDPI

Article

Worker Safety in High-Field NMR Spectroscopy Laboratories: Challenges and Risk Assessment

Alessandra Flori [1], Giuseppe Acri [2,*], Maria Antonietta D'Avanzo [3], Massimo Mattozzi [3] and Valentina Hartwig [4,*]

1 Bioengineering Unit, Fondazione Toscana G. Monasterio, Via G. Moruzzi 1, 56124 Pisa, Italy; alessandra.flori@ftgm.it
2 Department of Biomedical, Dental, and Image Sciences, University of Messina, Via Consolare Valeria, 98125 Messina, Italy
3 Department of Occupational and Environmental Medicine, INAIL, Via Fontana Candida 1, 00078 Rome, Italy; m.davanzo@inail.it (M.A.D.); m.mattozzi@inail.it (M.M.)
4 Institute of Clinical Physiology, CNR, Via G. Moruzzi 1, 56100 Pisa, Italy
* Correspondence: giuseppe.acri@unime.it (G.A.); valentina.hartwig@cnr.it (V.H.)

Abstract: Magnetic Resonance (MR) technology is extensively used in academic and industrial research laboratories and represents one of the most significant methodologies in clinical radiology. Although MR does not use ionizing radiation, it cannot be considered risk-free due to the strong static magnetic fields and time-varying electromagnetic fields employed in the technology. To mitigate risks for MR operators, the European Community and ICNIRP have established safety limits based on the existing literature, primarily related to diagnostic MR. However, the literature on occupational exposure in non-clinical nuclear magnetic resonance (NMR) spectroscopy is limited. Due to their specificity, non-medical NMR environments present unique challenges from the point of view of operator exposure. NMR spectrometers are characterized by extremely high static magnetic fields, reaching up to 28 T in commercial systems; moreover, routine activities performed near the magnet, where field gradients are highest, increase operator exposure. Such environments are not typically perceived as hazardous and are frequented by various types of personnel, often without specific training. This study aims to highlight the critical issues in managing a preclinical MR laboratory equipped with a high-field NMR spectrometer, discussing operator safety challenges and presenting risk assessment data.

Keywords: nuclear magnetic resonance spectroscopy; NMR; occupational exposure; risk assessment

1. Introduction

Before its widespread adoption in medicine as a diagnostic technique, magnetic resonance (MR) was predominantly used in fundamental laboratory research, food quality assessment, and molecular studies through nuclear magnetic resonance (NMR) spectroscopy. NMR spectroscopy provides a comprehensive understanding of molecular structure, dynamics, reaction states, and chemical environments [1–3]. Concurrently, there has been a rapid proliferation of high-field magnetic resonance imaging (MRI) scanners in research settings (both academic and non-academic), particularly for preclinical studies involving animal models, especially rodents [4].

Diagnostic MRI and NMR spectrometers share the same operating principles, involving three phases: the polarization of nuclear spins in a static magnetic field (B0); the

https://doi.org/10.3390/environments12040113

excitation of the sample with a radiofrequency (RF) magnetic field (B1) at the Larmor frequency; and the application of spatial magnetic field gradients for spin localization. NMR spectrometers generate extremely high magnetic fields (up to 28 T), which are typically well-confined near the instrument. Some risks associated with MR devices are documented in the literature and should not be underestimated, especially given the rapid development and dissemination of the technology [5,6].

In magnetic resonance environments, the primary exposure risks for workers stem from both static and spatially heterogeneous magnetic fields, as well as, in some cases, radiofrequency (RF) fields. Workers who move in close proximity to the magnet are additionally exposed to time-varying magnetic fields, which can induce electric currents within the body. If these currents reach sufficient strength, they may interact with the central nervous system (CNS), potentially leading to neurological effects, and can also stimulate peripheral nerves, causing sensations such as tingling or muscle contractions.

Recent research has documented various transient symptoms experienced by workers due to movement within these magnetic fields, including dizziness, nausea, visual disturbances, and a sensation of vertigo [7–12].

Recent studies have explored the neural impact of static magnetic fields and dynamic magnetic fields using animal models. Research on the influence of magnetic fields on cognitive functions such as learning and memory, as well as emotional behaviour, neuronal activity, and neurotransmitter dynamics, is steadily growing. However, due to variations in magnetic field parameters, experimental models, and study conditions, findings remain inconsistent [13,14].

As magnetic resonance technology advances and field strengths increase, further investigation into occupational safety measures and exposure limits is essential to mitigate potential health risks for personnel working in these environments.

To address these concerns, the European Union (EU) and the International Commission on Non-Ionizing Radiation Protection (ICNIRP) have established limits for the exposure of workers to the risks arising from physical agents (electromagnetic fields, EMF) [15–18]. Several studies evaluate health risks for workers in MR diagnostic environments [19–23]. Worker exposure to static magnetic fields and movements in fringe fields has been assessed and discussed for MRI scanners with field strengths from 0.25 T to 3.0 T [22,24–28].

However, there is limited research on occupational risk assessment for workers in NMR spectroscopy and, more broadly, in non-clinical magnetic resonance environments, such as preclinical or fundamental research laboratories. NMR spectrometers, operating at up to 28 T @ 1.2 GHz, are commonly found in universities and research centres. These instruments are also used by doctoral students and research fellows who are considered scientific users rather than workers. Although they may be proficient in the scientific applications of the technique, they often lack awareness of safety aspects and may mistakenly perceive NMR spectrometers as low-risk devices. In this context, it is crucial to educate workers on appropriate behaviour and movement control to prevent adverse events.

Given the nature of NMR equipment and considering that some operational tasks involve direct interaction with the devices, it is presumed that researchers working in spectrometry laboratories may experience daily exposure to relatively high levels of magnetic fields and/or EMF. However, these exposure levels and conditions have not yet been thoroughly analysed and require evaluation through targeted on-site measurements.

This study highlights the challenges of high-field NMR spectroscopy laboratories regarding magnetic field exposure and discusses risk assessment aspects for operators. Particular attention is given to workers at particular risk, such as operators with active implantable medical devices (AIMDs), a sensitive risk group requiring protection from electromagnetic field interference.

2. Materials and Methods

2.1. High-Field NMR Spectroscopy Laboratory

An NMR spectrometer (Bruker, Billerica, Massachusetts the manufacturer, city, and country) comprises a superconducting coil immersed in a liquid helium jacket surrounded by a liquid nitrogen jacket. At the centre of the spectrometer is an empty cylinder, known as the gantry, where the static magnetic field is generated. This bore accommodates the probe, a cylindrical container that holds the sample to be analysed. Depending on the experiment, different probes are used, which may be nucleus-specific or multinuclear, with variations in internal coil design determining specificity. Sample insertion operations are typically performed at the top of the equipment, accessible via ladders, or near the base of the magnet, requiring operators to crouch near the magnet.

A high-field NMR spectroscopy laboratory is a specialized environment housing the NMR spectrometer and essential components for its operation, including the cryogenic cooling system for the superconducting magnet with liquid helium and nitrogen tanks and the refilling system, the console and electronic components, and safety systems such as ventilation systems, quench piping, and oxygen sensors. Additional auxiliary systems (e.g., sample containers, ladders, and sample insertion/removal structures) and at least one workstation are typically present.

The NMR spectroscopy laboratories can house spectrometers of various generations. Older installations, with lower magnetic fields, often neglect manufacturer safety recommendations. For example, older NMR equipment typically lacks safety systems found in modern superconducting magnets used in medical imaging, such as quench piping to direct helium outside the laboratory, auxiliary safety devices (e.g., oxygen sensors), or ventilation systems to expel helium gas released within the laboratory during a quench event. Conversely, newer spectrometers, operating at higher fields and frequencies (up to 1200 MHz), necessitate advanced safety systems like cryogenic gas evacuation pipes and oxygen monitoring sensors. As a case in point, new-generation solid-state NMR spectrometers utilize ultra-high field pulses and decoupling power [29]. This may result in potential hazards relative to high-power RF fields, which may interfere with electronics and sensors within the NMR environment. It is imperative to ensure adequate RF shielding to prevent unintended exposure and to position sensitive equipment safely outside of high-field and high-RF zones. Manufacturers of modern equipment include detailed safety system guidelines in instruction manuals, outlining risk assessments and management strategies, which, if implemented, represent a significant safety improvement.

2.2. Potential Hazards and Specific Critical Points

In the context of NMR applications, it is hypothesized that workers may be exposed on a daily basis to relatively high levels of magnetic and/or RF fields. The primary source of exposure is the static magnetic field; as reported by Berlana and Ubeda [30], no detectable emissions of RF field were found in the surrounding environment, indicating that the electromagnetic radiation generated by the NMR remained confined within the devices. The potential hazards associated with magnetic fields can be classified as either direct or indirect. Direct risks manifest in the human body through biological effects, which can be sensory or health-related. Indirect risks are associated with magnetic fields, such as the projectile effect (attraction of ferromagnetic materials), a significant torque applied to objects, and potential interference with implanted medical devices.

In contrast to clinical MRI sites, the primary users of the NMR equipment consist of students, postgraduates, scholarship holders, and contract workers. These individuals do not qualify as employees but rather as scientific users, sometimes even occasional, often highly competent in the scientific application of technology but generally not very sensitive to safety aspects because they are unaware of the associated risks, having most often not been properly trained and made aware of these important aspects. Those with a greater familiarity with the operational situation may erroneously assume that the utilization of NMR spectrometers in the present context entails reduced exposure for operators. For example, the sample loading typically occurs over a significantly shorter time interval compared to other MRI applications. However, in the majority of cases, this process is carried out by approaching the instrument, either at the top or by crouching down with the arms positioned underneath the structure and the head placed very close to the instrument. Moreover, it should be noted that for NMR investigations, an additional level of exposure exists that is not present in other cases and is related to the tuning and matching procedure. This procedure must be performed for each type of sample introduced unless the analysis is repeated on the same types of samples. This underscores the significance of the dwell time at high levels of static magnetic field as a crucial factor in ensuring protection.

The NMR laboratory is typically a single room where the highest-risk exposure area (near the magnet) is easily accessible and not always marked with appropriate signage (such as the 5 Gauss line).

This also means that, in many NMR laboratories, the operators' workstation, the equipment controls area, and sometimes the chemical laboratory where the samples are prepared are situated within the same room as the NMR spectrometer or in close proximity. This configuration necessitates a comprehensive and detailed investigation into safety concerns.

2.3. *Regulatory Framework and Current Challenges*

Currently, there is a notable lack of a specific regulatory framework for NMR spectroscopy environments, resulting in limited awareness of safety requirements. In Europe, the primary regulatory reference is the Directive 2013/35/EU, which addresses worker exposure to electromagnetic fields, focusing on short-term effects while excluding long-term effects due to insufficient scientific evidence.

For general population protection, exposure limits are established by the European Recommendation 1999/519/EC, which sets a threshold of 40 mT for potential human risk (excluding indirect effects) [31].

According to current regulations, static magnetic fields are significant for operators when exposure exceeds 2 Tesla for sensory effects (transient sensory perception disturbances, nausea, vomiting, dizziness, and minor changes in brain functions) and 8 Tesla for health effects (thermal heating and/or the stimulation of nervous or muscular tissue).

It is important to note that these limits do not apply to individuals with specific contraindications to magnetic field exposure (e.g., wearers of active implantable devices), for whom the established threshold is significantly lower, at 0.5 mT (5 Gauss). With regard to passive implanted devices, current regulations do not set action values; therefore, an assessment must be conducted on a case-by-case basis. However, with regard to the projectile effect, European Recommendation 1999/519/EC establishes an action level of 3 mT (3 Gauss) [31].

In most NMR installations, the limits for direct effects—2 T for the body and 8 T for the limbs—remain confined within the equipment; consequently, workers are not directly exposed. Additionally, there are no exposures related to the radio frequencies emitted during the operation of the NMR. However, the 0.5 mT limit is probably exceeded in the vicinity of the NMR device. According to regulations, a colour-coded floor marking delineates the magnetic induction dispersion field, as outlined below:

Red/white line for 0.5 mT;
Yellow line for 0.4 mT;
Green line for 0.3 mT.

The 0.5 mT limit can only be exceeded by authorized personnel, who are trained, informed, and certified as fit for the specific task by the occupational physicians.

The ICNIRP guidelines published in 2014 provide recommendations for limiting exposure to static magnetic fields and time-varying magnetic fields below 1 Hz [18]. The primary objective of these guidelines is to prevent peripheral nerve stimulation (PNS) and reduce the likelihood of transient sensory effects caused by electric fields induced in the human body due to movements within spatially heterogeneous static magnetic fields. These effects can include sensations such as tingling, dizziness, or even muscle contractions, which may pose safety concerns in occupational and clinical settings. To ensure controlled exposure conditions, the ICNIRP has established specific safety thresholds. According to ICNIRP guidelines, a basic restriction is set at 1.1 V/m for peak-induced electric fields within the body. Additionally, a reference level of 2.7 T/s is defined for the time derivative of magnetic flux density (dB/dt), aiming to limit excessive exposure to rapidly changing magnetic fields that could exacerbate neuromuscular stimulation. These guidelines serve as an essential framework for safeguarding individuals working in or exposed to strong magnetic environments, such as those found in MRI facilities [18]. The basic restriction and reference levels for uncontrolled exposures (protection against magnetophosphenes and peripheral nerve stimulation) change as a function of 1/f (up to 0.66 Hz), where f is the frequency of motion-induced fields.

2.4. *Risk Assessment Procedure*

A correct risk assessment, linked to the presence of the static magnetic field in the NMR environment, must necessarily consider the construction characteristics of the equipment and the dispersion of the field around it in order to identify the areas of risk, the attention levels to be kept, and the operating procedures to be followed to minimize exposure and the possibility of the occurrence of risk scenarios. First of all, the 0.5 mT line should be identified to delineate the area restricted for unauthorized access, which is to be made accessible exclusively to authorized personnel (listed in a dedicated register). This is initiated by the precise measurement of the fringe field surrounding the NMR spectrometer.

Then, regarding the occupational exposure to time-varying magnetic fields, an estimation of the reference parameters should be conducted. In this evaluation, worker exposure is assessed as part of a comprehensive risk analysis, focusing on the induced electric field ($|E|$) and the time derivative of the magnetic flux density ($|dB/dt|$) to establish safe operating procedures. Special attention is devoted to individuals with active implantable medical devices (AIMDs), who represent a particularly vulnerable group requiring stringent protection from the risks associated with electromagnetic field interference [32].

We present here the risk assessment for a research NMR laboratory including a 7T (@300 MHz) spectrometer. First of all, the static magnetic field was mapped by positioning a three-axis Hall magnetometer (THM 1176, Metrolab Instruments SA, Plan-les-Ouates, Switzerland) at five different heights above the ground plane (z = 0 cm, 40 cm, 80 cm, 120 cm, and 160 cm). Measurements were taken along a predefined theoretical path extending from the console to the spectrometer and back, with a spatial resolution of 10 cm, as previously described in [27]. Based on these measurements, the fringe field distribution in the vertical (xz) plane was determined. Subsequently, the magnitude of the induced electric field $|E|$ was calculated for a trajectory representative of a worker's movement during routine sample processing operations. This calculation was performed using the analytical model outlined in the ICNIRP guidelines, allowing for an assessment of potential exposure risks associated with workplace activities in the presence of spatially varying magnetic fields [18]. By way of example, we considered the typical movement of an operator who, starting from a standing position, kneels down next to the NMR spectrometer (Figure 1a). The movement speed was set at 1 m/s along the entire movement [33]. Furthermore, a 90° torso flexion was also considered, with a maximum velocity of 4 rad/s (Figure 1b). For both of these movements, a point on the head (shown in Figure 1 as a red point) and a point on the torso corresponding to the heart (shown in Figure 1 as a black star), were designated as the reference points.

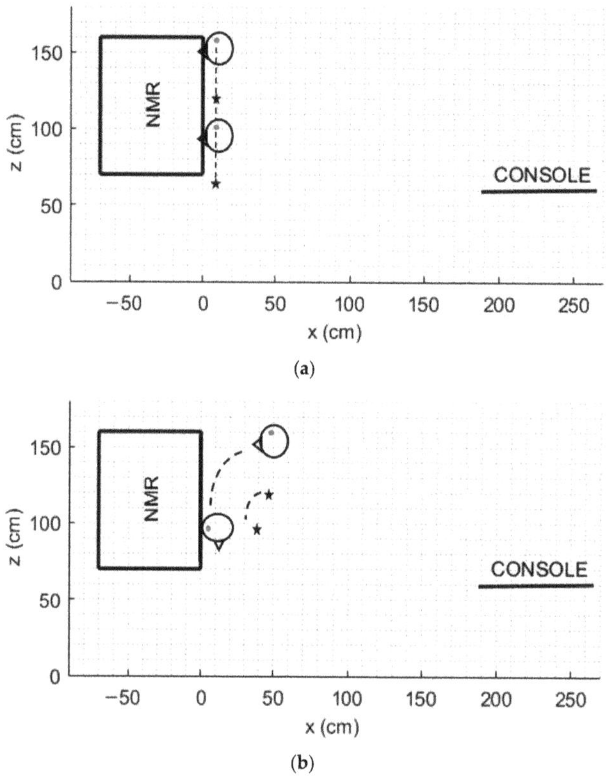

Figure 1. Schematization of the considered movements in the fringe field of a 7T NMR spectrometer: (**a**) linear movement along the z axis, (**b**) flexion movement of 90°. Red point: head reference point. Black star: torso reference point.

Finally, for both of the considered movements, we also calculated the maximum induced voltage (electromotive force, EMF) in an active device implanted in the torso (such as a pacemaker) by simplifying the Faraday–Neumann–Lenz law as reported in [32].

3. Results

Figure 2 shows the map of the fringe field on an xz plane $|B|_{xz}$ through the isocentre of the NMR spectrometer described previously, with the indication of the 0.5 mT line (dashed red line). Moreover, Figure 2 also shows the vector representation of the two-dimensional spatial gradient of the magnetic field $|B|_{xz}$ together with the contour plot of $|B|_{xz}$ around the NMR spectrometer.

For the considered xz plane, the maximum value of $|B|$ is 18.08 mT, the maximum value of $|dB/dx|$ is 58.8 mT/m, and the maximum value of $|dB/dz|$ is 19.35 mT/m.

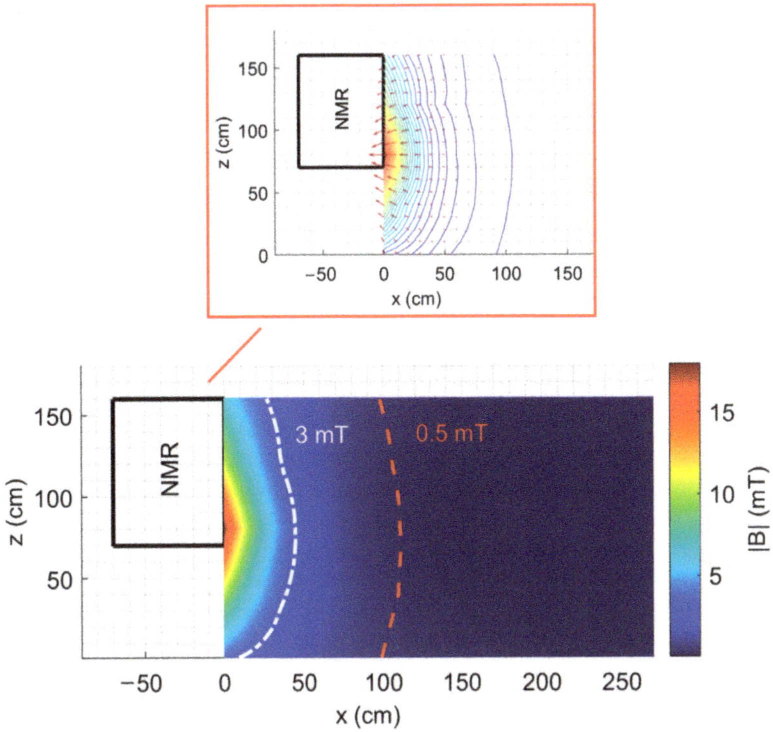

Figure 2. Map of the fringe field |B|xz with the indication of the 0.5 mT line and the representation of the two-dimensional spatial gradient around a 7 T NMR spectrometer.

Tables 1 and 2 present the peak values of the estimated parameters for the risk assessment relative to the linear movement along the z-axis and the flexion movement of 90°, considering the head and the thorax–heart reference points.

Table 1. Peak values of the estimated parameter for the risk assessment of a 7T NMR spectrometer: linear movement along the z-axis.

Linear Movement Along z Axis @v = 1 m/s	$\lvert B \rvert_{max}$ (mT)	$\lvert dB/dt \rvert_{max}$ (mT/s)	$\lvert E \rvert_{max}$ (mV/m)	EMF_{max} (mV)
Head	14.59	32.14	1.45	-
Thorax–Heart	18.00	32.93	5.27	0.74

Table 2. Estimated parameter for the risk assessment of a 7T NMR spectrometer: flexion movement of 90°.

Flexion Movement @90°, v = 4 rad/s	$\lvert B \rvert_{max}$ (mT)	$\lvert dB/dt \rvert_{max}$ (mT/s)	$\lvert E \rvert_{max}$ (mV/m)	EMF_{max} (mV)
Head	16.11	66.80	3.01	-
Thorax–Heart	7.48	17.88	2.86	0.40

4. Discussion

The occupational exposure literature in non-diagnostic NMR environments is currently sparse [30,34,35], particularly compared to the characterization of exposures for healthcare personnel working with MRI scanners [5,7,26,36–39]. However, well-established physical mechanisms describe interactions between electromagnetic fields and living tissues, responsible for acute and transient effects above exposure thresholds, leading to the establishment of exposure limits. For example, translational and rotational movements of operators within magnetic fields are the focus of numerous studies on occupational exposures in medical MRI environments, yielding insights into induced body currents and their effects on humans [7,40–43].

A classical NMR spectrometer generates a strong magnetic field that extends beyond the magnet itself, thereby creating a significant stray magnetic field around the instrument. This has the potential to interfere with nearby electronic devices and necessitates a dedicated, controlled environment to prevent unwanted interactions. The majority of new ultra-high field instruments (above 500 MHz) are ultra-shielded, with the design of these spectrometers being such that advanced shielding techniques are incorporated to minimize the stray magnetic field. In [30], the authors conducted a comparative analysis of the static magnetic field measurements obtained from both the classical and ultra-shielded NMR settings. It was established that all values were well below the exposure limits set by the European standard for workers' protection. However, the study revealed that ultra-shield technology can achieve a 20–65-fold reduction in the field strength received by the operator. This reduction in external magnetic field strength enables the instrument to be situated in a wider range of environments with fewer spatial constraints. However, this fact gives rise to another potential hazard, since the stray field strength is observed to increase in a direct and significant manner with decreasing distance from the magnet, both directly above and below it. This increase in the attractive forces exerted on magnetic items is a consequence of this phenomenon.

Up until today, little is known about the long-term effects of chronic occupational exposure to static magnetic fields, as the available epidemiological and experimental evidence remains limited and inconclusive [12,40,44]. This knowledge gap makes it difficult to establish definitive conclusions regarding potential health risks. Regarding the direct effects of magnetic fields, particularly for long-term exposures, the current body of literature does not provide enough evidence to draw definitive conclusions about the biological and health effects of exposure to weak static magnetic fields (SMF). A lack of consistency in the studied biological systems, the examined endpoints, and scientific rigour in many reviewed studies has weakened the credibility of reported findings. While direct effects of weak magnetic fields have been reliably reported, including effects on melatonin bio-synthesis, locomotor activity, blood pressure regulation, brain enzyme activities, or neurotransmitter levels [44], they remain insufficiently understood to be incorporated into existing safety standards. Despite the paucity of long-term risks and potential benefits observed in the majority of animal and human studies conducted to date [45], further research is required to comprehensively assess the exact long-term biological effects of various SMFs on different physiological and pathological conditions. A recent report by the Scientific Committee on Health, Environmental and Emerging Risks (SCHEER) updated the potential health effects of exposure to EMF with regard to frequencies between 1 Hz and 100 kHz [46]. The SCHEER report identified a lack of recent systematic reviews or meta-analyses on low-frequency EMF exposure to update the previous (2015) Scientific Committee on Emerging and Newly Identified Health Risks (SCENIHR) [40] assessment and concluded that there is no convincing evidence of a causal relationship between ELF magnetic field exposure and self-reported symptoms.

Furthermore, standardized procedures for assessing occupational exposure in MR and NMR environments have yet to be developed. The lack of uniform assessment methods complicates efforts to evaluate and mitigate risks, particularly for highly specialized workers in industrial and research settings where exposure to extremely strong static magnetic fields—reaching up to 28 T in some NMR applications—is common. In view of the challenges identified, further studies are imperative to enhance our understanding of exposure conditions and establish safety guidelines that are tailored to workers in high-field environments. This is of crucial importance, as the basis for effective guidelines and best practices lies in a clear understanding of the physical parameters involved.

This is a significant consideration for risk assessment, as non-medical MR environments present unique challenges, including the presence of personnel often inadequately trained about occupational exposure, the high intensity of static magnetic fields and field gradients (active shielding), and the need to perform routine operations (such as tuning or cryogen refilling) in close proximity to the instrument, where magnetic field intensity is highest.

In this paper, we discuss a pathway for acquiring risk awareness for NMR laboratories. The pathway is based on a risk management model that is both concrete and applicable (Figure 3).

As an example, a case study is presented in which mathematical models and algorithms are used to explore and characterize occupational exposure levels to magnetic fields generated by a 300 MHz (7 T) NMR spectrometer. The findings of this study indicate that the maximum magnetic field levels ($|B|$) and associated exposure levels were observed in the proximity of the spectrometer. The measurements of $|B|$, spatial distribution, and gradient indicate high-risk areas corresponding to zones with steep magnetic field gradients, where operators should exercise caution and move slowly.

Despite the selection of elevated values for motion velocity and areas exhibiting greater values for magnetic field spatial gradient (worst case), none of the calculated exposure parameters surpassed the relevant limits stipulated by the applicable guidelines [18], meaning that the considered exposure conditions remained in compliance with the stipulated restrictions. Nevertheless, it is not possible to generalize this conclusion due to the high variability of movements, particularly in terms of speed. This variability is contingent on the operator's habits and body size, as well as the working conditions (whether routine or emergency). It is therefore important to have a simple yet reliable tool for risk assessment under different exposure conditions.

NMR environments can present significant risks for workers with certain implants, particularly AIMDs or other electronic medical equipment. Exposure to electromagnetic fields in these settings can interfere with the functionality of such devices, potentially leading to malfunctions, degraded performance, loss of functionality, or unintended physiological responses. Our findings indicate that workers may be exposed to magnetic fields exceeding 0.5 mT, especially during tasks that require close proximity to the equipment or at heights corresponding to the typical positioning of active medical implants, such as pacemakers and defibrillators. Additionally, movement within the fringe field can induce voltages in the leads of AIMDs, potentially triggering inappropriate device responses. These risks highlight the need for stringent safety measures and exposure assessments for workers with implanted medical devices in high-field NMR environments.

Mattei and colleagues [26] demonstrated that pacemaker (PM) performance degradation can occur during rotational movements at approximately 2 rad/s in an MRI environment. Similarly, for an implantable cardioverter-defibrillator (ICD), movements with a maximum speed of 6 rad/s may lead to a misclassification of ectopic beats as ventricular fibrillation. To the best of our knowledge, a comparable study has not yet been conducted in NMR laboratory settings.

Our simulation results indicate that the voltage induced by typical worker movements near an NMR spectrometer—at positions representative of those for individuals wearing a PM or an ICD—does not exceed the programmed sensitivity threshold of these devices (typically 2 mV) [47,48] in a unipolar configuration. However, in a bipolar configuration, the induced voltage can surpass the lower threshold of 0.3 mV. It is important to note that this threshold is defined for a standardized stimulus with higher frequency components than those of the low-frequency voltage signal induced by movement within the NMR magnetic field, which is approximately 1 Hz [24].

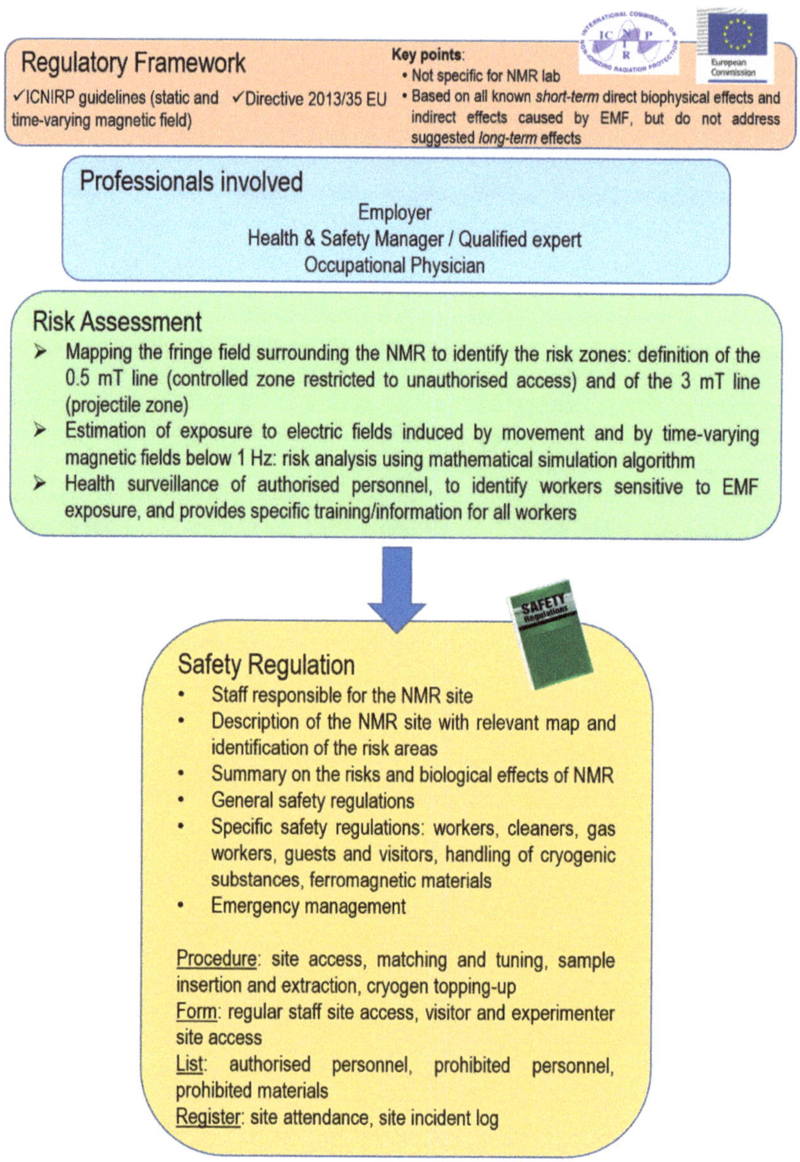

Figure 3. General overview of NMR laboratory safety management.

Additionally, comparing the computed maximum induced electric field (EMFmax) with the immunity levels required for PM/ICD compliance with international market-entry standards presents challenges. These immunity levels vary depending on frequency and generally do not account for signals below 16.6 Hz, making direct comparisons difficult.

5. Conclusions

The objective of this study was to enhance awareness of the necessity for safety measures in environments where they have yet to be implemented. The overarching aim is to ensure the safety of NMR environment workers and all other individuals involved. This work constitutes a rigorous attempt to provide original insights that address the critical gap in the extant literature regarding the safety of NMR laboratories. It also offers valuable implications for both research and practical applications.

In conclusion, it is essential to consider that technological advancements in NMR are pushing towards increasingly higher static magnetic field intensities and operating frequencies, significantly increasing the risk level for workers. The risk assessment process in NMR environments must involve all relevant stakeholders. Employers play a crucial role by ensuring that workers undergo medical examinations to certify their health suitability for tasks involving exposure to the spectrometer's magnetic fields. At the same time, workers must adhere to specific safety protocols and adopt appropriate behaviours, particularly when approaching the spectrometer, to minimize potential risks. Another critical aspect is the design and construction of NMR sites, which, in addition to incorporating necessary safety devices (e.g., quench pipes), must ensure adequate spaces for activities related to the spectrometer's use, minimizing occupational risks for workers.

With regard to the potential effects of chronic exposure, it is advisable to await further comprehensive knowledge and to adopt technical and operational strategies for exposure minimization. In the absence of substantial data regarding the potential consequences associated with long-term exposure to EMF, the adequacy of health risk assessments pertaining to MR workers remains questionable, particularly with respect to exposure levels that fall below the thresholds associated with acute effects [9]. Therefore, we strongly encourage further, more systematic research in this area. Future studies should specifically investigate the effects of SMF exposure on human biological functioning to determine whether SMF pose any significant health risks.

Finally, updating regulations to ensure safety is essential, particularly for laboratories with outdated equipment lacking advanced safety systems that may pose significant risks. Additionally, raising operator awareness of safety aspects, through specific training programs, for example, and systematically assessing risks using innovative tools and methods, is imperative.

Author Contributions: Conceptualization, V.H. and G.A.; methodology, V.H. and A.F.; software, V.H.; validation, G.A., M.M. and M.A.D.; investigation A.F.; resources, A.F.; data curation, V.H. and G.A.; writing—original draft preparation, V.H. and A.F.; writing—review and editing, G.A., M.A.D. and M.M.; visualization, A.F.; supervision, V.H. All authors have read and agreed to the published version of the manuscript.

Funding: This research was funded by INAIL (National Institute for Insurance against Accidents at Work), grant number Bric 2022 CUP: J43C22001390005.

Data Availability Statement: The data presented in this study are available on request from the corresponding author.

Acknowledgments: We acknowledge the Multi-Modal Molecular Imaging (MMMI) Italian Node of the Eurobioimaging Research Infrastructure for supporting the research activity at the 7 T high-field MRI facility at the "G. Monasterio" Foundation.

Conflicts of Interest: The authors declare no conflicts of interest.

References

1. Wong, K.C. Review of NMR Spectroscopy: Basic Principles, Concepts and Applications in Chemistry. *J. Chem. Educ.* **2014**, *91*, 1103–1104. [CrossRef]
2. Keeler, J. *Understanding NMR Spectroscopy*; John Wiley and Sons: Hoboken, NJ, USA, 2010; ISBN 9781119964933.
3. Acri, G.; Sansotta, C.; Ruello, E.V.; Denaro, L.; Salmeri, F.M.; Testagrossa, B. The Use of Time Domain NMR in Food Analysis: A Review. *Curr. Nutr. Food Sci.* **2020**, *17*, 558–565. [CrossRef]
4. Moser, E.; Laistler, E.; Schmitt, F.; Kontaxis, G. Ultra-high field NMR and MRI-the role of magnet technology to increase sensitivity and specificity. *Front. Phys.* **2017**, *5*, 33. [CrossRef]
5. Schaap, K.; Christopher-De Vries, Y.; Crozier, S.; De Vocht, F.; Kromhout, H. Exposure to static and time-varying magnetic fields from working in the static magnetic stray fields of MRI scanners: A comprehensive survey in the Netherlands. *Ann. Occup. Hyg.* **2014**, *58*, 1094–1110. [CrossRef] [PubMed]
6. Kim, S.J.; Kim, K.A. Safety issues and updates under MR environments. *Eur. J. Radiol.* **2017**, *89*, 7–13. [CrossRef]
7. De Vocht, F.; Batistatou, E.; Mölter, A.; Kromhout, H.; Schaap, K.; van Tongeren, M.; Crozier, S.; Gowland, P.; Keevil, S. Transient health symptoms of MRI staff working with 1.5 and 3.0 Tesla scanners in the UK. *Eur. Radiol.* **2015**, *25*, 2718–2726. [CrossRef] [PubMed]
8. Acri, G.; Inferrera, P.; Denaro, L.; Sansotta, C.; Ruello, E.; Anfuso, C.; Salmeri, F.M.; Garreffa, G.; Vermiglio, G.; Testagrossa, B. dB/dt evaluation in MRI sites: Is ICNIRP threshold limit (for workers) exceeded? *Int. J. Environ. Res. Public Health* **2018**, *15*, 1298. [CrossRef]
9. Hartwig, V.; Virgili, G.; Mattei, F.E.; Biagini, C.; Romeo, S.; Zeni, O.; Scarfì, M.R.; Massa, R.; Campanella, F.; Landini, L.; et al. Occupational exposure to electromagnetic fields in magnetic resonance environment: An update on regulation, exposure assessment techniques, health risk evaluation, and surveillance. *Med. Biol. Eng. Comput.* **2021**, *1*, 3. [CrossRef]
10. Bravo, G.; Modenese, A.; Arcangeli, G.; Bertoldi, C.; Camisa, V.; Corona, G.; Giglioli, S.; Ligabue, G.; Moccaldi, R.; Mucci, N.; et al. Subjective Symptoms in Magnetic Resonance Imaging Personnel: A Multi-Center Study in Italy. *Front. Public Health* **2021**, *9*, 699675. [CrossRef]
11. Bouisset, N.; Nissi, J.; Laakso, I.; Reynolds, R.F.; Legros, A. Is activation of the vestibular system by electromagnetic induction a possibility in an MRI context? *Bioelectromagnetics* **2024**, *45*, 171–183. [CrossRef] [PubMed]
12. König, A.M.; Pöschke, A.; Mahnken, A.H. Health risks for medical personnel due to magnetic fields in magnetic resonance imaging. *RöFo—Fortschritte auf dem Gebiet der Röntgenstrahlen und der Bildgeb. Verfahr.* **2024**, *197*, 135–143. [CrossRef]
13. Glans, A.; Wilén, J.; Lindgren, L.; Björkman-Burtscher, I.M.; Hansson, B. Health effects related to exposure of static magnetic fields and acoustic noise—Comparison between MR and CT radiographers. *Eur. Radiol.* **2022**, *32*, 7896–7909. [CrossRef]
14. Wang, X.; Ye, Y.; Zuo, H.; Li, Y. Neurobiological effects and mechanisms of magnetic fields: A review from 2000 to 2023. *BMC Public Health* **2024**, *24*, 3094. [CrossRef] [PubMed]
15. ICNIRP. Guidelines on Limits of Exposure To Static Magnetic Fields. *Health Phys.* **2009**, *96*, 504–514. [CrossRef]
16. ICNIRP. Guidelines for limiting exposure to time-varying electric and magnetic fields (1 Hz to 100 kHz). *Health Phys.* **2010**, *99*, 818–836. [CrossRef]
17. European Parliament and Council of the European Union. Directive 2013/35/EC on the minimum health and safety requirements regarding the exposure of workers to the risks arising from physical agents (electromagnetic fields). *Off. J. Eur. Union* **2013**, L179/1-21. Available online: https://eur-lex.europa.eu/legal-content/EN/ALL/?uri=celex:32013L0035 (accessed on 27 March 2025).
18. ICNIRP. Guidelines for limiting exposure to electric fields induced by and by time-varying magnetic fields below 1 Hz. *Health Phys.* **2014**, *106*, 418–425. [CrossRef]
19. Laakso, I.; Kännälä, S.; Jokela, K. Computational dosimetry of induced electric fields during realistic movements in the vicinity of a 3 T MRI scanner. *Phys. Med. Biol.* **2013**, *58*, 2625–2640. [CrossRef] [PubMed]
20. Zilberti, L.; Bottauscio, O.; Chiampi, M. Assessment of exposure to MRI motion-induced fields based on the International Commission on Non-Ionizing Radiation Protection (ICNIRP) guidelines. *Magn. Reson. Med.* **2016**, *76*, 1291–1300. [CrossRef] [PubMed]
21. Gurrera, D.; Gallias, K.K.; Spanò, M.; Abbate, B.F.; D'Alia, F.; Iacoviello, G.; Caputo, V. Moving across the static magnetic field of a 1.5 T MRI scanner: Analysing compliance with Directive 2013/35/EU. *Phys. Medica* **2019**, *57*, 238–244. [CrossRef]
22. Gurrera, D.; Leardini, A.; Ortolani, M.; Durante, S.; Caputo, V.; Gallias, K.K.; Abbate, B.F.; Rinaldi, C.; Iacoviello, G.; Acri, G.; et al. Experimental and Modeling Analyses of Human Motion Across the Static Magnetic Field of an MRI Scanner. *Front. Bioeng. Biotechnol.* **2021**, *1*, 613616. [CrossRef]
23. Roemer, P.B.; Wade, T.; Alejski, A.; Ertan, K.; McKenzie, C.A.; Rutt, B.K.; Lutz, F. Electric field calculation and peripheral nerve stimulation prediction for head and body gradient coils. *Magn. Reson. Med.* **2021**, *86*, 2301–2315. [PubMed]
24. Acri, G.; Testagrossa, B.; Causa, F.; Tripepi, M.G.; Vermiglio, G.; Novario, R.; Pozzi, L.; Quadrelli, G. Evaluation of occupational exposure in magnetic resonance sites. *Radiol. Medica* **2014**, *119*, 208–213. [CrossRef]
25. Sannino, A.; Romeo, S.; Scarfì, M.R.; Massa, R.; d'Angelo, R.; Petrillo, A.; Cerciello, V.; Fusco, R.; Zeni, O. Exposure Assessment and Biomonitoring of Workers in Magnetic Resonance Environment: An Exploratory Study. *Front. Public Health* **2017**, *5*, 344. [CrossRef]

26. Hartwig, V.; Virgili, G.; Ferrante Vero, L.F.; De Marchi, D.; Landini, L.; Giovannetti, G. Towards a Personalised and Interactive Assessment of Occupational Exposure To Magnetic Field During Daily Routine in Magnetic Resonance. *Radiat. Prot. Dosim.* **2018**, *182*, 546–554. [CrossRef]
27. Hartwig, V.; Biagini, C.; De Marchi, D.; Flori, A.; Gabellieri, C.; Virgili, G.; Ferrante Vero, L.F.L.F.; Landini, L.; Vanello, N.; Giovannetti, G. The Procedure for Quantitative Characterization and Analysis of Magnetic Fields in Magnetic Resonance Sites for Protection of Workers: A Pilot Study. *Ann. Work Expo. Health* **2019**, *63*, 328–336. [CrossRef] [PubMed]
28. Hartwig, V.; Biagini, C.; De Marchi, D.; Flori, A.; Gabellieri, C.; Virgili, G.; Fabiano, L.; Vero, F.; Landini, L.; Vanello, N.; et al. Analysis, comparison and representation of occupational exposure to a static magnetic field in a 3-T MRI site. *Int. J. Occup. Saf. Ergon.* **2022**, *28*, 76–85. [CrossRef] [PubMed]
29. Reif, B.; Ashbrook, S.E.; Emsley, L.; Hong, M. Solid-state NMR spectroscopy. *Nat. Rev. Methods Prim.* **2021**, *1*, 2. [CrossRef]
30. Berlana, T.; Úbeda, A. Occupational exposure of NMR spectrometrists to static and radiofrequency fields. *Radiat. Prot. Dosim.* **2017**, *177*, 397–406. [CrossRef]
31. Council of the European Communities. *CELEX1, 1999/519/EC: Council Recommendation of 12 July 1999 on the Limitation of Exposure of the General Public to Electromagnetic Fields (0 Hz to 300 GHz)*; Publications Office of the European Union: Luxembourg, 1999.
32. Mattei, E.; Censi, F.; Calcagnini, G.; Falsaperla, R.; Genovese, E.; Napolitano, A.; Cannatà, V. Pacemaker and ICD oversensing induced by movements near the MRI scanner bore. *Med. Phys.* **2016**, *43*, 6621–6631. [CrossRef]
33. Shimizu, H.; Tsujita, K. Control strategy of human the sit-to-stand movement. In Proceedings of the 2021 60th Annual Conference of the Society of Instrument and Control Engineers of Japan (SICE), Tokyo, Japan, 8–10 September 2021; pp. 144–149.
34. Decat, G. Occupational Exposure Assessment of the Static Magnetic Flux Density Generated by Nuclear Magnetic Resonance Spectroscopy for Biochemical Purposes. *PIERS Online* **2007**, *3*, 513–516. [CrossRef]
35. Hartwig, V.; Sansotta, C.; Morelli, M.S.; Testagrossa, B.; Acri, G. Occupational Exposure Assessment of the Static Magnetic Field Generated by Nuclear Magnetic Resonance Spectroscopy: A Case Study. *Int. J. Environ. Res. Public Health* **2022**, *19*, 7674. [CrossRef] [PubMed]
36. De Vocht, F.; Liket, L.; De Vocht, A.; Mistry, T.; Glover, P.; Gowland, P.; Kromhout, H. Exposure to alternating electromagnetic fields and effects on the visual and visuomotor systems. *Br. J. Radiol.* **2007**, *80*, 822–828. [CrossRef] [PubMed]
37. McRobbie, D.W. Occupational exposure in MRI. *Br. J. Radiol.* **2012**, *85*, 293–312. [CrossRef] [PubMed]
38. Acri, G.; Testagrossa, B.; Vermiglio, G. Personal Time-Varying Magnetic Fields Evaluation During Activities in MRI Sites. In Proceedings of the IFMBE Proceedings, Toronto, ON, Canada, 7–12 June 2015; Volume 51, pp. 741–744.
39. Hartwig, V.; Romeo, S.; Zeni, O. Occupational exposure to electromagnetic fields in magnetic resonance environment: Basic aspects and review of exposure assessment approaches. *Med. Biol. Eng. Comput.* **2018**, *56*, 531–545. [CrossRef] [PubMed]
40. SCENIHR (Scientific Committee on Emerging and Newly Identified Health Risks). *Potential Health Effects of Exposure to Electromagnetic Fields (EMF)*; European Commission: Brussels, Belgium, 2015.
41. Heinrich, A.; Szostek, A.; Nees, F.; Meyer, P.; Semmler, W.; Flor, H. Effects of static magnetic fields on cognition, vital signs, and sensory perception: A meta-analysis. *J. Magn. Reson. Imaging* **2011**, *34*, 758–763. [CrossRef] [PubMed]
42. Schaap, K.; Portengen, L.; Kromhout, H. Exposure to MRI-related magnetic fields and vertigo in MRI workers. *Occup. Environ. Med.* **2016**, *73*, 161–166.
43. Walker, M.; Fultz, A.; Davies, C.; Brockopp, D. Symptoms Experienced by MR Technologists Exposed to Static Magnetic Fields. *Radiol. Technol.* **2020**, *91*, 316–323.
44. Driessen, S.; Bodewein, L.; Dechent, D.; Graefrath, D.; Schmiedchen, K.; Stunder, D.; Kraus, T.; Petri, A.K. Biological and health-related effects of weak static magnetic fields (<1 mT) in humans and vertebrates: A systematic review. *PLoS ONE* **2020**, *15*, e0230038. [CrossRef]
45. Zhang, X. *Biological Effects of Static Magnetic Fields*, 2nd ed.; Springer: Singapore, 2023; ISBN 9789811988691.
46. SCHEER (Scientific Committee on Health Environmental and Emerging Risks). *Potential Health Effects of Exposure to Electromagnetic Fields (EMF): Update with Regard to Frequencies Between 1 Hz and 100 kHz—Preliminary Opinion*; European Commission: Brussels, Belgium, 2024.
47. *UNI EN 45502-2-1:2005*; Active Implantable Medical Devices—Part 2-1: Particular Requirements for Active Implantable Medical Devices Intended to Treat Bradyarrhythmia (Cardiac Pacemakers). UNI: Roma, Italia, 2005.
48. *UNI EN 45502-2-2:2008*; Active implantable Medical Devices—Part 2-2: Particular Requirements for Active Implantable Medical Devices Intended to Treat Tachyarrhythmia (Includes Implantable Defibrillators). UNI: Roma, Italia, 2008.

environments

MDPI

Article

Young Workers and Lifestyles in a Mediterranean Cultural Context: What Is the Contribution of Occupational Health Promotion?

Elpidio Maria Garzillo [1], Anna Rita Corvino [2,*], Giuseppe Porciello [2], Daniele Guida [2], Marco Spasiano [2], Nadia Miraglia [2] and Monica Lamberti [2]

1 Department of Prevention, Abruzzo Local Health Unit No. 1, 67100 L'Aquila, Italy; egarzillo@asl1abruzzo.it
2 Department of Experimental Medicine -Hygiene, Occupational, and Forensic Medicine Division-Occupational Forensic Area, University of Campania "Luigi Vanvitelli", 80138 Naples, Italy; giuseppe.porciello@studenti.unicampania.it (G.P.); daniele.guida1@studenti.unicampania.it (D.G.); marco.spasiano@unicampania.it (M.S.); nadia.miraglia@unicampania.it (N.M.); monica.lamberti@unicampania.it (M.L.)
* Correspondence: annarita.corvino@unicampania.it

Abstract: Adherence to a healthy diet and an active lifestyle is now a key component of workplace health promotion (WHP) programs. The primary objective of the study is the assessment of the need for the implementation of corrective WHP interventions aimed at improving the lifestyle in students belonging to health-related degree programs. A prospective observational epidemiological study through the recruitment of a sample of 242 young adult-equated workers at the Vanvitelli University in Naples was conducted. Two questionnaires were administered, one related to Mediterranean diet adherence (PREDIMED) and one concerning daily physical activity (IPAQ). A total of 56.6% of the participants were in the intermediate level of adherence to the Mediterranean diet, 24.0% low and 19.4% in the high level, with highly significant differences in the distribution between the groups. The chi-square test revealed a statistically significant association between groups and physical activity level ($p = 0.0166$). A statistically significant association was also found between gender and physical activity level (men showing high levels of physical activity). The analysis showed significant differences in adherence to the Mediterranean diet between the different students' groups, with no gender-related differences. This study highlighted the need for a systematic and differentiated approach to WHP, differentiating the various groups.

Keywords: workplace health promotion (WHP); PREDIMED; Mediterranean diet; corrective interventions; epidemiological study

1. Introduction

The World Health Organization (WHO) has identified the workplace as an ideal setting for health promotion because it provides a prime environment for influencing people's health behaviors. Even in countries with high unemployment rates, most of the adult population is still employed, making the workplace a strategic platform for improving public health [1,2]. Since 2003, the National Institute for Occupational Safety and Health (NIOSH) has supported the integration of measures to protect occupational safety and health with interventions to promote the health and well-being of workers. Adherence to proper nutrition and active lifestyle is, to date, a key part of workplace health promotion

 https://doi.org/10.3390/environments12050147

(WHP) programs. In Italy, the National Strategic Plan for Prevention drafted for the five-year period 2020–2025 calls for the need to adopt more effective intervention models for strengthening the overall health of workers, such as the WHO Healthy Workplace Model and the NIOSH Total Worker Health Model. The evolution of the WHP concept led, in 2011, to the creation of the Total Worker Health® (TWH) program. The Total Worker Health® approach is defined as a set of policies, programs and practices that integrate protection from occupational safety and health hazards with the promotion of injury and illness prevention initiatives to improve worker well-being. Worker well-being is an integrative concept that characterizes quality of life in relation to individual health and work-related environmental, organizational and psychosocial factors [3]. Poor nutrition is a modifiable and preventable risk factor that can lead to the onset or worsening of some chronic non-communicable diseases. As is well known, habitual consumption of unhealthy foods can result in weight gain and subsequent obesity [4], which in turn influence the development of chronic diseases, such as cardiovascular problems and diabetes [5,6]. Adherence to a proper diet is therefore, to date, a key part of workplace health promotion programs. The Mediterranean diet, recognized by UNESCO as an intangible heritage of humanity, represents a healthy eating pattern, rich in fruits, vegetables, legumes, whole grains, fish, olive oil and moderate consumption of wine. Adherence to the Mediterranean diet is associated with numerous health, socio-cultural, economic and environmental benefits [7] that make it one of the healthiest and most sustainable food models [8]. Adherence to the Mediterranean diet also results in lower mortality from cardiovascular and neoplastic diseases [9], and in addition to health effects, additional benefits include low environmental impact, biodiversity of products consumed, high socio-cultural value of foods and support for the local economy [10]. Sedentariness is a condition that can be fostered by the type of work performed, but it can also be a habit maintained in leisure time [11]. In Europe, it is estimated that more than 35 percent of people sit for more than 7 h a day [2]. In Italy, sedentary behavior, determined by long periods spent standing or sitting, throughout the day, is also widespread among the active adult population. According to the PASSI survey in the two-year period 2021–2022, among adults living in Italy, the "physically active" are 47% of the population, the "partially active" 24% and the "sedentary" 29% [12]. Existing scientific evidence shows that physical activity is a protective factor for health. The level of exercise is inversely related to mortality risk and thus associated with longer life expectancy [13]. Regular practice of adequate aerobic physical activity has been shown to act as a protective factor against high-incidence diseases in the general population, such as cardiovascular disease. For example, compared with inactive individuals, those who exercise for an average of 92 min per week or 15 min a day had a 14% reduced risk of all-cause mortality (0·86, 0·81–0·91) and had a 3-year longer life expectancy [14]. The primary purpose of this study is to assess the need for corrective health promotion interventions aimed at improving the lifestyle of young adults. Given that Italian university students engaged in internships are regarded as workers when exposed to health and safety risks, the occupational context represents an ideal setting for health promotion. Specifically, the study seeks to examine the dietary habits and metabolic health of young adults enrolled in health-related degree programs at Vanvitelli University in Naples, with a focus on adherence to the Mediterranean diet, the intensity of daily physical activity and body mass index (BMI).

2. Materials and Methods

A prospective observational epidemiological study was conducted to assess proper lifestyles in terms of adherence to the Mediterranean diet and performance of physical activity in a population of young adults enrolled in health-related degree programs. The study involved the administration of questionnaires during preventive visits carried out as part of the University's Health Surveillance Program as well as the direct detection of participants' weight and height. The study population is represented by students in the first year of the degree courses of the following health professions of the "Luigi Vanvitelli" University: Dentistry and Dental Prosthetics, Physiotherapy, Speech Therapy, Psychiatric Rehabilitation Technique, Neuropsychomotricity Therapy, Biomedical Laboratory Techniques, Orthotics, Medical Radiology Techniques, Dental Hygiene and Prevention Techniques in the Environment and Workplaces, and students attending the third year of the degree course in Medicine and Surgery.

Inclusion criteria were students equated with workers under Article 2 of Legislative Decree 81/2008 and belonging to the 18–34 age group. Exclusion criteria included the following: (1) the presence of known chronic diseases that affect metabolism or appetite; (2) the presence of pathologies or disabilities that prevent a proper active lifestyle; (3) pregnancy status; (4) taking medications that affect body weight or physical activity; and (5) failure to sign the informed consent. Indeed, the subjects involved in the study are students attending health study courses, subjected to preventive visits carried out as part of the University Health Surveillance Program, prior to the commencement of their internships and clinical placements. Therefore, recruitment was planned during the scheduled preventive visits. An information sheet on data processing for experimental purposes and an explanatory sheet on the contents and objectives of the study were distributed during the students' access to the University Health Surveillance Service. Informed consent was then collected using the forms prepared for data collection, processing and publication. Two questionnaires, one related to adherence to the Mediterranean diet (PREDIMED) and one to daily physical activity (IPAQ), were administered during the medical examination, and body weight and height measurements were taken with standardized instruments for calculating BMI.

2.1. PREDIMED and IPAQ Questionnaires

The PREDIMED (PREvención con DIeta MEDiterránea) questionnaire was designed to assess adherence to the Mediterranean diet. It is mainly used in the PREDIMED study, a major clinical trial that analyzed the effects of the Mediterranean diet on cardiovascular disease prevention [15]. The questionnaire contains 14 questions that address the consumption of specific foods (e.g., fruits, vegetables, legumes, fish, olive oil), indicating frequency, portions and eating habits (e.g., use of fat from seasoning). The result of the PREDIMED questionnaire is a score (varying between 1 and 14), the interpretation of which involves division into 3 classes: 1–5, poor adherence; 6–9 medium adherence; and greater than 10, good adherence.

The International Physical Activity Questionnaire (IPAQ) is designed to measure adults' physical activity in various settings and is used to quantify physical activity level to assess adherence to international physical activity recommendations and to correlate physical activity levels with various health conditions. For this study, the IPAQ-S (Short Form), a short questionnaire about physical activity performed in the past 7 days, was used. It consists of 7 questions and measures time spent in physical activities of different intensities (light, moderate and vigorous) and time spent sitting [16]. The result of the IPAQ questionnaire is reported in MET (Metabolic Equivalent of Task), which is the unit of measurement that estimates the amount of energy used by the human body during an activity compared to when at rest. Based on the frequency of activity during the past 7 days, a subject is described as inactive (<700 METs), sufficiently active (701–2519 METs) and active (>2520 METs).

2.2. Statistical Analysis

Each participant was assigned an anonymous ID to comply with the principles established by the GDPR. The collected data were organized into a structured database using Microsoft Excel (Office 365 version), where each row represented an individual participant and the columns contained the variables of interest. The database was exported for statistical analysis conducted with JASP software 0.19.3, while Julius AI, a specialized artificial intelligence system utilizing Python 3.11.6-based data science libraries (pandas for data manipulation, matplotlib and seaborn for visualization and scipy/statsmodels for statistical validation), was employed to generate graphical visualizations and validate the accuracy of statistical analyses. To ensure the integrity and quality of the data, periodic checks were conducted for completeness and accuracy, and any changes or corrections were documented.

3. Results

3.1. Descriptive Statistics and Sample Characteristics

The study involved a sample of 242 young adults equated within 11 health professions degree programs: Nursing (67, 27.7% of the total sample), Medicine and Surgery (36, 14.9%), Nursing and Midwifery Sciences (24, 9.9%), Speech Therapy (24, 9.9%), Medical Radiology Technicians (20, 8.2%) and the remaining percentage equally distributed at the lower levels represented by Biomedical Laboratory Technicians, Physiotherapy, Dental Hygiene, Environmental and Workplace Prevention Technicians, Orthoptics and Ophthalmic Care and Psychiatric Rehabilitation Technicians. The sample shows a prevalence of females (162, 66.9 percent) compared to males (80, 33.1 percent), with a heterogeneous distribution among the different degree programs. The mean age of participants is 22.5 years (SD $\pm$ 4.1) with a range of 18 to 34 years. Specifically, the highest mean age was found in Nursing and Midwifery (29.1 years) and Medicine and Surgery (26.0 years) courses, while the courses with the lowest mean age and least variability were Nursing (20.1 years) and Psychiatric Rehabilitation Techniques (20.0 years). Regarding BMI, the sample mean value of 23.7 kg/m^2 (SD $\pm$ 3.8) falls within the range considered as normal weight according to WHO (18.5–24.9 kg/m^2); however, it should be noted that 61.6% (149) of the participants fell into the category of normal weight, 8.3% (20) had a BMI above 30 kg/m^2, falling into the category of obesity; 23.1% (56) had a BMI above 25 kg/m^2, classifying as overweight; and 7.0% (17) had a BMI below 18.5 kg/m^2, a category of underweight. Inferential analysis was conducted to reveal whether there were differences in adherence to the Mediterranean diet, physical activity habit and BMI between study programs and genders. To optimize the statistical analysis, a reorganization of the sample was proposed, grouping participants according to their specialty. This division led to the creation of four main groups (Table 1):

Table 1. Distribution of students across the four groups of healthcare degree courses (N = 242).

Degree Course	Sample Size	Mean Age	% Male	Mean BMI
Group 1—Medicine	36 (14.9%)	26.0 $\pm$ 2.3	41,67	23.0 $\pm$ 3.9
Group 2—Nursing	67 (27.7%)	20.1 $\pm$ 2.8	26,87	24.2 $\pm$ 4.3
Group 3—Nursing and Midwifery	24 (9.9%)	29.1 $\pm$ 3.1	16,67	23.1 $\pm$ 3.2
Group 4—Other Health Professions	115 (47.5%)	21.5 $\pm$ 3.2	37,39	23.7 $\pm$ 3.6

Medicine (Group 1) and Nursing and Midwifery (Group 3) degrees were analyzed as distinct groups due to their significantly higher mean ages (26.0 $\pm$ 2.3 and 29.1 $\pm$ 3.1 years, respectively), as confirmed by one-way ANOVA with post hoc Tukey HSD tests ($F = 27.34$, $p < 0.001$). Nursing (Group 2) was maintained as a separate category given its substantial sample size (n = 67, 27.7%) and its unique professional training pathway. The grouping approach also accounted for differences in clinical exposure during internships and ensured adequate statistical power. Group 4 aggregated allied health professions that share comparable theoretical and practical training frameworks within the health sciences.

3.2. Analysis of Mediterranean Diet Adherence Based on PREDIMED Questionnaire Data

Analysis of adherence levels to the Mediterranean diet in the equated groups showed differences in the distribution of adherence categories (poor, average/sufficient, good). The results showed that 56.6 percent of participants were in the intermediate level of adherence, 24.0 percent in the low level and 19.4 percent in the high level. Analyzing the data broken down by the four main groups, as follows:

- Group 1—Medicine: Most participants (63.9%) reported sufficient adherence, followed by good adherence (19.4%) and poor adherence (16.7%).
- Group 2—Nursing: Reported the highest percentage of poor adherence (32.8%) and the lowest percentage of good adherence (3.0%), with 64.2% of participants falling into the sufficient adherence category.
- Group 3—Nurses and Midwives: The majority (75.0%) showed sufficient adherence, with a low percentage of poor adherence (8.3%) and good adherence of 16.7%.
- Group 4—Other Health Professionals: This group shows an intermediate distribution with 67.8% of participants showing adequate adherence, 24.3% poor adherence and 7.8% good adherence.

Inferential analysis revealed a statistically significant association between group membership and level of adherence to the Mediterranean diet ($\chi^2 = 14.54$; $p = 0.024$). Test for normality indicated that the data do not follow a normal distribution (Shapiro–Wilk test: $W = 0.975$, $p = 0.0004$); so, a Kruskal–Wallis test (Figure 1) was conducted on the total PREDIMED scores, showing highly significant differences between groups ($p = 0.00004$). To better understand these differences, a post hoc analysis was conducted using Dunn's test with Bonferroni correction, which revealed a significant difference between Group 1 and Group 2 ($p = 0.0031$); a significant difference between Group 1 and Group 4 ($p = 0.0258$); a significant difference between Group 2 and Group 3 ($p = 0.0008$); and a significant difference between Group 3 and Group 4 ($p = 0.0059$).

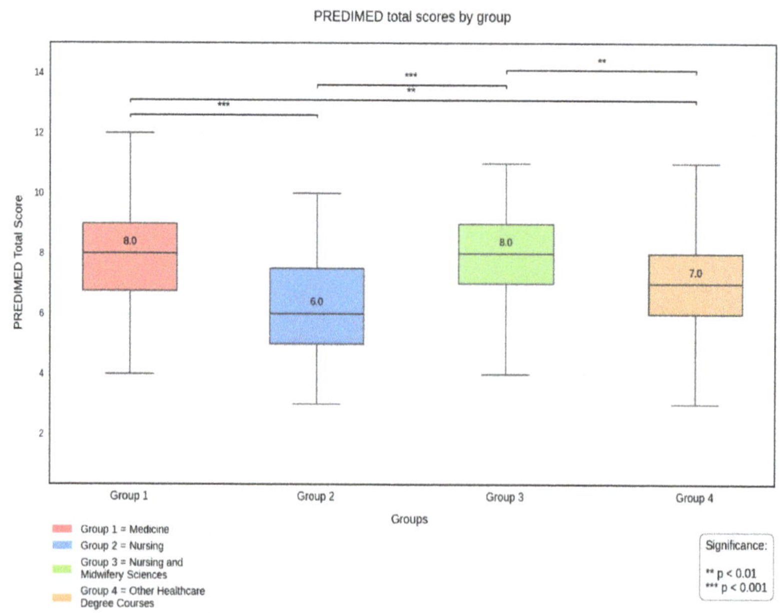

Figure 1. Results of the analysis of the total scores of the PREDIMED questionnaires administered.

Regarding the relationship between gender and adherence level, the chi-square test showed no statistically significant differences in the total population under study ($\chi^2 = 1.23$; $p = 0.54$). Instead, statistical analysis showed a positive correlation between the level of adherence to the Mediterranean diet and BMI by the Kruskal–Wallis test (test = 12.415; $p = 0.002$), which was confirmed by post hoc analysis, with a significant difference especially between poor and good adherence ($F = 5.9796$; $p = 0.015$) (Figure 2).

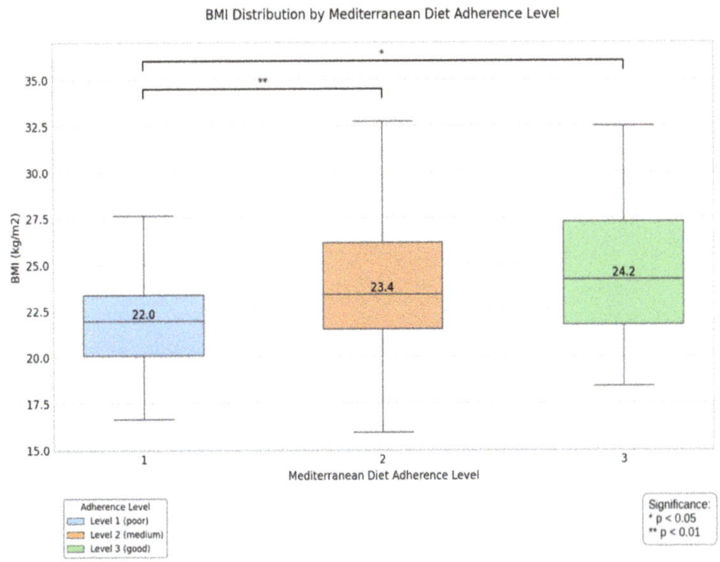

Figure 2. Box plots of BMI in relation to levels of adherence to the Mediterranean diet.

3.3. Analysis of Physical Activity Levels Based on IPAQ Questionnaire Data

The analysis of physical activity levels, based on the IPAQ questionnaire and classified into three categories (low, sufficient, good), showed that 43.4% was in the intermediate level, 33.5% in the high level and 23.1% in the low level. Significant differences emerged in the distribution of levels between the four groups:

- Group 1—Medicine: 44.4% of the participants reported a sufficient level of physical activity, while another 44.4% achieved a good level of physical activity. Only 11.2% of the participants fell into the poor physical activity category.
- Group 2—Nurses: The majority (55.2%) showed a sufficient level of physical activity, while 28.4% reported a poor level of physical activity and 16.4% a good level of physical activity.
- Group 3—Nurses and Midwives: This group shows a balanced distribution, with 41.7% of the participants falling into the categories of sufficient and good physical activity and 16.7% with poor physical activity.
- Group 4—Other Health Professions: 36.5% showed a sufficient level of physical activity, 38.3% good physical activity and 25.2% poor activity.

This performed analysis showed that men had a greater tendency towards high levels of physical activity, with almost 49% achieving a 'good' level compared to 26% of women. Moreover, the percentage of low physical activity is slightly higher in women (24.7%) than in men (20.0%).

Inferential analysis revealed a statistically significant association between peer group membership and physical activity level ($\chi^2 = 15.51$; $p = 0.0166$). Figure 3 shows the box plot of the distribution of total MET scores by degree groups. Due to non-normal distribution, confirmed by the Shapiro–Wilk test (W = 0.97, p = 0.001), a non-parametric Kruskal–Wallis test was conducted, which demonstrated significant differences in total METs between groups (p = 0.004).

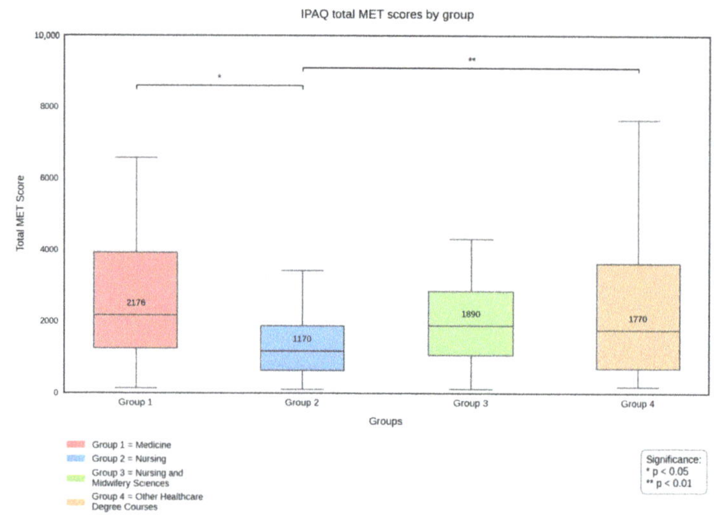

Figure 3. Results of the analysis of the IPAQ questionnaires broken down by total MET scores among the various groups.

A statistically significant association was also found between gender and physical activity level (Figure 4), confirmed by both the chi-square test (χ^2 = 12.90; p = 0.0016) and T-test on total MET (t = −2.26; p = 0.025). The assessment of levels and quality of physical activity performed cannot be separated from the analysis of sedentary habits. The results obtained showed significantly different patterns among the equated groups, both during working days (p < 0.001) and, to a lesser extent, during rest days (p = 0.005) (Figure 5).

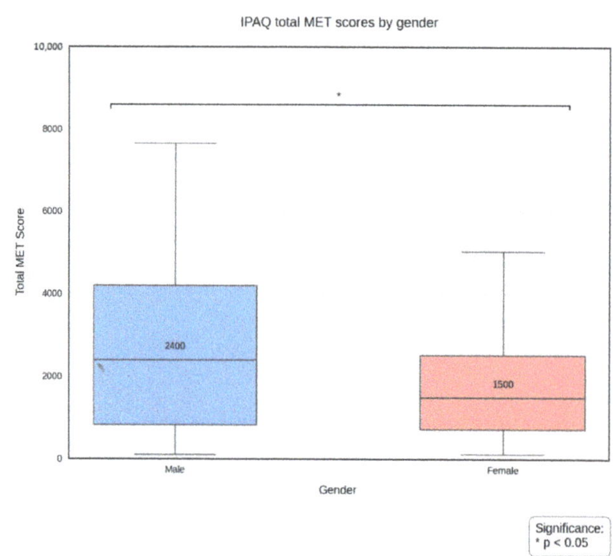

Figure 4. Results of the analysis of the participants' total MET scores in relation to their gender.

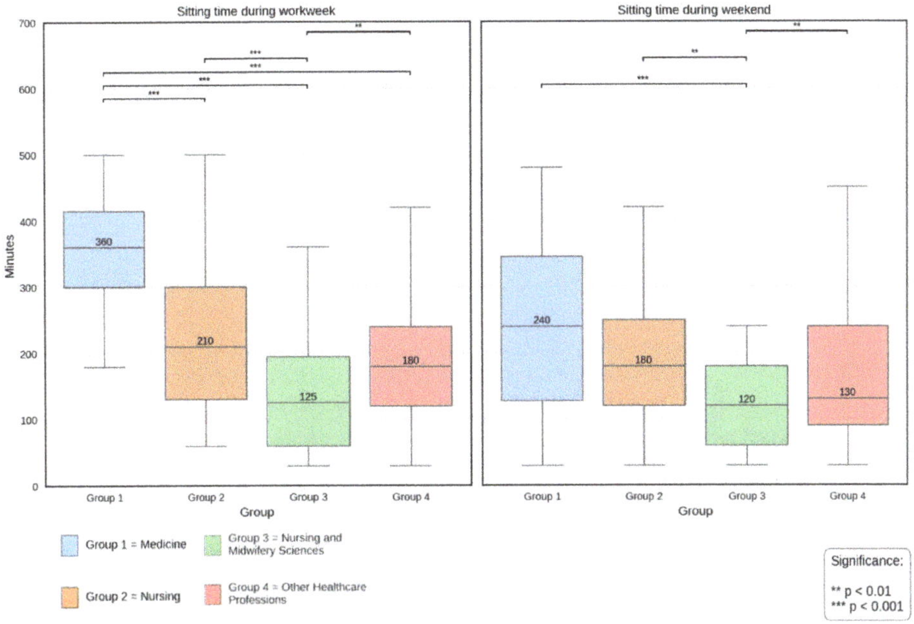

Figure 5. Results of the analysis of sedentariness on work days (left) and rest days (right) by groups.

4. Discussion

Italian Legislative regarding Health and Safety at Work has put trainees, interns and apprentices on the same footing as workers, recognizing their rights and protections in the workplace. This legislation is particularly important for a segment of the population that is going through a delicate phase of the life cycle, marked by fundamental choices such as the completion of studies, entry into the world of work and the development of social and territorial relations. Consequently, it is crucial to understand their state of well-being and monitor its evolution over time, as these challenges can profoundly affect not only their psychological health, but also their lifestyles, including diet and physical activity. In fact, as reported in the previous paragraph, while numerous studies demonstrate the positive impact of healthy eating habits on general health, research shows a progressive abandonment of the Mediterranean diet among young Italians, despite its documented benefits for the prevention of chronic diseases and for psychophysical well-being [17]. Young adults face intense life rhythms and social pressures that often lead them to prefer convenience and processed foods, which meet their needs for convenience but do not fully satisfy their nutritional needs [18]. In addition, there is a growing tendency towards physical inactivity, often sacrificed due to stress and study or workloads [19].

The analysis conducted in this work revealed significant differences in adherence to the Mediterranean diet between the different groups of healthcare workers, while no gender-related differences emerged. In particular, Group 2 (nurses) showed lower scores than the other groups, suggesting the need for possible targeted interventions for this group. The analysis of the individual responses to the questions of the PREDIMED questionnaire revealed interesting patterns in the distribution of positive responses among the participants (where 'positive' refers to the response indicating greater adherence to the Mediterranean diet). The questions with the highest rate of positive responses were those on the use of extra virgin olive oil (95.5%), less use of butter or margarine (90.5%) and low consumption of sugary drinks (81.4%). On the other hand, the questions with the lowest rate of positive answers were those on the consumption of wine (1.2%), fruit (10.3%) and fish (23.6%). Also interesting were the data on the consumption of vegetables (two or more portions per day for only 44.6%) and red meat and sausages (more than one portion per day for 41.3%). While virtuous behavior is observed in the use of healthy fats (extra virgin olive oil) and in limiting saturated fats (butter and margarine), significant criticism emerges in the low consumption of fundamental foods of the Mediterranean diet such as fruit, vegetables and fish, as well as in the excessive consumption of red meat and sausages for a good percentage of participants. It should be remembered that even the most recent WHO recommendations indicate the introduction in the diet of at least five portions of fruit and vegetables per day and two to three portions of fish per week and the reduction in red meat to once a week, while sausages should be avoided.

Concerning wine consumption, the latest scientific evidence is challenging the traditional paradigm of the benefits of moderate alcohol consumption. In particular, a meta-analysis published in 2023 [20] provided significant results that contradict previous beliefs on the subject, demonstrating the absence of a statistically significant correlation between moderate alcohol consumption and reduced mortality in general, thus disproving previously accepted assumptions about the supposed cardioprotective effects and other health benefits of alcohol taken in low doses. This new perspective finds further support in the official WHO position: there is no threshold of alcohol consumption that can be considered completely safe for an individual's health. These findings are particularly important in the context of the Mediterranean diet, whose moderate consumption of wine is historically considered one of its defining elements. Thus, the very low percentage of daily wine drinkers revealed in the study seems to be positive and not negative. The study shows that the surveyed population generally has a good propensity for moderate physical activity, especially when compared to regional data (17.3% partially active and 34.4% active). Taking the WHO guidelines for physical activity as a reference [11], to achieve substantial health benefits, adults should perform 150 to 300 min of moderate aerobic activity per week, 75 to 150 min of intense aerobic activity per week or an equivalent combination of both within the week. In general, the majority of students in all groups exceed the WHO minimum recommendations, with a relatively low percentage (between 8.3% and 12.5% depending on the graduating class group) not reaching the minimum recommended levels.

Examination of the four groups by degree course, however, revealed significant differences in the distribution of physical activity levels. Contingency table analysis showed a statistically significant association between occupational group and level of physical activity, while analysis of variance for total METs revealed significant differences between Group 2 (Nursing) compared to students in Medicine and other degree courses. The observed differences could be attributed to various factors, including workloads, schedules and the specific characteristics of each health profession, but it is clear that nursing students/workers are again a group worthy of attention for possible health promotion interventions. Similarly, the results regarding gender-related physical activity levels suggest that particular attention should be paid to the female gender when designing interventions to promote physical activity. Despite the sample being predominantly female (66.9%), 49% of men reached a level of physical activity, compared to 26% of women, indicating a greater male propensity for engaging in regular and high-intensity physical activity. On the other hand, the percentage of individuals with poor physical activity levels was higher among women (24.7%) compared to men (20.0%). Previous studies have demonstrated significant gender differences in physical activity levels among university students [21], with females generally engaging in less vigorous physical activity than their male counterparts. These differences may be influenced by multiple factors, including socio-cultural barriers, psychological aspects and environmental constraints. Eventual gender-specific barriers and motivators should be carefully considered when designing workplace health promotion programs.

The assessment of the level and quality of physical activity performed cannot be separated from the analysis of sedentary habits. This analysis is based on the separate examination of time spent sitting on working days and days off (questions from the IPAQ questionnaire). In particular, Group 1 (Medicine) shows the highest levels of sedentariness during the working day (365.0 ± 124.0 min), followed by Group 2 (Nursing) with 245.6 ± 170.3 min and Group 4 (Other Health Professions) with 224.1 ± 144.3 min. Group 3 (Nursing and Midwifery) presents the lowest levels of sedentary work. On rest days, a trend towards a reduction in sedentary time is observed in all groups, with Group 1 maintaining the highest values, while Group 3 confirms the lowest levels. Interestingly, the differences between the groups decrease on rest days, suggesting a homogenization of behavior outside the work environment. Since there is moderate evidence that correlates a sedentary lifestyle with increased mortality from all causes (cardiovascular diseases and cancer in particular), but there are no minimum levels at which sedentariness is not considered harmful, it is advisable to raise awareness among the population to remain as active as possible in their free time, since exceeding the recommended minimum levels of moderate-to-intense physical activity established by the WHO may reduce the negative effects associated with sedentariness. The positive correlation between the level of adherence to the Mediterranean diet and BMI on the Kruskal–Wallis test, with a significant difference especially between poor and good adherence, would seem to be counterintuitive to traditional expectations of the benefits of the Mediterranean diet; in reality, this suggests the presence of more complex dynamics in the relationship between dietary patterns and body composition. The surveyed population generally has a good propensity for moderate physical activity, especially when compared to regional data (17.3% partially active and 34.4% active), with significant differences in the distribution of physical activity levels.

Although the PREDIMED questionnaire is a validated tool for assessing adherence to the Mediterranean diet, it has inherent limitations. In particular, it does not consider the amounts of food actually consumed, but relies primarily on the frequency of food intake. This methodological feature could mask substantial differences in total caloric intake between individuals who instead show similar adherence scores. In addition, interpretation of the results must take into account an important confounding factor: overweight people very often tend to seek the advice of nutrition professionals and adopt healthier eating patterns, such as the Mediterranean diet. This could explain the seemingly counterintuitive correlation between higher BMI and greater dietary adherence. However, in the absence of information on the duration and timing of nutrition initiation, it is impossible to determine the causal direction of this relationship.

Regarding physical activity level, the Kruskal–Wallis test shows that there are no statistically significant differences in BMI values ($p = 0.0698 > 0.05$), although level 2 (Sufficient) shows slightly higher BMI values, but this difference is not statistically significant. Finally, it is interesting to note that there is a weak but significant positive correlation between the parameters of physical activity levels and adherence to the Mediterranean diet ($r = 0.16$; $p = 0.01$; $\chi^2 = 11.98$; $p = 0.017$). This may suggest that there is a tendency, albeit modest, to associate higher levels of physical activity with greater adherence to the Mediterranean diet and vice versa, and that targeted health promotion interventions aimed at filling individual gaps in terms of information and education on these issues could be effective tools for improving lifestyles in general. Based on the analysis of the data collected, the discrepancy between some WHO recommendations and detected eating habits suggests the need to implement nutrition education programs for young health workers, focusing particularly on the nursing graduating class. It would be absolutely strategic to develop strategies to encourage general consumption of fruits, vegetables and fish and, at the same time, promote greater awareness of the importance of following international nutritional guidelines. The analysis of adherence to the Mediterranean diet showed different dietary patterns among the professional groups examined, with the nursing student group showing lower average adherence values than the other groups examined. In addition, the discrepancy observed between the eating habits of all participants and the WHO nutritional recommendations regarding the consumption of certain foods underscores the need for targeted educational interventions.

Regarding physical activity, the results showed a general propensity for moderate physical activity, with a relatively low percentage of individuals not reaching the minimum levels recommended by WHO. However, the significant differences found between occupational groups and between genders suggest the need for a differentiated approach in the design of physical activity promotion interventions. In particular, the nursing student group showed significantly lower levels of total physical activity, a finding that, combined with lower adherence to the Mediterranean diet, configures a risk profile that requires special attention. The assessment of sedentary behaviors also revealed significant differences between the groups, with the medical group showing the highest levels of sedentariness during the workday. This finding underscores the importance of implementing strategies to reduce time spent sitting, considering that it is an independent risk factor for many chronic diseases.

Finally, a weak but significant positive correlation was found between the parameters of physical activity levels and adherence to the Mediterranean diet, suggesting that there is a tendency, albeit modest, to associate higher levels of physical activity with greater adherence to the Mediterranean diet and vice versa, and that could target health promotion interventions. Another interesting finding from the study is the positive, albeit weak, correlation between adherence to the Mediterranean diet and body mass index (BMI). This seemingly counterintuitive result could be explained by several factors. The PREDIMED score, while validated for assessing Mediterranean diet adherence, may not fully capture the quantitative aspects of food consumption or other lifestyle factors that influence BMI. Additionally, it is possible that subjects with a higher BMI have already undertaken lifestyle modifications, including the adoption of healthier eating patterns, as a response to their condition. However, the cross-sectional nature of the study does not allow causal relationships to be established.

Strengths and Limitations

Our recruitment strategy through preventive health visits, while systematic, may have introduced selection bias: our sample of students belonging to health-related degree programs might represent a more health-conscious subset of the student population. Additionally, while participation was voluntary, those who chose to participate might have been more interested in health-related behaviors, potentially leading to self-selection bias. However, our achieved sample size (242) exceeded the minimum required sample size (174) calculated through G*Power analysis ($\alpha = 0.05$, power = 0.80, medium effect size = 0.25), suggesting adequate statistical power for our analyses.

The use of self-administered questionnaires to assess eating habits and physical activity may be subject to bias; the PREDIMED questionnaire, while a validated instrument, focuses on frequency of food consumption rather than actual quantities, limiting the ability to assess total caloric intake. Another limitation concerns the PREDIMED questionnaire's score regarding wine consumption, as future studies might benefit from modified scoring systems that better align with contemporary public health recommendations. Furthermore, although possible causal relationships between the variables are suggested, the cross-sectional design used does not allow for causal inferences to be drawn. Despite these limitations, the results provide important insights into health promotion for the University of Campania peer group. In particular, the following recommendations emerge: it would be necessary to implement specific nutrition education programs for different professional groups, with particular attention to nursing students. These programs should focus not only on the transmission of theoretical knowledge but also on the development of practical skills for the adoption of proper Mediterranean alimentation. In addition, physical activity promotion interventions should be differentiated according to gender and occupational group. Particular attention should be paid to reducing sedentary behavior during working hours.

5. Conclusions

The study highlighted the need for a systematic and differentiated approach to workplace health promotion, with special attention to the specifics of different occupational groups. It is desirable to implement a system of continuous monitoring radiation of eating habits and physical activity, possibly through the use of objective instruments and detailed food diaries. Integrating personalized dietary and physical activity assessment and counseling into routine occupational health surveillance would allow for early identification of individuals at risk and provide opportunities for personalized intervention. This could involve the use of validated questionnaires during periodic health checks and the provision of tailored advice. Targeted awareness campaigns should be developed to educate healthcare students about the benefits of regular physical activity, with particular attention to gender-specific barriers and motivators. In addition, for future research, longitudinal studies should be conducted to assess the temporal evolution of eating habits and physical activity. Furthermore, the relationship between Mediterranean diet adherence and BMI in young adult students may be influenced by factors not captured in our study, such as total caloric intake, portion sizes or the timing of meals—variables that should be considered in future investigations. It would also be necessary to expand the sample to include a more representative population of all equated workers and to adopt an integrated approach that considers not only individual behavioral aspects but also environmental and organizational factors that may influence workers' health choices. Even the understanding of the level of awareness regarding health risks associated with unhealthy lifestyles among healthcare students is crucial. Future studies should assess risk perception and health literacy concerning dietary habits and physical activity, as these factors may significantly influence behavior change and also influence the rate of participation in specific WHP initiatives.

Author Contributions: Conceptualization, M.L. and N.M.; methodology, E.M.G. and A.R.C.; formal analysis, G.P. and N.M.; investigation, G.P., D.G. and M.S.; data curation, E.M.G., A.R.C. and G.P.; writing—original draft preparation, E.M.G., G.P. and N.M.; writing—review and editing, E.M.G.; supervision, M.L. All authors have read and agreed to the published version of the manuscript.

Funding: This research received no external funding.

Data Availability Statement: The data presented in this study are available on request from the corresponding author.

Conflicts of Interest: The authors declare no conflicts of interest.

References

1. Andersen, L.L. Health Promotion and Chronic Disease Prevention at the Workplace. *Ann. Rev. Public. Health* **2024**, *45*, 337–357. [CrossRef] [PubMed]
2. WHO; Burton. WHO Healthy Workplace Framework and Model: Background and Supporting Literature and Practices. 2010. Available online: https://iris.who.int/bitstream/handle/10665/113144/9789241500241_eng.pdf (accessed on 7 October 2024).

3. Antonaci, F.G.; Olivetti, E.C.; Marcolin, F.; Castiblanco Jimenez, I.A.; Eynard, B.; Vezzetti, E.; Moos, S. Workplace Well-Being in Industry 5.0: A Worker-Centered Systematic Review. *Sensors* **2024**, *24*, 5473. [CrossRef]
4. Elizabeth, L.; Machado, P.; Zinöcker, M.; Baker, P.; Lawrence, M. Ultra-Processed Foods and Health Outcomes: A Narrative Review. *Nutrients* **2020**, *12*, 1955. [CrossRef] [PubMed]
5. Ejtahed, H.S.; Mardi, P.; Hejrani, B.; Mahdavi, F.S.; Ghoreshi, B.; Gohari, K.; Heidari-Beni, M.; Qorbani, M. Association between junk food consumption and mental health problems in adults: A systematic review and meta-analysis. *BMC Psychiatry* **2024**, *24*, 438. [CrossRef]
6. The GBD 2015 Obesity Collaborators. Health Effects of Overweight and Obesity in 195 Countries over 25 Years. *N. Engl. J. Med.* **2017**, *377*, 13–27. [CrossRef]
7. Mattavelli, E.; Olmastroni, E.; Bonofiglio, D.; Catapano, A.L.; Baragetti, A.; Magni, P. Adherence to the Mediterranean Diet: Impact of Geographical Location of the Observations. *Nutrients* **2022**, *14*, 2040. [CrossRef]
8. Serra-Majem, L.; Tomaino, L.; Dernini, S.; Berry, E.M.; Lairon, D.; Ngo de la Cruz, J.; Bach-Faig, A.; Donini, L.M.; Medina, F.-X.; Belahsen, R.; et al. Updating the Mediterranean Diet Pyramid towards Sustainability: Focus on Environmental Concerns. *Int. J. Environ. Res. Public. Health* **2020**, *17*, 8758. [CrossRef]
9. Finicelli, M.; Di Salle, A.; Galderisi, U.; Peluso, G. The Mediterranean Diet: An Update of the Clinical Trials. *Nutrients* **2022**, *14*, 2956. [CrossRef]
10. Obeid, C.A.; Gubbels, J. S.; Jaalouk, D.; Kremers, S.P.J.; Oenema, A. Adherence to the Mediterranean diet among adults in Mediterranean countries: A systematic literature review. *Eur. J. Nutr.* **2022**, *61*, 3327–3344. [CrossRef]
11. Bull, F.C.; Al-Ansari, S.S.; Biddle, S.; Borodulin, K.; Buman, M.P.; Cardon, G.; Carty, C.; Chaput, J.-P.; Chastin, S.; Chou, R.; et al. World Health Organization 2020 guidelines on physical activity and sedentary behaviour. *Br. J. Sports Med.* **2020**, *54*, 1451–1462. [CrossRef] [PubMed]
12. Epicentro Istituto Superiore di Sanità. 2022. Available online: https://www.epicentro.iss.it/passi/ (accessed on 15 December 2024).
13. Smith, S.S. NCHS Dataline. *Public. Health Rep.* **2014**, *129*, 200–202. [CrossRef]
14. Wen, C.P.; Wai, J.P.; Tsai, M.K.; Yang, Y.C.; Cheng, T.Y.; Lee, M.C.; Chan, H.T.; Tsao, C.K.; Tsai, S.P.; Wu, X. Minimum amount of physical activity for reduced mortality and extended life expectancy: A prospective cohort study. *Lancet* **2011**, *378*, 1244–1253. [CrossRef] [PubMed]
15. Fernández-Lázaro, C.I.; Ruiz-Canela, M.; Martínez-González, M.Á. Deep dive to the secrets of the PREDIMED trial. *Curr. Opin. Lipidol.* **2021**, *32*, 62–69. [CrossRef] [PubMed]
16. Sember, V.; Meh, K.; Sorić, M.; Starc, G.; Rocha, P.; Jurak, G. Validity and Reliability of International Physical Activity Questionnaires for Adults across EU Countries: Systematic Review and Meta Analysis. *Int. J. Environ. Res. Public. Health* **2020**, *17*, 7161. [CrossRef] [PubMed]
17. Veronese, N.; Notarnicola, M.; Cisternino, A.M.; Inguaggiato, R.; Guerra, V.; Reddavide, R.; Donghia, R.; Rotolo, O.; Zinzi, I.; Leandro, G.; et al. MICOL study group. Trends in adherence to the Mediterranean diet in South Italy: A cross sectional study. *Nutr. Metab. Cardiovasc. Dis.* **2020**, *30*, 410–417. [CrossRef] [PubMed]
18. Braune, T.; Kudlek, L.; Xiao, C.; Tang, H.; Demers-Potvin, É.; Harris, H.A.; Fitzsimons-West, E.; Adams, J.; Winpenny, E.M. Interpersonal determinants of diet quality and eating behaviors in people aged 13-30 years: A systematic scoping review. *Obes. Rev.* **2025**, *26*, e13835. [CrossRef]
19. Huang, Z.; Liu, Y.; Zhou, Y. Sedentary Behaviors and Health Outcomes among Young Adults: A Systematic Review of Longitudinal Studies. *Healthcare* **2022**, *10*, 1480. [CrossRef] [PubMed]
20. Zhao, J.; Stockwell, T.; Naimi, T.; Churchill, S.; Clay, J.; Sherk, A. Association Between Daily Alcohol Intake and Risk of All-Cause Mortality: A Systematic Review and Meta-analyses. *JAMA Netw. Open* **2023**, *6*, e236185. [CrossRef] [PubMed]
21. McCarthy, C.; Warne, J.P. Gender differences in physical activity status and knowledge of Irish University staff and students. *Sport. Sci. Health* **2022**, *18*, 1283–1291. [CrossRef]

environments

MDPI

Article

Impact of Environmental Pollutants on Otorhinolaryngological Emergencies in the COVID-19 Era

Tommaso Saccardo [1,*], Elisa Masetto [2], Elia Biancoli [1], Anna Rachel Colombo [1], Antonio Daloiso [1], Alessandra Deretti [1], Francesco Benvegnù [1], Maria Angiola Crivellaro [3], Marco Marani [4], Piero Nicolai [1], Rosario Marchese Ragona [1], Gino Marioni [1], Bruno Scarpa [2] and Giancarlo Ottaviano [1]

1 Department of Neurosciences, Otolaryngology Section, University of Padova, 35122 Padova, Italy
2 Department of Statistical Sciences, University of Padova, 35122 Padova, Italy
3 Department of Cardiac Thoracic Vascular Sciences and Public Health, University of Padova, 35128 Padua, Italy
4 Department of Civil and Environmental Engineering, University of Padova, 35131 Padua, Italy
* Correspondence: tommaso.saccardo@unipd.it

Abstract: Air pollution (AP) is a critical environmental factor influencing public health, with well-documented associations with upper respiratory tract (URT) diseases. This study investigates the relationship between ENT emergency department (ENT-ED) visits at Azienda Ospedale Università di Padova (AOPD) and daily concentrations of environmental pollutants during the first year of the COVID-19 pandemic (March 2020–March 2021), compared to pre-pandemic data from 2017. The study focuses on patients diagnosed with URT inflammatory diseases, excluding those with COVID-19 infection, who sought care at the AOPD ENT-ED. Environmental data, including meteorological variables, air pollutants, and major aeroallergen levels, were collected from regional monitoring stations. A total of 4594 patients were admitted in 2020/2021, marking a 37% reduction from 2017, with URT inflammatory admissions decreasing by 52%. A significant decline in PM10, NO_2 and *Alternaria* levels was observed, whereas *Betullaceae* and *Corylaceae* concentrations significantly increased. Multivariate analyses revealed strong associations between aeroallergen exposure and ENT admissions, particularly for *Alternaria*, which had a notable impact on total admissions ($p < 0.001$) and was significantly linked to cases of otitis media and tonsillitis. PM10 concentrations on specific days preceding ED visits were associated with increased incidences of pharyngitis and rhinosinusitis ($p < 0.05$). These findings reinforce the connection between environmental pollutants and ENT emergency visits, highlighting the adverse effects of AP and climate variables on URT diseases, even during a pandemic when enhanced airway protection measures were in place. This study underscores the necessity of stringent air quality regulations and interdisciplinary strategies to mitigate environmental health risks and inform future public health policies.

Keywords: pollution; upper respiratory tract; emergency; pollens; particulate matter; COVID-19; air quality; environment

1. Introduction

The World Health Organization (WHO) officially declared COVID-19 a global pandemic on 11 March 2020 [1]. Governments around the world implemented massive travel restrictions (through the so called "lockdown"—partial or total) to mitigate the spread of this global infection [2]. These decisions brought sudden and immense changes to human activities: not only a reduction in traveling, but also a decrease in access to medical care for reasons unrelated to COVID-19 [3]. Healthcare providers reduced their routine activities, such as surgery or other medical services that were not considered "essential" or urgent, to provide treatment for COVID-19 cases [4]. Furthermore, people reduced their access to health institutions for fear of exposing themselves to the viral infection.

In the General Emergency Departments of the Veneto Region, Italy, an absolute decrease in hospitalizations was described during the lockdown periods, with some of them, such as those due to traumas, accidents at work and road accidents, declining due to lower risk exposure [5]. In other cases, a different perception of urgency in such a dramatic situation often caused patients to avoid seeking medical evaluation even when in need [6,7].

The forced reduction in human activity in cities resulted in a subsequent decrease in air pollution derived from vehicular traffic and industrial activity. In Italy, measurements and comparisons have been conducted on the concentration of environmental pollutants such as particulate matter (PM), carbon monoxide (CO), ozone (O_3) and nitrogen dioxide (NO_2), showing a significant decline in these pollutants during the restrictions [8,9]. Variations in air pollutants (AP), pollen concentration and climatic variations may have an impact on upper respiratory tract (URT) pathology, especially in pollen-allergic patients [10].

The impact of these variables on accesses to the Ear, Nose and Throat (ENT) Emergency Department (ED) admissions in the Azienda Ospedale Università di Padova (AOPD) has already been investigated in the pre-COVID era [11]. The correlation between air quality and human health is receiving increasing attention, yet its connection to ENT urgencies during the COVID-19 pandemic has remained relatively unexplored.

In this study, we aim to describe new data that may contribute to a deeper understanding of environmental impacts on otorhinolaryngological pathologies during the pandemic and provide useful insights for managing future health emergencies.

We examined the impact of the pandemic on ENT ED admissions in the AOPD (I), focusing on variations in the number and typology of admissions during restriction periods. We also conducted an analysis on the changes in environmental pollutants such as PM, chemicals and pollens in the same timeframe (II). Through a comparison with the pre-pandemic period, we aimed to identify trends and substantial changes in the patterns of ENT ED admission in our center (III), as well as to assess the potential role of environmental pollutants in this context (IV).

2. Materials and Methods

This is a retrospective study conducted at the ENT ED of the AOPD, Italy. The data analyzed were provided in reference to two timeframes: from 1 January 2017 to 31 December 2017 and from 9 March 2020 (beginning of Italian lockdown) to March 8th 2021. Both periods therefore cover the duration of one year and refer to two different circumstances: the first timeframe refers to a situation of normality, whereas the second refers to the first year of the COVID-19 pandemic.

The study was conducted in accordance with the ethical standards of the Helsinki Declaration. Data were examined in agreement with the Italian privacy and sensitive data laws and the internal regulations of the AOPD. Informed consent on personal data collection and use for research purpose was obtained from each subject.

2.1. Population Considered

The AOPD is a tertiary teaching hospital in the Italian region of Veneto that covers a population of roughly 350,000 people and records more than 85,000 referrals to the Emergency Department every year.

In this study, only patients admitted to the ED with a negative nasopharyngeal swab and then referred to the ENT emergency room during the aforementioned time frames were considered. All patients underwent high-sensitivity nasopharyngeal swab testing for SARS-CoV-2 upon ED admission, as soon as such tests became available. Those with signs or symptoms suggestive of COVID-19 followed a dedicated triage pathway. Only patients with confirmed negative results and no clinical suspicion of infection were eligible for ENT evaluation.

For each patient, we recorded the date of the ED admission, sex, date of birth, main diagnosis and comorbidities.

Patients with URT disorders (including pharyngitis, laryngitis, otitis, rhinosinusitis, tonsillitis and tracheitis) were included in the study group while those referred for facial trauma or foreign body inhalation formed the control group, as previously described by Ottaviano et al. [11].

2.2. Pollution and Meteorological Data

Daily AP concentration (NO_2, O_3 and PM10 expressed in $\mu g/m^3$), rainfall depth (mm), air temperature (°C), minimum and maximum relative humidity (%) and the concentration (g/m^3) of the most common aeroallergens in the Padua urban area were obtained from environmental monitoring stations operated by the Regional Agency for Environmental Protection and Prevention of the Veneto Region (ARPAV).

The aeroallergens considered were the following:

- *Alternaria*: A genus of fungi widely distributed in the environment, particularly in decaying vegetation and soil. It is a major source of outdoor mold allergens.
- *Betulaceae*: A family of trees including birch (*Betula* spp.), which are significant pollen producers in temperate regions, especially in the spring season.
- *Compositae* (*Asteraceae*): A large family of flowering plants including ragweed, mugwort, and others. These produce highly allergenic pollen particularly in late summer and autumn.
- *Corylaceae*: A botanical family that includes hazel (*Corylus* spp.) and hornbeam. Pollen from these trees is prevalent in early spring.
- *Gramineae* (*Poaceae*): The grass family, a major source of allergenic pollen worldwide. Grass pollens are typically abundant in late spring and early summer.

For O_3 and NO_2, the daily maximum value was considered, for humidity, the daily maximum and minimum values were considered and for all other variables, the average of 24-hourly measurements in the same day were used. To account for temporal trends and delayed effects, we also considered the moving average of mean values over four consecutive days [ma], as well as the lagged effects at one and two days [lag 1] and [lag 2].

2.3. Statistical Analysis

Descriptive statistics are represented by the median (interquartile range) for continuous variables and absolute values (percentage) for categorical variables. An exploratory analysis of environmental variables was carried out by studying the pairwise correlations (Pearson correlation coefficient).

The univariate analyses, which explored the relationships between response variables and risk factors, were carried out by generalized models with Poisson linkage, both in the linear (GLM—Generalized Linear Model) and additive (GAM—Generalized Additive Model) versions.

The model structure for generalized model is

$$g(\mu) = \alpha + \Sigma_j f_j (X_j)$$

where g is the link function (in the case of the Poisson model, the link function is the logarithmic function), α is the model intercept, μ is the mean of the response variable conditioned on the explanatory variables and X_j; f_j are the linear functions in the case of the GLM and non-parametric smoothing functions in the case of the GAM.

Multivariate analyses, considering the adjustment for potential confounders (climate variables: temperature, maximum and minimum humidity and rainfall), were carried out with the additive models to consider the possible presence of non-parametric effects. Interactions between timeframes and risk factors were examined with a non-parametric approach using GAMs. This approach was also used to assess the differences between temporal distribution of environmental variables and number of total admissions in the two timeframes.

It is important to note that the use of non-parametric methods, such as GAMs, helps reduce the influence of extreme values (outliers) on the analysis. These values were intentionally retained, as they may represent genuine extreme environmental events that are highly relevant to the objectives of this study.

p-Values were calculated, and 5% was considered the critical level of significance. All analyses were performed using R, a language and environment for statistical computing (R Foundation for Statistical Computing, Vienna, Austria) [12].

3. Results

3.1. Emergency Department Admissions

The total number of admissions in 2017 and 2020/2021 were 7278 and 4594, respectively.

Figure 1 shows the time series of total visits throughout the two years, with the interpolating curves fitted by the GAM.

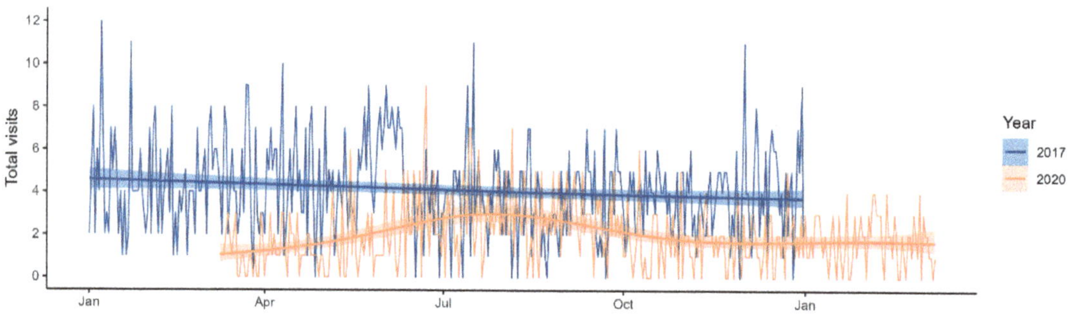

Figure 1. Number and temporal trends of emergency room admissions in 2017 and 2020/2021.

Table 1 displays the descriptive statistics of ENT emergency room admissions.

In 2020/2021, there was a reduction in total admissions of 37%. Focusing only on URT inflammatory disease admissions, there was a 52% reduction, decreasing from a total of 1502 admissions in 2017 to 726 in the 2020–2021 timeframe. In both cases, the reduction in admissions in the second timeframe was statistically significant (p-value < 0.001). When considering only admissions for URT inflammations, it was found that in 2017, the disease causing more admissions was otitis (29% of URT admissions), and this percentage decreased to 22% in 2020/2021, being surpassed by pharyngitis (37% of URT admissions).

Considering trauma and foreign bodies, in 2020/2021, there was a 35.6% reduction, decreasing from 4866 to 3137.

Table 1. Absolute distribution (percentage) by gender and main diagnosis of emergency room admission; median (IQR) by age.

	2017	2020/2021
Sex		
Female	3674 (50%)	2220 (48%)
Male	3604 (50%)	2374 (52%)
Age (years)	47 (29, 67)	52 (31, 71)
Diagnosis		
Pharyngitis	210 (3%)	272 (6%)
Laryngitis	273 (3.7%)	91 (2%)
Otitis	433 (6%)	158 (3.4%)
Rhinosinusitis	229 (3.1%)	84 (1.8%)
Tonsillitis	353 (4.8%)	112 (2.4%)
Tracheitis	4 (0.1%)	9 (0.2%)
Traumas	910 (12.5%)	731 (16%)
Others	4866 (66.8%)	3137 (68.2%)
Total admissions	7278 (100%)	4594 (100%)

Figure 2 highlights the percentage reduction in 2020/2021 compared to 2017 of URT admissions and traumas admissions, respectively.

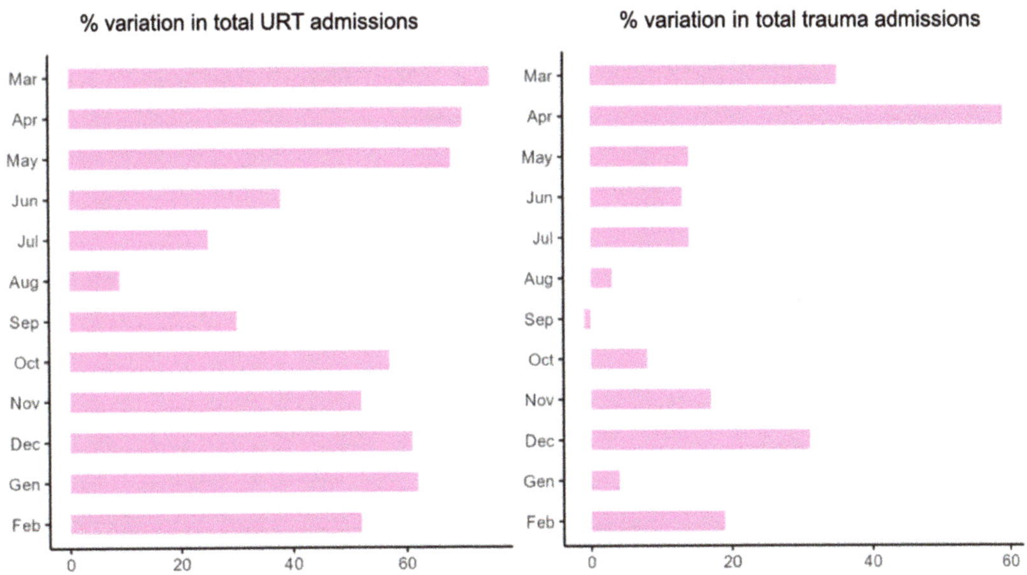

Figure 2. Percentage reduction in 2020/2021 compared to 2017 of total URT admissions and trauma admissions during 2020/2021.

3.2. Environmental Variables

The distributions of environmental variables have been depicted through box plots in Figure 3. For allergens and precipitation, the graph focuses on non-zero values for better interpretability. The significance of the difference in the distributions of the two timeframes was assessed based on the temporal trends, as follows.

Figures 4–6 compare the temporal trend of allergens, climatic variables and pollutants, respectively.

In 2020/2021, levels of *Alternaria* appeared significantly lower compared to 2017 (p-value < 0.001), especially during summer, when the concentration peaked. The release of *Betullaceae* and *Corylaceae* occurred later in the year, reaching higher peaks compared to those recorded in 2017 (p-value < 0.001). The concentrations of *Compositae* and *Gramineae* were essentially the same in both periods (p-value = 0.471 and p-value = 0.656, respectively).

No significant differences were detected in the two timeframes for temperature, minimum humidity and rainfall time trends. Maximum humidity was significantly higher in 2020/2021 compared to 2017 (p-value = 0.003). Regarding PM10 levels (Figure 6), the concentration was significantly lower in 2020/2021 compared to 2017 (p-value < 0.001), especially in the months between April and October. The same behavior was observed for NO_2, showing a significantly lower concentration in 2020/2021 (p-value < 0.001). O_3 levels remained substantially unchanged, similarly to the pattern observed for temperature (p-value = 0.284).

Figure 7 shows the scatter plots amongst the environmental variables with significant correlations in 2020/2021 (p-value < 0.05). PM10 results were negatively associated with temperature (correlation = −0.51), whilst they were positively correlated with NO_2 (correlation = 0.61). O_3 was positively associated with temperature and negatively with PM (correlation of 0.83 and −0.54, respectively). *Alternaria* concentration was positively correlated with temperature (correlation = 0.75), and *Betullaceae* concentration was positively associated with *Corylaceae* concentration (correlation = 0.82).

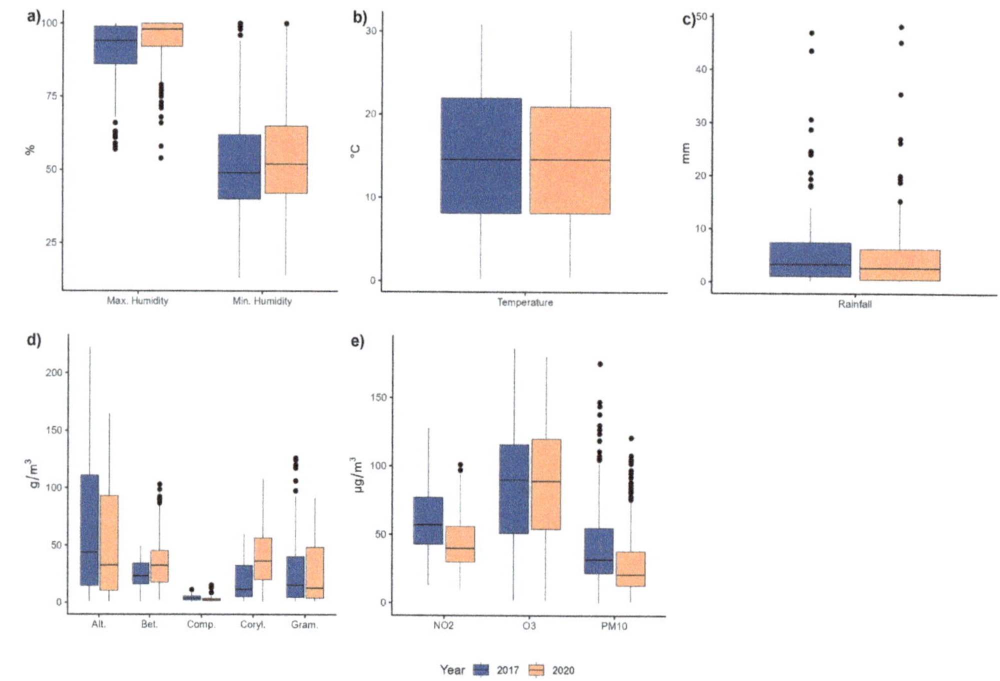

Figure 3. Distributions of environmental variables (**a**,**b**), precipitations (**c**), allergens (**d**) and AP (**e**) in 2017 and 2020/2021.

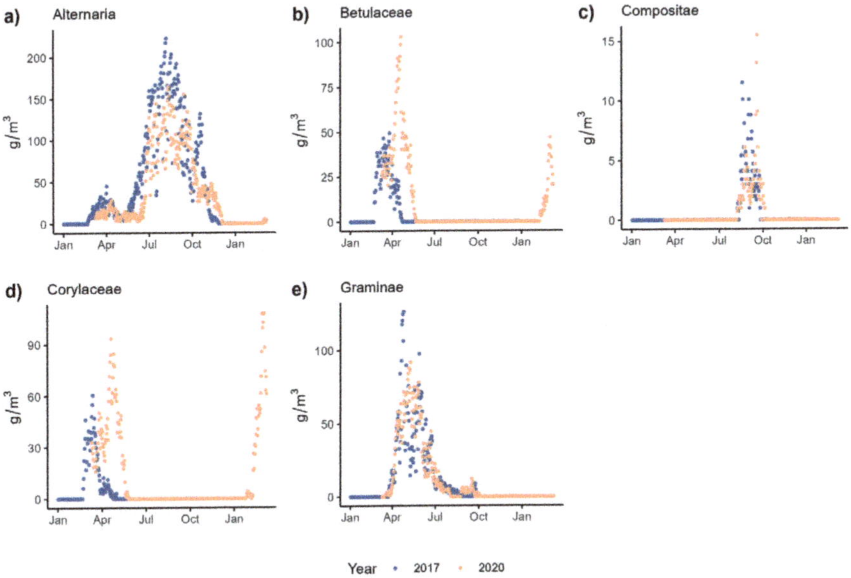

Figure 4. Temporal trends of allergens as measured by local environmental monitoring stations in 2017 and 2020/2021.

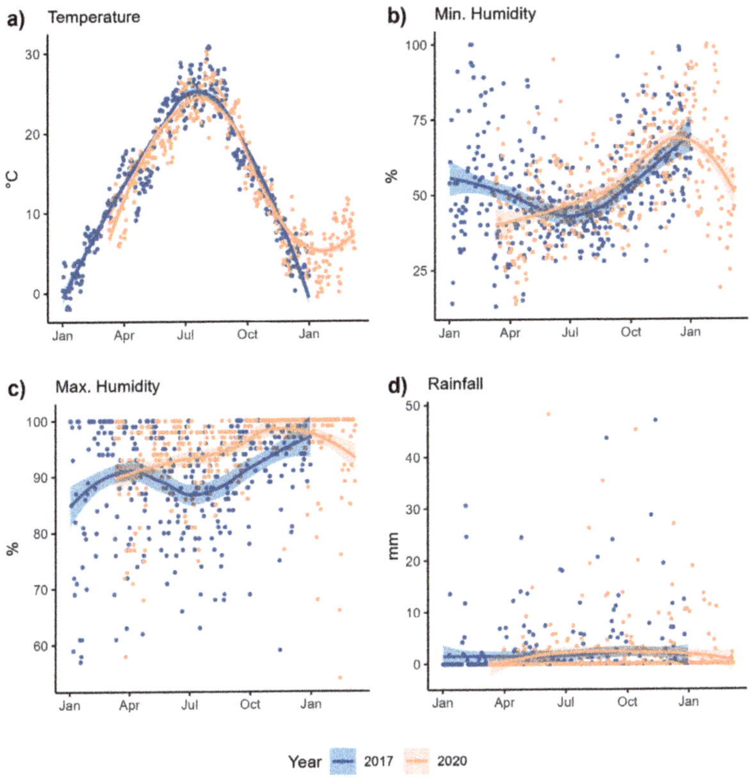

Figure 5. Temporal trends of climatic variables as measured by local environmental monitoring stations in 2017 and 2020/2021.

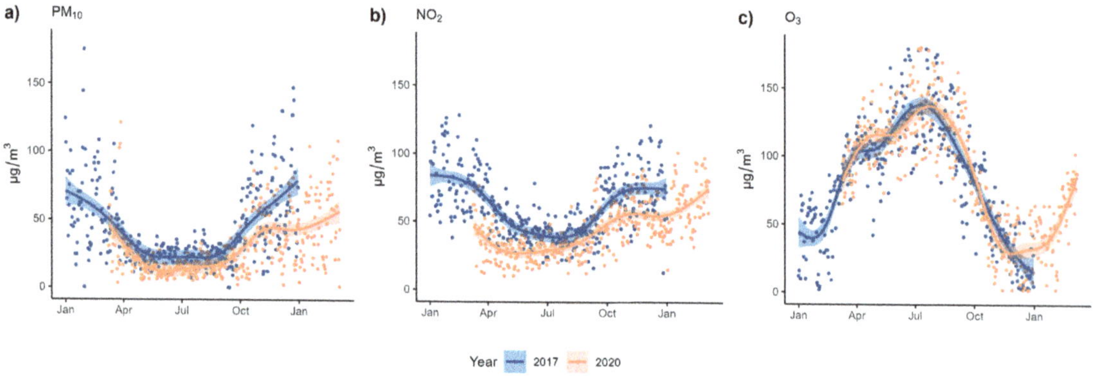

Figure 6. Temporal trends of AP in 2017 and 2020/2021.

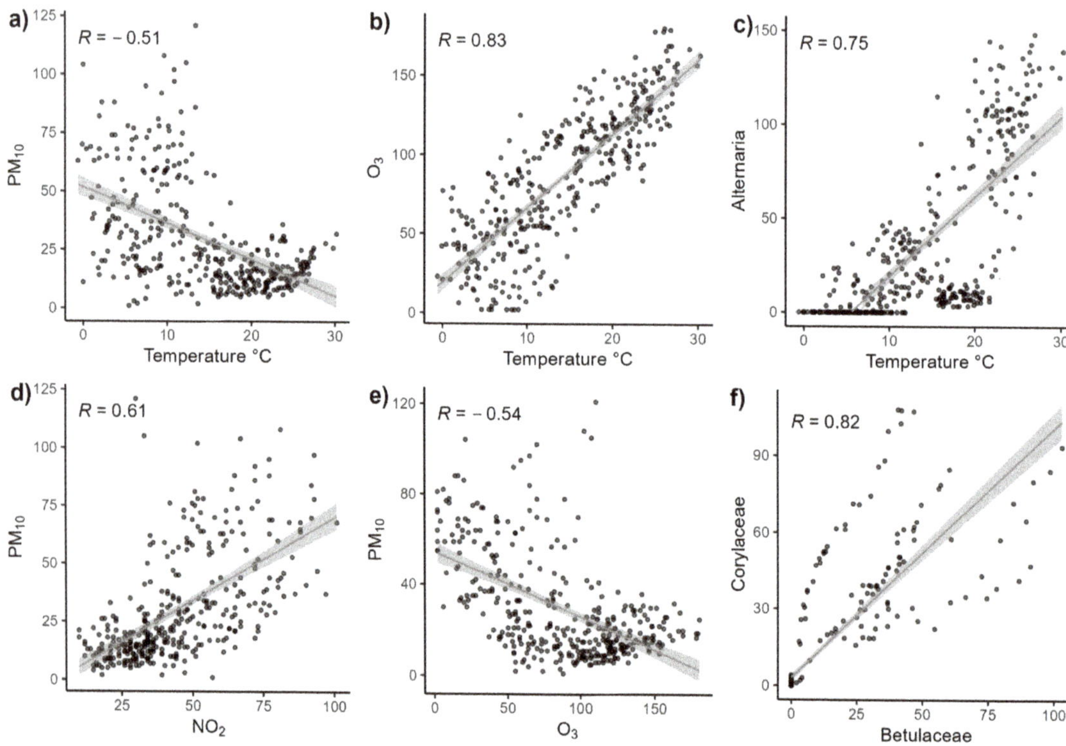

Figure 7. Scatter plots illustrating the relationships between the environmental variables with significant correlation in 2020/2021. Regression line with 95% confidence interval; R represents the Pearson correlation coefficient (all p-values < 0.001).

3.3. Environment and URT Admissions

The influence of environmental factors on the daily number of emergency room admissions in 2020/2021 was analyzed. To capture any non-linear effects, while maintaining good interpretability of the results, univariate Poisson-type GAMs were adapted. Table 2 shows the p-values associated with each non-parametric effect. For each model, graphs showing the significant effects are presented in Supplementary Materials Figure S1.1–S1.6.

Table 2. *p*-Values of the effects obtained from univariate GAMs.

	Total URT	Otitis	Rhino-Sinusitis	Pharyngitis	Laryngitis	Tonsillitis
Alternaria	**<0.001**	**<0.001**	0.108	**0.024**	**0.018**	**<0.001**
Betulaceae	**<0.001**	**0.001**	0.275	**<0.001**	0.314	**0.003**
Compositae	**0.002**	0.636	**0.004**	0.219	0.295	**0.003**
Corylaceae	**<0.001**	**0.042**	0.109	**0.002**	0.300	**0.003**
Gramineae	**0.001**	0.377	0.468	**<0.001**	0.840	**0.017**
PM10	**0.003**	0.407	0.155	**0.014**	0.992	0.354
O_3	**<0.001**	0.075	0.233	**0.004**	0.072	0.943
NO_2	**0.003**	0.083	0.960	0.055	0.184	0.265
Temperature	**<0.001**	**0.007**	**0.047**	**<0.001**	0.113	0.113
Max. Humidity	0.685	0.749	0.316	0.152	0.533	0.640
Min. Humidity	**0.046**	**0.034**	0.116	0.113	**0.004**	0.149
Rainfall	0.443	0.252	0.465	0.086	0.522	0.113

From the univariate analysis, it emerged that *Alternaria* had a positive and linear effect on admissions for middle ear infection, pharyngitis, laryngitis and URT diseases, while the effect of *Corylaceae* showed a decreasing and then increasing trend starting at approximately 60 g/m^3 (30 g/m^3 for middle ear infection). *Betullaceae* pollen had an increasing effect after about 40 g/m^3 on middle ear infection and respiratory system-related admissions; for the latter, *Gramineae* pollen started to have an increasing effect at around 50 g/m^3. *Compositae* pollen was a risk factor for sinusitis, tonsillitis and URT admissions up to approximately 5 g/m^3.

Regarding pollutants, there was a positive effect of O_3 on total admissions, URT-related admissions and pharyngitis, while NO_2 showed a nearly constant trend. Fine particulate matter had a negative effect on URT-related admissions and pharyngitis.

3.4. Multivariate Analysis

To investigate the effect of pollutants in greater detail, GAMs were fitted for each type of admission and separately for each pollutant, also considering delayed effects of the pollutant and adjustment for possible confounders (climate variables). In order to simplify the model, the non-parametric effects were converted to parametric if the effect was linear, and a stepwise backward selection procedure was adopted. The significant results are displayed in Table 3. For parametric effects, results are expressed as Incidence Rate Ratios (IRRs) with 95% confidence intervals (CIs), indicating the multiplicative change in the mean number of ED admissions per 10-unit increase in the exposure variable. When effects were non-parametric, they could not be summarized as IRRs and are instead graphically represented in the Supplementary Materials (Figure S2).

A significant effect of the cumulative mean value of PM10 was found for pharyngitis. The effect showed an increasing trend from around 30 $\mu g/m^3$. A positive, linear effect of the PM10 delayed at day 1 for rhinosinusitis was found, too (an increase of 10 $\mu g/m^3$ of PM10 delayed at day 1 is associated with an 35.4% [0.30–78.1] increase in the average number of rhinosinusitis admissions). A positive and linear effect of *Alternaria* was observed for tonsillitis and otitis admissions (increase of 15.1% [0.7–24.0] and 11.4% [0.5–18.5], respectively), confirming the results of the univariate analysis. Otitis was also positively influenced by the concentration of *Betulaceae* starting around 30 g/m^3, as were URT admissions. *Corylaceae* showed a positive effect on pharyngitis and URT admissions starting around 60 g/m^3.

Table 3. Significant effects obtained from multivariate GAMs are expressed as Incidence Rate Ratios, if parametric; (*p*) = non-parametric effect was turned into parametric; [ma] = mobile average, mean values in four consecutive days. Graphs showing the non-parametric effect are presented in Supplementary Materials Figure S2.

Risk Factor	Response	Incidence Rate Ratio [95% CI]	*p*-Value
O_3 lag 2 (*p*)	Pharyngitis	0.879 [0.776; 0.996]	0.042
O_3 lag 2 (*p*)	URT	0.959 [0.927; 0.991]	0.013
PM10 [ma]	Pharyngitis		0.017
PM10 lag 1 (*p*)	Rinosinusitis	1.354 [1.030; 1.781]	0.035
NO_2 [ma]	Pharyngitis		0.015
Alternaria (*p*)	Otitis	1.114 [1.046; 1.185]	<0.001
Alternaria (*p*)	Tonsillitis	1.151 [1.068; 1.240]	<0.001
Alternaria (*p*)	Pharyngitis	0.944 [0.904; 0.985]	0.008
Gramineae (*p*)	Otitis	0.894 [0.804; 0.994]	0.038
Gramineae (*p*)	Tonsillitis	0.804 [0.681; 0.948]	0.009
Gramineae	Pharyngitis		0.025
Betulaceae	URT		0.032
Betulaceae	Otitis		0.011
Corylaceae	URT		0.036
Corylaceae	Pharyngitis		0.008

3.5. Model Comparison Between 2017 and 2020/2021

A further comparison of the multivariate models investigating the effects of pollutants including the interaction between timeframe and risk factor was performed. The models were constructed by initially including lagged effects and confounders; they were then simplified by removing non-significant terms. The significant results are displayed in Table 4. The parametric effects are presented as IRRs. When effects were non-parametric, they could not be summarized as IRRs and are instead graphically represented in the Supplementary Materials Figure S3.

Table 4. Models that consider 2017 and 2020/2021 data by including the interaction between timeframe and risk factor. Significant effects obtained from multivariate GAM are expressed as Incidence Rate Ratioa, if parametric; (*p*) = non-parametric effect was turned into parametric; [ma] = mobile average, mean values in four consecutive days. Graphs showing the non-parametric effect are presented in Supplementary Materials Figure S3.

Risk Factor	Response	Incidence Rate Ratio 2017 [95% CI]	Incidence Rate Ratio 2020/2021 [95% CI]	*p*-Value 2017	*p*-Value 2020/2021
PM10 [ma]	URT			**0.037**	0.159
PM10 [ma] (*p*)	Otitis media	**1.047 [1.001; 1.094]**	0.939 [0.857; 1.030]	**0.046**	0.181
PM10 [ma]	Pharyngitis			0.347	**0.001**
PM10 [ma] (*p*)	Tonsillitis	**1.209 [1.054; 1.388]**	**1.234 [1.041; 1.463]**	**0.007**	**0.015**
NO_2 (*p*)	Otitis media	**1.067 [1.017; 1.120]**	0.923 [0.843; 1.009]	**0.009**	0.078
Alternaria (*p*)	URT	**0.971 [0.958; 0.983]**	**1.032 [1.013; 1.051]**	**<0.001**	**0.001**
Alternaria (*p*)	Otitis media	**0.958 [0.934; 0.983]**	**1.047 [1.008; 1.088]**	**0.001**	**0.018**
Alternaria (*p*)	Rinosinusitis	0.992 [0.959; 1.026]	**1.064 [1.009; 1.123]**	0.652	**0.023**
Alternaria (*p*)	Pharyngitis	**0.940 [0.910; 0.971]**	0.974 [0.940; 1.008]	**<0.001**	0.131
Alternaria (*p*)	Tonsillitis	0.987 [0.962; 1.013]	**1.079 [1.035; 1.125]**	0.314	**<0.001**
Betulacee	URT			**0.033**	**<0.001**
Betulacee	Otitis media			**0.001**	**<0.001**
Corylaceae	URT			**0.005**	**<0.001**

Table 4. *Cont.*

Risk Factor	Response	Incidence Rate Ratio 2017 [95% CI]	Incidence Rate Ratio 2020/2021 [95% CI]	*p*-Value 2017	*p*-Value 2020/2021
Corylaceae	Otitis media			**<0.001**	0.064
Corylaceae	Pharyngitis			0.978	**0.003**
Corylaceae	Tonsillitis			0.870	**0.007**

Regarding pollutants, the cumulative mean value of PM10 maintained its positive effect on tonsillitis in both time periods analyzed, while its effect on pharyngitis was detected only during the 2020/2021 period. The NO_2 effect on otitis media was not confirmed in the second timeframe, while it presented a positive linear effect in 2017.

Alternaria showed a significant positive linear effect in 2020/2021 on most URT-related admissions. *Betullaceae* concentration presented a risk effect for middle ear infection and URT-related admissions in 2020/2021 after about 50 g/m^3, while in 2017, the effect was almost linear. *Corylaceae* retained their effect on the total number of admissions in the two periods: in 2017, the effect was linear, whilst in 2020/2021, it showed a decreasing and then increasing trend starting around approximately 60 g/m^3.

4. Discussion

4.1. Reduction in ENT ED Accesses

Our research primarily examined how the Italian COVID-19 lockdown affected the number of admissions for ENT-related disorders at a tertiary emergency department in the Veneto Region. As expected, we found a consistent overall reduction in the number of patients admitted to our ED: the number of overall admissions was reduced by over a third while the number of specific admissions for inflammatory diseases of the URT was reduced by over half. This was in line with the previous findings in other tertiary referral centers in Italy that described a reduction in ENT-related ED admissions between 62.16 and 71.5% [13,14]. These studies, however, only focused on the earlier months of the pandemic. Similar trends have also been described in the pediatric population, with a significant decrease in patients' attendance to the pediatric ED, especially in cases caused by ENT-related disorders [15].

It was challenging to find a comprehensive explanation for the effect of the pandemic on ENT-emergencies. However, we had to consider that at the onset of the pandemic, the Veneto Region implemented healthcare policies aimed at discouraging non-urgent visits to hospital clinics and in-person visits to family practitioners. This might have resulted in several patients not seeking medical treatment for minor issues. The reduction could also be due to the fear of contracting the virus in hospitals or outpatient clinics. These elements, along with restricted access to consultations and the increased use of telemedicine [16], might have led to two outcomes: a reduction in the total number of ENT-ED admissions and the selection of only the most complex cases. Similar scenarios have already been described in previous investigations by Pontillo et al. [17] and Gallo et al. [18], emphasizing the increase in complex or late-diagnosed cases and emergency/urgent surgeries.

4.2. Environmental Pollutants and URT Manifestations

In parallel with the reduction in admissions to the ED, there was a significant reduction in AP, in particular PM and NO_2. Road traffic was the major anthropic component that showed a clear reduction relative to the lockdown period. The Italian national travelling reduction was approximately 80% compared to the pre-COVID-19 period for light vehicles and approximately 40% for heavy vehicles [19]. However, road traffic is only one source of particulate matter production. Other significant emissions, such as those from domestic heating systems, agricultural activities and animal farms were not affected by restrictions and were not as strongly regulated as road traffic [20].

Considering PM, which had lower concentrations in 2020/2021 than in 2017, it is reasonable to assume that lower PM10 levels probably resulted in milder manifestations of upper respiratory tract diseases. In fact, their incremental effect on total admissions and otitis media was not confirmed in 2020/2021. Nevertheless, the effect of increasing admissions for tonsillitis and pharyngitis remained, particularly when PM10 concentrations exceeded 40 $\mu g/m^3$. This was in line with a recent meta-analysis that confirmed how larger particles might trigger upper respiratory infections more than smaller ones [21]. On the other hand, O_3 concentrations were similar in the two years and the impact of this pollutant on URT diseases seemed limited. NO_2 levels were lower in 2020/2021 and their role in otitis media was not confirmed by the multivariate analysis in this timeframe.

4.3. Aeroallergens and URT Manifestations

Regarding aeroallergens, it is interesting to note that *Alternaria* levels appeared lower in 2020/2021. *Alternaria* is usually present in lower atmospheric concentrations compared to other allergenic airborne spores but is responsible for the highest rate of sensitization amongst atopic patients [22,23]. Exposure to *Alternaria* primarily occurs outdoors since fungal spores largely originate from agricultural lands. Seasonal variations are influenced by climate [24]. However, its presence as an indoor pollutant should not be overlooked, as it remains a dominant indoor fungus, alongside *Cladosporium* and *Penicillium* [25].

Urban areas typically have higher pollution levels and may also influence spore production and allergenicity. Increased levels of PM10 are linked to a rise in airborne fungi [26], and elevated CO_2 concentrations can triple the spore production of *Alternaria* species, doubling the number of allergenic proteins [27].

During the pandemic, reduced pollution in urban areas likely contributed to lower *Alternaria* levels in Padua. Despite this, it is worth noting that home confinement and mask usage only partly diminished *Alternaria*'s role in URT diseases. It emerged as a significant independent factor in conditions such as otitis media, tonsillitis and URT related diseases. Differently from *Alternaria*, *Gramineae* and *Compositae* levels did not have a significant change in the first year of the COVID-19 pandemic. Their pollens are a major cause of seasonal allergies in temperate climates, affecting up to 30% of the population in Western countries [28]. Although the levels of these allergens did not decrease as much as AP, the increased use of masks and indoor activities might be an explanation for the significant reduction in rhinitis/rhinosinusitis (over 60% in our series) and the reason for the decreasing trend of allergic rhinitis found during this period [29]. The protective effect of confinement, however, might have been mitigated in the case of *Betulaceae* and *Corylaceae* in view of the higher levels of pollen that were recorded. Their peculiar effect on total URT, tonsillitis and pharyngitis admissions could be partially explained by the trend in the spring and summer months: in fact, both had higher and later peaks in 2020/2021. In particular, the delayed peak in their pollen's concentrations observed in 2020/2021 compared to 2017 could plausibly be attributed to a slight delay in the seasonal rise in temperatures, which plays a key role in triggering pollen release for both families. The fact that they reached higher levels during a period of loosening of the restrictions, albeit with an almost constant use of masks even outdoors, may have contributed to the peculiar distributions of their effect, which appear to be decreasing up to a certain critical threshold and then reach significantly higher incremental trends when compared to 2017.

Social distancing and isolation, the use of masks and implemented hand hygiene measures were responsible for the significant decrease in new diagnoses of otitis media during the lockdown periods as recently demonstrated in a meta-analysis by Warner et al. [30]. In our cohort, we observed a reduction of almost two-thirds in the number of otitis admissions when compared to 2017. When looking at the effect of pollutants on otitis, it is interesting to highlight that only *Alternaria* and *Betullaceae* maintained their significant effect in the multivariate analysis in 2020/2021, whilst the other allergens and APs lost their level of significance, probably mitigated by the reduction in AP levels and the aforementioned behavioral measures.

The aim of the comparison between the two years was to determine whether different living conditions, in this case markedly changed due to the pandemic, lead to different associations between pollutants and admissions to emergency rooms. Although it was not easy to unambiguously determine what caused the differences that emerged, the present study supports the current literature and confirms the harmful effects of pollution on health. While climatic factors, such as temperature and humidity, are not directly controllable by human activity, it is possible to act on other elements that have an influence on public health. In addition to carefully choosing the trees that will be placed in the city to avoid harmful aeroallergens as much as possible, it is important to take measures to reduce air pollution and to raise awareness among the population for responsible behavior that may limit the anthropogenic impact on the environment, also in the interest of our own health.

The interplay between environmental changes, public health and clinical outcomes underscores the need for interdisciplinary collaboration. To better understand the environmental factors influencing public health, it is essential to foster cooperation among medical professionals, public health providers, environmental researchers and experts in animal health. Such an integrated approach would enable a more comprehensive analysis of how human activities and environmental modifications contribute to health outcomes, paving the way for evidence-based interventions and sustainable solutions.

Moreover, although this study focused on otorhinolaryngological pathologies, future research could expand the scope by applying the same statistical approach to other health domains, particularly cardiovascular diseases. There is increasing evidence that air pollutants (especially particulate matter) may contribute to cardiovascular morbidity [31,32]. Including these conditions in future analyses could provide a broader understanding of the impact of air pollution on human health and further strengthen the public health relevance of environmental monitoring.

The main limitations of the present study are its retrospective and monocentric design and the lack of comparison with data collected from other ENT emergency departments. Considering different time frames over several years and with different ENT centers could lead to more robust results.

5. Conclusions

The COVID-19 lockdown in the Veneto Region of Italy led to a significant decrease in the number of patients admitted to the emergency department (ED) for ENT-related disorders. This reduction was consistent with findings from other regions in Italy and was particularly notable for URT inflammatory diseases. The lockdown also resulted in decreased air pollution, particularly in PM and NO_2 levels. While certain allergens such as *Alternaria* showed lower levels during the lockdown, they continued to play a significant role in ENT disorders such as otitis media and tonsillitis. Other allergens, such as *Betulaceae* and *Corylaceae*, had higher peaks compared to 2017 and showed a significant and independent effect particularly regarding the total number of URT accesses, tonsillitis and pharyngitis. Social distancing, mask-wearing and enhanced hygiene practices likely contributed to a significant decrease in URT infections, especially in otitis media during the lockdown period.

These findings highlight the harmful effects of pollution on health even during global pandemic and underline the importance of reducing air pollution and promoting responsible behavior to minimize anthropogenic environmental impacts for better public-health outcomes.

Moreover, this study supported the value of integrating clinical data with environmental monitoring and advanced statistical modeling to elucidate complex cause–effect relationships in selected settings. This can contribute to the growing body of evidence supporting the inclusion of environmental health indicators in public health planning. In light of these findings, there is a rationale for deeply investigating the adoption of long-term strategies aimed at reducing pollutant emissions, regulating allergenic vegetation in urban planning and maintaining certain protective behaviors. Public health campaigns should also aim to raise awareness about the environmental determinants of ENT diseases.

While the study was limited by its retrospective, monocentric design and focused on a specific geographic area, its results lay the groundwork for broader investigations. Future research should aim to confirm these findings in other populations and expand the scope to other environmentally sensitive health conditions, such as cardiovascular and respiratory diseases or animal well-being. Multi-center, longitudinal studies with integrated environmental and clinical datasets would be instrumental in shaping evidence-based policy and reinforcing the environmental dimension of public health.

Supplementary Materials: The following supporting information can be downloaded at: https://www.mdpi.com/article/10.3390/environments12040115/s1, Figures S1.1–S1.6, S2 and S3.

Author Contributions: Conceptualization, T.S., R.M.R., G.M. and G.O.; methodology, T.S., E.M., G.M., B.S. and G.O.; software, E.M. and B.S.; validation, T.S., E.M., E.B., A.R.C., A.D. (Antonio Daloiso), A.D. (Alessandra Deretti), F.B., M.A.C., M.M., P.N., R.M.R., G.M., B.S. and G.O.; formal analysis, T.S., E.B., A.R.C., A.D. (Antonio Daloiso), A.D. (Alessandra Deretti) and F.B.; investigation, T.S., E.M., G.M., B.S. and G.O.; data curation T.S., E.M., E.B., A.R.C., A.D. (Antonio Daloiso), A.D. (Alessandra Deretti) and F.B.; writing—original draft preparation, T.S., E.M., E.B. and A.R.C.; writing—review and editing, T.S., E.M., G.M. and G.O.; visualization, T.S., E.M., E.B., A.R.C., A.D. (Antonio Daloiso), A.D. (Alessandra Deretti), F.B., M.A.C., M.M., P.N., R.M.R., G.M., B.S. and G.O.; supervision, P.N., G.M. and G.O. All authors have read and agreed to the published version of the manuscript.

Funding: This research received no external funding.

Institutional Review Board Statement: The study was conducted in accordance with the ethical standards of the Helsinki Declaration. Data were examined in agreement with the Italian privacy and sensitive data laws, and the internal regulations of AOPD.

Informed Consent Statement: Informed consent on personal data collection and use for research purpose was obtained from each subject.

Data Availability Statement: The datasets generated and analyzed during the current study are available on reasonable request.

Conflicts of Interest: The authors declare no conflicts of interest.

References

1. Cucinotta, D.; Vanelli, M. WHO Declares COVID-19 a Pandemic. *Acta Biomed.* **2020**, *91*, 157–160. [CrossRef] [PubMed]
2. Linka, K.; Peirlinck, M.; Sahli Costabal, F.; Kuhl, E. Outbreak Dynamics of COVID-19 in Europe and the Effect of Travel Restrictions. *Comput. Methods Biomech. Biomed. Eng.* **2020**, *23*, 710–717. [CrossRef]
3. Núñez, A.; Sreeganga, S.D.; Ramaprasad, A. Access to Healthcare during COVID-19. *Int. J. Environ. Res. Public Health* **2021**, *18*, 2980. [CrossRef]
4. Buja, A.; Paganini, M.; Fusinato, R.; Cozzolino, C.; Cocchio, S.; Scioni, M.; Rebba, V.; Baldo, V.; Boccuzzo, G. Health and Healthcare Variables Associated with Italy's Excess Mortality during the First Wave of the COVID-19 Pandemic: An Ecological Study. *Health Policy* **2022**, *126*, 294–301. [CrossRef]

5. Paganini, M.; Barbiellini Amidei, C.; Valastro, M.F.; Favaro, A.; Saia, M.; Buja, A. Adult Emergency Department Visits during the COVID-19 Pandemic in Veneto Region, Italy: A Time-Trend Analysis. *Intern. Emerg. Med.* **2022**, *17*, 285–289. [CrossRef] [PubMed]
6. Wheaton, M.G.; Prikhidko, A.; Messner, G.R. Is Fear of COVID-19 Contagious? The Effects of Emotion Contagion and Social Media Use on Anxiety in Response to the Coronavirus Pandemic. *Front. Psychol.* **2021**, *11*, 567379. [CrossRef] [PubMed]
7. Ferry, A.V.; Keanie, C.; Denvir, M.A.; Mills, N.L.; Strachan, F.E. Chest Pain Presentations to Hospital during the COVID-19 Lockdown: Lessons for Public Health Media Campaigns. *PLoS ONE* **2021**, *16*, e0249389. [CrossRef]
8. Collivignarelli, M.C.; Abbà, A.; Bertanza, G.; Pedrazzani, R.; Ricciardi, P.; Carnevale Miino, M. Lockdown for CoViD-2019 in Milan: What Are the Effects on Air Quality? *Sci. Total Environ.* **2020**, *732*, 139280. [CrossRef]
9. Vultaggio, M.; Varrica, D.; Alaimo, M.G. Impact on Air Quality of the COVID-19 Lockdown in the Urban Area of Palermo (Italy). *Int. J. Environ. Res. Public Health* **2020**, *17*, 7375. [CrossRef]
10. Berger, M.; Bastl, M.; Bouchal, J.; Dirr, L.; Berger, U. The Influence of Air Pollution on Pollen Allergy Sufferers. *Allergol. Sel.* **2021**, *5*, 345–348. [CrossRef]
11. Ottaviano, G.; Pendolino, A.L.; Marioni, G.; Crivellaro, M.A.; Scarpa, B.; Nardello, E.; Pavone, C.; Trimarchi, M.V.; Alexandre, E.; Genovois, C.; et al. The Impact of Air Pollution and Aeroallergens Levels on Upper Airway Acute Diseases at Urban Scale. *Int. J. Environ. Res.* **2022**, *16*, 42. [CrossRef]
12. R Core Team. *R: A Language and Environment for Statistical Computing*; R Foundation for Statistical Computing: Vienna, Austria, 2020.
13. Elli, F.; Turri-Zanoni, M.; Arosio, A.D.; Karligkiotis, A.; Battaglia, P.; Castelnuovo, P. Changes in the Use of Otorhinolaryngology Emergency Department during the COVID-19 Pandemic: Report from Lombardy, Italy. *Eur. Arch. Otorhinolaryngol.* **2020**, *277*, 3525–3528. [CrossRef] [PubMed]
14. Campagnoli, M.; Cerasuolo, M.; Renna, M.; Dell'Era, V.; Valletti, P.A.; Garzaro, M. ENT Referral From Emergency Department During COVID-19: A Single-Center Experience. *Ear Nose Throat J.* **2023**, *102*, NP95–NP98. [CrossRef]
15. Torretta, S.; Cantoni, B.; Bertolozzi, G.; Capaccio, P.; Milani, G.P.; Pignataro, L.; Aleo, S.; Marchisio, P. Has Otitis Media Disappeared during COVID-19 Pandemic? A Fortuitus Effect of Domestic Confinement. *J. Clin. Med.* **2021**, *10*, 2851. [CrossRef]
16. Brotto, D.; Sorrentino, F.; Favaretto, N.; Bovo, R.; Trevisi, P.; Martini, A. Pediatric Hearing Loss Management in the COVID-19 Era: Possible Consequences and Resources for the Next Future. *Otolaryngol.–Head Neck Surg.* **2022**, *166*, 217–218. [CrossRef]
17. Pontillo, V.; Iannuzzi, L.; Petrone, P.; Sciancalepore, P.I.; D'Auria, C.; Rinaldi, M.; Graziano, G.; Quaranta, N. ENT Surgical Emergencies during the COVID-19 Outbreak. *Acta Otorhinolaryngol. Ital.* **2020**, *40*, 399–404. [CrossRef]
18. Gallo, O.; Locatello, L.G.; Orlando, P.; Martelli, F.; Bruno, C.; Cilona, M.; Fancello, G.; Mani, R.; Vitali, D.; Bianco, G.; et al. The Clinical Consequences of the COVID-19 Lockdown: A Report from an Italian Referral ENT Department. *Laryngoscope Investig. Otolaryngol.* **2020**, *5*, 824–831. [CrossRef] [PubMed]
19. Gualtieri, G.; Brilli, L.; Carotenuto, F.; Vagnoli, C.; Zaldei, A.; Gioli, B. Quantifying Road Traffic Impact on Air Quality in Urban Areas: A Covid19-Induced Lockdown Analysis in Italy. *Environ. Pollut.* **2020**, *267*, 115682. [CrossRef] [PubMed]
20. Pivato, A.; Pegoraro, L.; Masiol, M.; Bortolazzo, E.; Bonato, T.; Formenton, G.; Cappai, G.; Beggio, G.; Giancristofaro, R.A. Long Time Series Analysis of Air Quality Data in the Veneto Region (Northern Italy) to Support Environmental Policies. *Atmos. Environ.* **2023**, *298*, 119610. [CrossRef]
21. Ziou, M.; Tham, R.; Wheeler, A.J.; Zosky, G.R.; Stephens, N.; Johnston, F.H. Outdoor Particulate Matter Exposure and Upper Respiratory Tract Infections in Children and Adolescents: A Systematic Review and Meta-Analysis. *Environ. Res.* **2022**, *210*, 112969. [CrossRef]
22. Lehmann, S.; Sprünken, A.; Wagner, N.; Tenbrock, K.; Ott, H. Clinical Relevance of IgE-Mediated Sensitization against the Mould *Alternaria Alternata* in Children with Asthma. *Ther. Adv. Respir. Dis.* **2017**, *11*, 30–39. [CrossRef] [PubMed]
23. Arbes, S.J., Jr.; Gergen, P.J.; Elliott, L.; Zeldin, D.C. Prevalences of Positive Skin Test Responses to 10 Common Allergens in the US Population: Results from the Third National Health and Nutrition Examination Survey. *J. Allergy Clin. Immunol.* **2005**, *116*, 377–383. [CrossRef] [PubMed]
24. Skjøth, C.A.; Damialis, A.; Belmonte, J.; De Linares, C.; Fernández-Rodríguez, S.; Grinn-Gofroń, A.; Jędryczka, M.; Kasprzyk, I.; Magyar, D.; Myszkowska, D.; et al. Alternaria Spores in the Air across Europe: Abundance, Seasonality and Relationships with Climate, Meteorology and Local Environment. *Aerobiologia* **2016**, *32*, 3–22. [CrossRef]
25. Chen, Y.; Liang, Z.; Li, G.; An, T. Indoor/Outdoor Airborne Microbiome Characteristics in Residential Areas across Four Seasons and Its Indoor Purification. *Environ. Int.* **2024**, *190*, 108857. [CrossRef]
26. Roy, S.; Chakraborty, A.; Maitra, S.; Bhattacharya, K. Monitoring of Airborne Fungal Spore Load in Relation to Meteorological Factors, Air Pollutants and Allergic Symptoms in Farakka, an Unexplored Biozone of Eastern India. *Environ. Monit. Assess.* **2017**, *189*, 370. [CrossRef]
27. Wolf, J.; O'Neill, N.R.; Rogers, C.A.; Muilenberg, M.L.; Ziska, L.H. Elevated Atmospheric Carbon Dioxide Concentrations Amplify *Alternaria Alternata* Sporulation and Total Antigen Production. *Environ. Health Perspect.* **2010**, *118*, 1223–1228. [CrossRef]

28. Ojeda, P.; Barjau, M.C.; Subiza, J.; Moreno, A.; Ojeda, I.; Solano, E.; Alonso, A.; Caballero, R.; Del Pozo, S.; Gómez-Perosanz, M.; et al. Grass Pollen Allergoids Conjugated with Mannan for Subcutaneous and Sublingual Immunotherapy: A Dose-Finding Study. *Front. Immunol.* **2024**, *15*, 1431351. [CrossRef]
29. Dayal, A.K.; Sinha, V. Trend of Allergic Rhinitis Post COVID-19 Pandemic: A Retrospective Observational Study. *Indian J. Otolaryngol. Head Neck Surg.* **2022**, *74*, 50–52. [CrossRef]
30. Warner, B.K.; Durrant, F.G.; Nguyen, S.A.; Meyer, T.A. Global Otitis Media Incidence Changes During the COVID Pandemic: Systematic Review and Meta-Analysis. *Laryngoscope* **2024**, *134*, 2028–2037. [CrossRef]
31. Brown, J.R.G.; Baptiste, P.J.; Hajmohammadi, H.; Nadarajah, R.; Gale, C.P.; Wu, J. Impact of Neighbourhood and Environmental Factors on the Risk of Incident Cardiovascular Disease: A Systematic Review and Meta-Analysis. *Eur. J. Prev. Cardiol.* **2025**. [CrossRef]
32. GBD 2021 HAP Collaborators Global, Regional, and National Burden of Household Air Pollution, 1990-2021: A Systematic Analysis for the Global Burden of Disease Study 2021. *Lancet* **2025**, *405*, 1167–1181. [CrossRef] [PubMed]

MDPI AG
Grosspeteranlage 5
4052 Basel
Switzerland
Tel.: +41 61 683 77 34

Environments Editorial Office
E-mail: environments@mdpi.com
www.mdpi.com/journal/environments

Enzyme Production Using Industrial and Agricultural By-Products

Enzyme Production Using Industrial and Agricultural By-Products

Guest Editors

Heitor B. S. Bento

Ana Karine F. Carvalho

MDPI • Basel • Beijing • Wuhan • Barcelona • Belgrade • Novi Sad • Cluj • Manchester

Guest Editors

Heitor B. S. Bento
Department of Engineering of Bioprocess and Biotechnology
São Paulo State University
Araraquara
Brazil

Ana Karine F. Carvalho
Department of Basic and Environmental Sciences
University of São Paulo
Lorena
Brazil

Editorial Office
MDPI AG
Grosspeteranlage 5
4052 Basel, Switzerland

This is a reprint of the Special Issue, published open access by the journal *Processes* (ISSN 2227-9717), freely accessible at: https://www.mdpi.com/journal/processes/special_issues/0M26MJQXZZ.

For citation purposes, cite each article independently as indicated on the article page online and as indicated below:

Lastname, A.A.; Lastname, B.B. Article Title. *Journal Name* **Year**, *Volume Number*, Page Range.

ISBN 978-3-7258-7657-0 (Hbk)
ISBN 978-3-7258-7658-7 (PDF)
https://doi.org/10.3390/books978-3-7258-7658-7

Contents

About the Editors

Heitor B. S. Bento

Heitor B. S. Bento is an Assistant Professor at São Paulo State University, affiliated with the Department of Engineering of Bioprocess and Biotechnology at the School of Pharmaceutical Sciences. His research interests lie in biotechnology and chemical engineering, with emphasis on bioprocess development, microbial lipid production, and the use of agro-industrial residues as renewable feedstocks. He is involved in projects focused on the production and purification of bioproducts, as well as the scale-up of biotechnological processes, including work with genetically modified microorganisms for enzyme production. His expertise also includes chemical and biochemical reactors, chemical and enzymatic catalysis, enzyme immobilization, and material characterization. He holds a BSc and MSc in Chemical Engineering from the University of São Paulo, and a PhD in Industrial Biotechnology, with a focus on applied microbiology, also from the University of São Paulo. He additionally completed a postdoctoral project at São Paulo State University, working on the scale-up of L-asparaginase production.

Ana Karine F. Carvalho

Ana Karine F. Carvalho is a faculty member at the University of São Paulo, affiliated with the Department of Basic and Environmental Sciences at the School of Engineering of Lorena. Her research interests focus on bioprocess engineering, renewable energy systems, and biosystems, with particular emphasis on the development of integrated biorefinery platforms. She is involved in projects that combine microbiology, molecular biology, food technology, catalysis, and energy resources to design sustainable and efficient processes. Her work includes the application of chemical and biochemical reactors for the valorization of agro-industrial residues, aiming at the production of biofuels, fine chemicals, and biomaterials. She holds a degree in Food Engineering from the Federal University of Ceará, as well as an MSc in Chemical Engineering and a PhD in Industrial Biotechnology from the University of São Paulo, and has previously held academic positions at the University of São Paulo and the Federal University of Alfenas.

processes

MDPI

Editorial

Special Issue: Enzyme Production Using Industrial and Agricultural By-Products

Heitor B. S. Bento [1,*] and Ana Karine F. Carvalho [2]

1 Department of Bioprocess Engineering and Biotechnology, School of Pharmaceutical Sciences, São Paulo State University-UNESP, Araraquara 14800-903, Brazil
2 Department of Basic and Environmental Sciences, Engineering School of Lorena, São Paulo University, Lorena 12602-810, Brazil; anacarvalho@usp.br
* Correspondence: heitor.bento@unesp.br

The transition toward a circular bioeconomy has intensified the search for more sustainable and cost-effective strategies for enzyme production. Enzymes are essential biocatalysts across multiple industrial sectors, yet their large-scale production is still largely dependent on refined substrates, contributing significantly to overall process costs. In this context, the use of industrial and agricultural by-products as alternative feedstocks has emerged as a promising solution to simultaneously address economic and environmental challenges [1,2].

This Special Issue consolidates recent advances in this field by presenting a diverse set of studies that explore the production of enzymes using low-cost and abundant residues. The published works collectively demonstrate the feasibility of utilizing lignocellulosic materials, agro-industrial wastes, and other underutilized biomass streams as substrates for microbial cultivation and enzyme synthesis. These contributions reinforce a key paradigm shift in industrial biotechnology, where waste streams are increasingly regarded as valuable raw materials rather than disposal burdens.

A clear trend emerging from the Special Issue is the diversification of both substrates and microbial platforms. The studies encompass the production of cellulases, hemicellulases, lipases, oxidoreductases, and other industrially relevant enzymes using bacteria, filamentous fungi, and yeasts, highlighting the adaptability of different biological systems to heterogeneous feedstocks. In parallel, several works emphasize process optimization through statistical experimental design and cultivation strategies, contributing to improved yields and productivity under both submerged and solid-state fermentation systems.

Another important aspect addressed by the collected articles is the integration of enzyme production with downstream applications. Enzymes produced from by-products were successfully applied in biomass hydrolysis, biotransformation processes, and environmental remediation, supporting the broader concept of integrated biorefineries. This alignment between upstream production and practical application is essential for improving overall process feasibility and industrial relevance [3,4].

Despite these advances, it is important to highlight persistent challenges. One of the most critical limitations remains the scalability of these processes [5]. While laboratory-scale results are promising, the transition to industrial production requires addressing substrate variability, process control, and reactor design. Agro-industrial residues are inherently heterogeneous, and this variability can significantly impact microbial performance and enzyme yields. In addition, downstream processing remains a major bottleneck, as enzyme recovery, purification, and stabilization continue to contribute substantially to production costs [1,6].

Another gap identified is the limited integration of techno-economic and environmental assessments. Although the sustainability argument for waste-based enzyme production

 https://doi.org/10.3390/pr14081187

is compelling, quantitative analyses such as life cycle assessment and techno-economic evaluation are still scarce, yet they are essential for guiding industrial implementation [4]. Furthermore, opportunities associated with advanced biotechnological tools remain underexplored in the context of complex waste-derived substrates, including metabolic engineering, omics approaches, and synthetic biology.

Within this framework, the present Special Issue contributes by advancing the understanding of how diverse by-products can be effectively converted into high-value enzymatic systems, while also demonstrating optimized cultivation strategies and application-oriented approaches. The studies collectively strengthen the foundation for integrating enzyme production into circular and biorefinery-based models.

Looking ahead, future research should move toward stronger integration of feedstock characterization, process optimization, and application development. Greater emphasis on scale-up studies, process robustness, and continuous operation will be necessary to bridge the gap between laboratory findings and industrial deployment. At the same time, combining enzyme production with other biorefinery processes can enhance resource efficiency and economic viability. Advances in strain engineering and data-driven process optimization are expected to play a key role in overcoming current limitations, while the development of efficient enzyme recovery and immobilization strategies will be crucial to improving process sustainability [1,7,8].

In conclusion, the contributions gathered in this Special Issue clearly demonstrate that enzyme production using industrial and agricultural by-products is a rapidly evolving field with significant potential to support sustainable bioprocessing. By aligning waste valorization with enzyme biotechnology, these studies contribute to the development of more resilient and resource-efficient industrial systems. Continued interdisciplinary efforts will be essential to translate these advances into scalable and economically viable solutions within the global bioeconomy.

Conflicts of Interest: The authors declare no conflicts of interest.

References

1. Lima, C.A.; Contato, A.G.; de Oliveira, F.; da Silva, S.S.; Hidalgo, V.B.; Irfan, M.; Gambarato, B.C.; Carvalho, A.K.F.; Bento, H.B.S. Trends in enzyme production from Citrus by-products. *Processes* **2025**, *13*, 766. [CrossRef]
2. Khan, P.A.; Singh, T.; Lal, B.; Singh, R.; Syed, A.; Verma, M.; Mishra, P.K.; Wong, L.S.; Ahmad, I.; Srivastava, N. Valorization of Coconut Shell and Blue Berries Seed Waste into Enhance Bacterial Enzyme Production: Co-fermentation and Co-cultivation Strategies. *Indian J. Microbiol.* **2025**, *65*, 741–748. [CrossRef] [PubMed]
3. Kabir, M.; López-Cortés, I.; Ferrer-Gisbert, C.; Moposita-Vasquez, D.-D.; Velázquez-Martí, B. From Upstream Assessment to Downstream Energy Conversion: A Systematic Review of Advances in Biomass Residue Utilization Techniques. *Biomass* **2026**, *6*, 24. [CrossRef]
4. Khandelwal, N.; Kumari, S.; Poduval, S.; Behera, S.K.; Kumar, A.; Gedam, V.V. Life-cycle assessment of three biorefinery pathways across different generations. *Sci. Rep.* **2025**, *15*, 13135. [CrossRef] [PubMed]
5. Fit, C.G.; Clauser, N.M.; Felissia, F.E.; Area, M.C. Biorefinery design from agroindustrial by-products and its scaling-up analysis. *Bioresour. Technol. Rep.* **2025**, *31*, 102175. [CrossRef]
6. Liu, T.; He, M.; Shi, R.; Yin, H.; Luo, W. Biofuel–Pharmaceutical Co-Production in Integrated Biorefineries: Strategies, Challenges, and Sustainability. *Fermentation* **2025**, *11*, 312. [CrossRef]
7. Ragini, Y.P.; Karishma, S.; Kamalesh, R.; Saravanan, A.; TajSabreen, B.; Eswaar, D.K. Sustainable biorefinery approaches in the valorization of agro-food industrial residues for biofuel production: Economic and future perspectives. *Sustain. Energy Technol. Assess.* **2025**, *75*, 104239. [CrossRef]
8. Hassan, M.E.; Zhu, X.; de Souza, E.F.; Elnashar, M.M.; Lu, F. Enzyme immobilization advances: A key to unlocking renewable bioenergy potential. *Green Chem.* **2025**, *27*, 11289–11311. [CrossRef]

 https://doi.org/10.3390/pr14081187

processes

MDPI

ticle

.PS from Activated Sludge: Prospection of Bioflocculation and :atalytic Properties

ıra Jaramillo Arvilla [1,2], Grazieli Pereira da Silva [1], Ismael Hernandes Pereira, Júnior [1], Sofia Kremer de Souza [1], ıarolina Gommersbach [1], Guilherme Urbano [1], Rodrigo de Almeida Mohedano [1], Paulo Belli Filho [1], ɛjane Helena Ribeiro da Costa [1] and Nelson Libardi, Junior [1,*]

1 Department of Sanitary and Environmental Engineering, Federal University of Santa Catarina, Florianópolis 88040-970, SC, Brazil; hsu.guilherme09@gmail.com (G.U.); rejanehcosta@gmail.com (R.H.R.d.C.)

2 EIDENAR School, Faculty of Engineering, Universidad del Valle, Santiago de Cali 76001, Colombia

* Correspondence: nelson.libardi@ufsc.br

Abstract

The recovery of extracellular polymeric substances (EPS) from activated sludge (AS) represents a promising strategy to transform wastewater treatment plants (WWTPs) into resource recovery facilities within a circular economy framework. In this study, EPS was extracted from an AS process in a full-scale WWTP, highlighting its catalytic and bioflocculant properties, which represent an innovation in the valorization of this biopolymer. The EPS was subsequently characterized in terms of polysaccharides, proteins, and enzymatic activities (amylase and lipase). The bioflocculation performance of the EPS was evaluated using activated sludge mixed liquor. Results showed that EPS recovery yields using 50 °C and 80 °C were 196.3 ± 38.2 mg EPS/g sludge and 283.5 ± 85.4 mg EPS/g sludge, respectively. Enzymatic assays confirmed amylase activity ranging from 100 to 350 U/g sludge according to the extraction temperature. Lipolytic activity (20 U/g sludge) was comparable to values reported in the literature for EPS from biological sludge. The addition of EPS significantly improved the sludge settling velocity (from 0.86 to 4.48 m/h) and the sludge volume index (from 118.6 to 35.5). However, EPS application also increased the resistance to filtration by 50% and reduced cellular respiration by approximately 40%. Overall, the findings demonstrate that EPS from activated sludge acts as an effective bioflocculant with relevant catalytic properties, highlighting its potential as a high-value biotechnological product while also pointing to operational challenges that require further optimization.

Keywords: amylase; lipase; extracellular polymeric substances; activated sludge; bioflocculation; resource recovery

1. Introduction

An increasingly studied and implemented strategy to enhance the relevance and value of wastewater treatment processes is to reconceptualize wastewater treatment plants (WWTPs) as resource recovery facilities (RRFs) rather than merely as treatment systems. Stricter regulations regarding effluent treatment levels and the need for self-sufficient or even energy- and resource-positive plants are the primary drivers for the research and development of new WWTP configurations [1]. New concepts in wastewater treatment, sometimes referred to as "biorefineries" or resource recovery facilities (RRFs), encompass circular economy principles and enable the creation and production of high-value-added co-products from residual biomass, which can meet niche market demands [2].

The extraction and recovery of biopolymers from biological sludge is a potential route for obtaining bioproducts, as described by several authors. In The Netherlands, two large-scale demonstration systems are already in operation to showcase the economic feasibility of biopolymer recovery [3]. These biopolymers have similar properties to alginate, which has various pharmaceutical, food, and textile industry applications. For biopolymers extracted from granular sludge, other applications arise, such as in the composition of construction materials, as flame retardants, bioflocculants, and biocatalysts. Their application directly at the WWTP can increase their economic potential, for example, by being used as a bioflocculant or adsorbent with catalytic activity, replacing commercial products, or as an adsorbent material for pollutant removal from water or for nutrient recovery, such as nitrogen and phosphorus [4].

According to Schambeck et al. [5], there is potential for biopolymer recovery from flocculent biomass in activated sludge systems due to the high sludge production of these systems. The extraction of biopolymers from the residual biomass of wastewater treatment systems emerges as an option for recovering a high-value-added product with a wide range of applications [6]. Biopolymer recovery represents an innovative concept for valorizing carbonaceous material instead of converting it into energy. According to the bioproduct recovery value pyramid, biomass should ideally first be transformed and recovered as a biomaterial (highest value) before being destined for final energy use (lowest value), such as its conversion into biogas or other forms of energy [7].

Studies, including those by Sun et al. [8] and Zhang et al. [9], have shown that residual activated sludge can be an effective source of EPS with bioflocculant properties, offering a low-cost and sustainable alternative for wastewater treatment. This approach has been considered an alternative to conventional inorganic and synthetic organic flocculants, such as alum, PAC, and commercial polymers, which are associated with drawbacks, including aluminum-related health concerns, the generation of chemically contaminated sludge, and potential toxic or carcinogenic effects from polymeric residues. In contrast, EPS-based bioflocculants are biodegradable, non-toxic, and do not cause secondary pollution, reinforcing their potential as environmentally favorable flocculation agents. Beyond their bioflocculation potential, EPS recovered from activated sludge can also act as a functional matrix for immobilized enzymes, enabling simultaneous pollutant adsorption and catalytic bioconversion.

More recent studies have been exploring the biomolecules present in EPS produced in activated sludge and aerobic granular sludge reactors. EPS produced by biological sludge consists mainly of proteins, humic compounds, polysaccharides, lipids, and nucleic acids. Adsorption and enzymatic bioconversion are the two main phenomena involved in pollutant removal by activated sludge, both of which occur within the EPS matrix. The diversity of functional groups present in EPS facilitates the adsorption of nutrients, organic micropollutants, heavy metals, and other pollutants of interest. The adsorption of these pollutants also increases their concentration and brings these molecules closer to the active sites of extracellular enzymes, facilitating enzymatic catalysis and their bioconversion [10].

Frølund et al. [11] studied the enzymatic activity contained in the EPS of activated sludge and found that extracellular enzymes are considered an integral part of this polymeric matrix, where they remain immobilized. Large molecular substrates/pollutants such as cellulose, starch, polypeptides, lipoproteins, glycoproteins, and fats are degraded upon contact with the matrix and can be absorbed by the microbial biomass. EPS not only protects enzymes against degradation but also allows proximity between their active sites and substrates. EPS acts as an immobilization agent for extracellular enzymes

 https://doi.org/10.3390/pr1403054

produced by the microbial biomass. These extracellular enzymes are retained within the EPS, interacting with polysaccharides and becoming immobilized, which increases their thermal stability and resistance to proteolysis [12]. Enzyme immobilization in the EPS matrix prevents their loss to the surrounding medium (mixed liquor), where they could be easily degraded by environmental conditions. Extracellular enzymes also appear to play an important role in degrading the EPS structure itself, to some extent, to maintain its porosity and, consequently, its high capacity for pollutant adsorption. Recovering EPS while preserving enzymatic activity can support the development of biotechnological products such as bioflocculants or catalytic adsorbents for environmental applications. According to Wasmund et al. [13] and Flemming et al. [14], carbohydrate-active enzymes, proteases, and lipases are key constituents of the EPS matrix.

Nabarlatz et al. [15] evaluated the activity of lipase extracted from activated sludge, using ultrasonication as an extraction method. The authors obtained 21 U/g sludge, highlighting that the obtained enzymatic extract could be used as an additive to enhance anaerobic digestion processes for biogas production. Liu and Smith [16] suggested that enzymes extracted from residual biomass from biological treatment processes could serve as an alternative and low-cost enzyme source for various environmental and industrial applications. The authors identified cellulase (13.5 U/g sludge), protease (8.4 U/g sludge), lipase (21 U/g sludge), and amylase activities (39 U/g sludge), using ultrasonication as the extraction method. Toja Ortega et al. [17] evaluated the hydrolytic activity of enzymes responsible for the hydrolysis of complex substrates during the anaerobic phase of a full-scale sequencing batch reactor. The authors state that the hydrolysis of particulate COD is the rate-limiting step for the bioconversion of complex substrates. According to these authors, flocculent sludge has higher hydrolytic activity compared to granular sludge.

Despite the well-documented bioflocculation capacity and enzymatic activity of EPS, these properties have so far been investigated separately, limiting the development of multifunctional bioproducts for wastewater treatment applications. In this context, the objective of this study was to recover EPS extracted from activated sludge of a full-scale WWTP and evaluate its potential as a bioflocculant with catalytic properties, aiming at a bioproduct applicable to sludge flocculation and biodegradation.

2. Materials and Methods

2.1. Materials

For the extraction of EPS, anhydrous sodium carbonate (purity 98.5%), supplied by Êxodo Científica (Sumaré, Brazil), was used. The evaluation of amylase enzymatic activity was carried out using isopropyl alcohol (isopropanol, purity 99.5%), 3,5-dinitrosalicylic acid (DNS, purity 99%), soluble starch (purity 99%), sodium chloride (purity 99%), glucose (purity 99%, supplied by LAFAN, São Paulo, Brazil), and maltose (purity 92%), with all reagents supplied by Êxodo Científica, unless otherwise specified. For buffer solution preparation, dipotassium phosphate (purity 92%), phosphoric acid (purity 85%), and sodium hydroxide (purity 98%, supplied by ALPHATEC, Rio de Janeiro, Brazil) were employed. The evaluation of lipase enzymatic activity was performed using p-nitrophenyl palmitate (purity 98%, supplied by Sigma-Aldrich, Waltham, MA, USA), together with Triton™ X-100 (purity 90%), tris(hydroxymethyl)aminomethane (Tris, purity 99%), and gum arabic (purity 99.5%), all supplied by Êxodo Científica.

2.2. EPS and ALE Recovery from Residual Biomass

Activated sludge (AS) samples were obtained from the aerobic treatment unit of a municipal WWTP operated by CASAN (Santa Catarina Sanitation Company, Florianópolis,

 https://doi.org/10.3390/pr14030547

Brazil). The facility, known as the Lagoa da Conceição WWTP, is located in Florianópolis, Santa Catarina, and is designed to treat a flow of 50–73 L/s. The biological process consists of a continuous-flow oxidation ditch activated sludge system configured for extended aeration. The mixed liquor sample was collected in the aeration tank and further centrifuged to remove the water. EPS was recovered following a modified version of the alkaline extraction protocol described by Felz et al. [18]. Briefly, 7.5 g of sludge was suspended in 150 mL of a sodium carbonate solution prepared with 0.625 g of Na_2CO_3 and subjected to constant agitation at 400 rpm at temperatures of 50 °C and 80 °C. After 35 min of extraction, the mixture was cooled to room temperature and subsequently centrifuged at 3000 rpm for 25 min; the supernatant containing solubilized EPS was collected while the solid fraction was discarded. The extracted EPS was subsequently used for physicochemical characterization, enzyme activity assessment, and bioflocculation experiments

Gelation tests were conducted to assess the hydrogel-forming capacity of alginate-like extracellular polymers (ALE) extracts obtained from EPS recovered at 50 °C and 80 °C. ALE was extracted via alkaline extraction with Na_2CO_3, followed by centrifugation (2150× g, 25 min) and dialysis. The dialyzed extract was acidified with 1 M HCl under gentle stirring (100 rpm, room temperature) to a final pH of 2.2 ± 0.05, yielding acidic ALE, which was subsequently recovered by centrifugation (4000× g, 4 °C, 20 min). The acidic gel was neutralized with 0.5 M NaOH to pH 8.5 to obtain Na-ALE. Ionic hydrogel formation was evaluated by slowly dripping the Na-ALE solution into a 2.5% (w/v) $CaCl_2$ solution. The formation of spherical Ca^{2+}–ALE beads was taken as evidence of ionic hydrogel formation [5].

2.3. Enzyme Activity Analyses

EPS samples collected on different dates were used for EPS extraction and for the evaluation of amylase activity. Lipase activity was assessed in a single EPS sample as a preliminary screening. Lipase activity was determined [19] through a spectrophotometric assay, employing p-nitrophenyl palmitate (p-NPP) as the substrate. During the reaction, the hydrolysis of p-NPP by the extracellular lipase promotes the release of p-nitrophenol, which, in an alkaline medium, exhibits a characteristic yellow coloration.

Amylase activity was determined based on starch hydrolysis and the quantification of reducing sugars released using the 3,5-dinitrosalicylic acid (DNS) colorimetric method. Initially, the buffers, the substrate solution, and a maltose standard curve were prepared and used as references for the analysis. For the evaluation of enzyme stability, a portion of the EPS was stored at 5 °C for six months. After this period, the EPS was brought to room temperature, and the amylase enzymatic activity was evaluated by incubating the enzyme with the starch solution at 37 °C for 10 min, followed by the addition of the DNS reagent as the colorimetric agent. The samples were boiled, cooled, diluted in distilled water, and analyzed at 540 nm using a spectrophotometer (DR3900, HACH, Jundiaí, Brazil). Amylase activity analysis was performed in triplicate.

Experiments were performed in triplicate ($n = 3$), and the results were expressed as mean values. Statistical analyses were carried out using analysis of variance (ANOVA), and mean comparisons were conducted using Tukey's test at a 5% significance level ($p < 0.05$). All statistical procedures were performed using Origin® 2017 software.

2.4. Polysaccharide and Protein Concentration in EPS

The concentration of polysaccharides in the extracted EPS was quantified by an adapted colorimetric assay using anthrone reagent [20]. Calibration curves were prepared using glucose (neutral sugars) and glucuronic acid (uronic acids) as standards. EPS samples were diluted (1:10) and analyzed in triplicate. Absorbance readings were performed in a spectrophotometer (HACH DR3900, Brazil) at 560 and 620 nm, and results were

 https://doi.org/10.3390/pr14030547

expressed as glucose equivalents (mg GLU/g sludge) and glucuronic acid equivalents (mg GLA/sludge).

Protein content in the EPS was determined using the modified Lowry method [21]. Calibration curves were prepared with bovine serum albumin (BSA) for protein quantification and humic substances to account for potential interference. EPS samples were analyzed in triplicate with a 1:10 dilution factor. Absorbance was measured at 750 nm in a spectrophotometer (HACH DR3900, Brazil). Final protein concentrations were expressed in mg BSA/g sludge after correction for humic substance interference [21].

2.5. Bioflocculation Properties of EPS

The jar tests were performed using six square-based jars with a volume of 2 L, each with six rotating propellers providing equal agitation and rest conditions for all jars. The experimental procedure for each jar test began with an intense mixing phase at 120 rpm for 15 s, followed by slow mixing at 50 rpm for 30 min, and subsequently a 15 min settling period. After the settling time, supernatant and settled solids samples were collected for further analysis.

Each jar was loaded with 1 L of activated sludge mixed liquor, which exhibited an initial pH of 6.73 and a temperature of 25.7 °C. The EPS volumes applied in the jars varied as follows: 0, 50, 100, 150, 200 and 250 mL.

Sludge settling velocity was determined by transferring 1 L of homogenized sample from each jar into graduated cylinder and monitoring the sludge blanket height at fixed time intervals (0–30 min). The sludge volume index (SVI) was calculated according to Standard Methods [22].

The Buchner funnel test was performed according to Lo et al. [23] and Zhang et al. [9]. This test is used to determine the Specific Resistance to Filtration (SRF) and the Filtration Time (FT) in order to identify dewatering characteristics of the treated effluent.

The oxygen uptake rate (OUR) test was performed to evaluate the impact of EPS on microbial respiration and on potential oxygen transfer limitations in the activated sludge mixed liquor, given that one possible application of EPS is its use as an additive to improve activated sludge bioflocculation. OUR measurements were conducted as described in [24]. For this procedure, the mixed liquor sample was aerated for 24 h without the addition of an exogenous substrate in order to reach the endogenous respiration phase. Glucose ($C_6H_{12}O_6$, 100 mg/L) and NH_4Cl (50 mg/L) were used as substrates for heterotrophic and autotrophic biomass, respectively, and allylthiourea was added as an inhibitor of autotrophic bacteria. Biomass fractionation was calculated according to Activated Sludge Model 1 (ASM1) [25].

3. Results and Discussion

3.1. EPS Recovery Yield and Biochemical Composition

The EPS extraction yields using 50 °C and 80 °C were 196.3 ± 38.2 mg EPS/g sludge and 283.5 ± 85.4 mg EPS/g sludge, respectively. The reduction in the recovery yields suggests that the extraction temperature influences recovery efficiency. Although higher temperatures increase the recovery yields, labile biomolecules like enzymes would suffer denaturation, and this was hypothesized in this work.

Schambeck et al. [5] found recovery yields for activated sludge flocs of 472 mg EPS/g sludge using the same extraction procedure at 80 °C. Higher recovery yields were found by the authors using aerobic granular sludge (495 mg EPS/g sludge), which is inherent to the structure of granules compared to activated sludge.

De Bruin et al. [26] analyzed the recovery of EPS from 16 Activated Sludge reactors located in 13 countries using the same alkaline extraction protocol with 80 °C used in

https://doi.org/10.3390/pr14030547

this work and found yields varying from 28.1 to 185 mg EPS/g sludge. Li et al. [27] presented EPS and biopolymer recovery yields from 90 to 190 mg EPS/g sludge from activated sludge biomass. Future improvements could include adjustments in extraction temperature, pH control, or sequential recovery steps aimed at enhancing the solubilization of high-molecular-weight biopolymers without compromising their structural integrity.

Besides higher extraction yield, higher temperature (80 °C) also favored the polysaccharide and protein concentration (Figure 1). The glucuronic acid is the monomer responsible for the hydrogel properties, and its concentration increased 1.5 times when the temperature was higher. According to the hydrogel test shown in Figure 2, EPS beads extracted at 80 °C were more compact and structurally stable than those extracted at 50 °C, supporting the influence of glucuronic acid concentration. Polysaccharides, quantified as glucose and glucuronic acid equivalents, constituted a significant fraction of the EPS composition. This composition is consistent with previous studies reporting the prevalence of proteins and uronic sugars in EPS matrices. Schambeck et al. [5], using a comparable EPS extraction procedure at 80 °C, reported concentrations of 137 mg/g sludge for proteins, 18 mg/g sludge for glucose, and 48 mg/g sludge for glucuronic acid in activated sludge biomass.

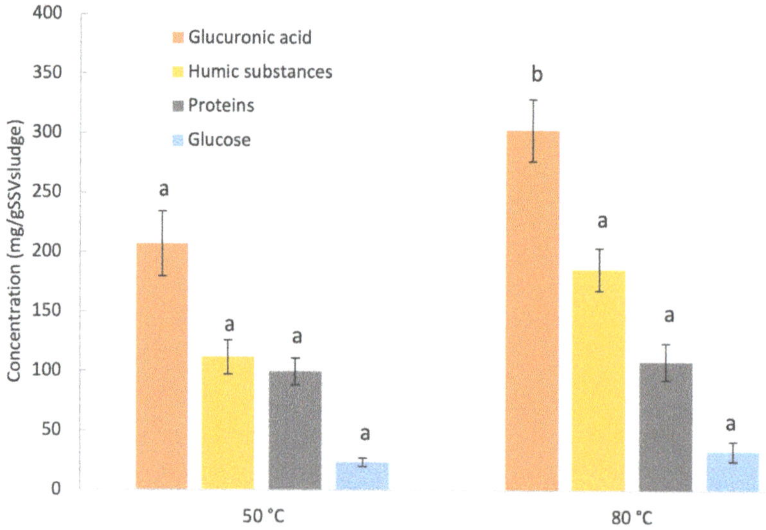

Figure 1. EPS biochemical composition from activated sludge after extraction at 50 °C and 80 °C. Bars represent mean values ± standard deviation (n = 3). Different letters indicate statistically significant differences between extraction temperatures according to Tukey's test ($p < 0.05$).

https://doi.org/10.3390/pr1403054

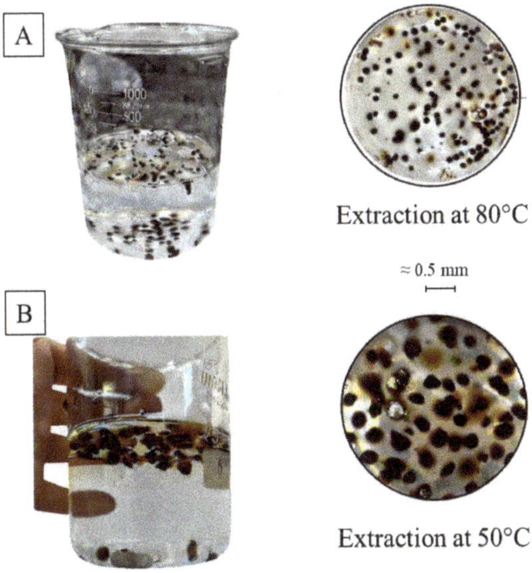

Figure 2. Hydrogel-forming properties of EPS recovered from activated sludge after extraction at 80 °C (**A**) and 50 °C (**B**).

One-way ANOVA revealed a significant effect of extraction temperature on glucuronic acid concentration ($p < 0.05$), with higher values obtained at 80 °C. No significant differences were observed for glucose or protein concentrations between temperatures ($p > 0.05$). Humic substances showed a borderline effect of temperature ($p \approx 0.05$), indicating a tendency toward higher values at 80 °C.

The ability of the extracted EPS to form hydrogels in the presence of divalent cations was demonstrated by the formation of stable beads upon contact with calcium chloride solution. This gelation behavior confirms the presence of alginate-like exopolymers (ALE), which are known to play a key role in EPS structuring and flocculation performance. The identification of ALE is particularly relevant to this study, as these polymers are directly associated with calcium-mediated cross-linking mechanisms that enhance particle aggregation and sludge settleability. Moreover, the extraction temperature significantly influenced the biopolymer composition and, consequently, the physicochemical properties of the recovered EPS. The predominance of proteins suggests an enhanced binding capacity through amino and amide functional groups, which promote electrostatic interactions and polymer bridging during bioflocculation. In parallel, the presence of humic substances may contribute to additional structural stability, given their resistance to biodegradation and their role in increasing EPS persistence within sludge systems [5]. From a functional perspective, humic substances may also affect the enzymatic activity associated with the EPS matrix, as these compounds are known to bind extracellular enzymes, stabilizing them while partially reducing their catalytic efficiency [28]. Overall, the combined presence of ALE, proteinaceous components, polysaccharides, and humic substances provides a coherent explanation for the observed bioflocculation performance of the EPS, supporting its potential application as a multifunctional bioproduct in wastewater treatment systems.

3.2. Enzyme Activity

Enzymatic analyses can help determine whether reducing the extraction temperature is an effective strategy to preserve the biological activity of proteins embedded within the EPS matrix. At a 5% significance level, the ANOVA and Tukey test results indicate that varying

https://doi.org/10.3390/pr14030547

the temperature between 50 °C and 80 °C does not promote statistically significant changes in amylase activity. A high degree of intragroup variability was observed, which may have contributed to the absence of a significant temperature effect. Moreover, extraction at 80 °C did not reduce enzyme activity as would be expected due to thermal denaturation. Instead, amylase exhibited a degree of thermostability, given the absence of significant differences among replicates and between the 50 °C and 80 °C extraction temperatures.

This apparent thermostability of amylase, evidenced by the lack of significant differences between the 50 °C and 80 °C extraction temperatures (Figure 3), is consistent with previous findings reported in the literature. Liu and Smith [29] evaluated the use of ultrasonication for the extraction of amylase, protease, and cellulase from waste activated sludge and reported a maximum amylase activity of 52.2 U/g VS in samples collected from the aeration tank. Notably, comparable enzymatic activities were also observed in samples obtained from other stages of the treatment line, such as the thickening belt. These results support the hypothesis that enzymes remain protected within the EPS matrix throughout the treatment process, which may mitigate thermal and operational stresses and enable effective enzyme recovery even from thickened sludge. Florianópolis

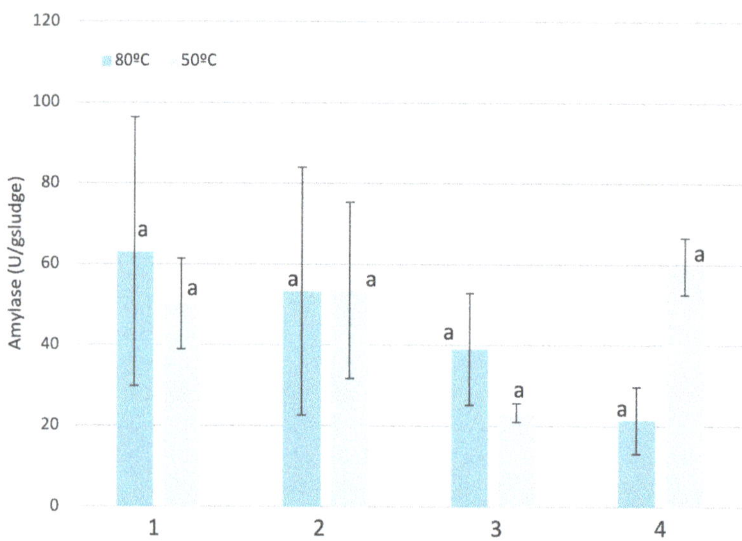

Figure 3. Specific amylase activity measured in EPS fractions extracted at 50 and 80 °C. Bars represent mean values ± standard deviation ($n = 3$). Same letters indicate not statistically significant differences between extraction temperatures according to Tukey's test ($p < 0.05$).

Yu et al. [30] evaluated several enzyme extraction procedures for activated sludge biomass, including ultrasonication, EDTA, formaldehyde, formaldehyde combined with ultrasonication, formaldehyde combined with NaOH, and cation-exchange resin. The authors reported amylase activities ranging from 11.4 to 14.9 U/g VS. Most of the amylase activity was recovered in the loosely bound EPS fraction, suggesting that carbohydrates present in the bulk liquid are adsorbed and subsequently degraded by amylases located in this compartment. These amylase activities were related to the loosely bound EPS obtained after the extraction procedure, similar to that obtained in this work.

Ortega and co-workers [31] studied amylase and protease activities in aerobic granular sludge through fluorescent activity assays. Amylase enzyme activity was identified in the outer layer of granules, indicating their relation to the substrates that will be hydrolyzed and the substrate mass transfer limitations.

https://doi.org/10.3390/pr14030547

The EPS was stored frozen for six months, after which the stability of the amylase was evaluated. According to Figure 4, approximately 55% of the enzyme activity was lost during the freezing period for the EPS extracted at 50 °C, and about 45% was lost for the EPS extracted at 80 °C. The thawing process may have caused EPS precipitation and potentially exposed the amylase enzymes to denaturation.

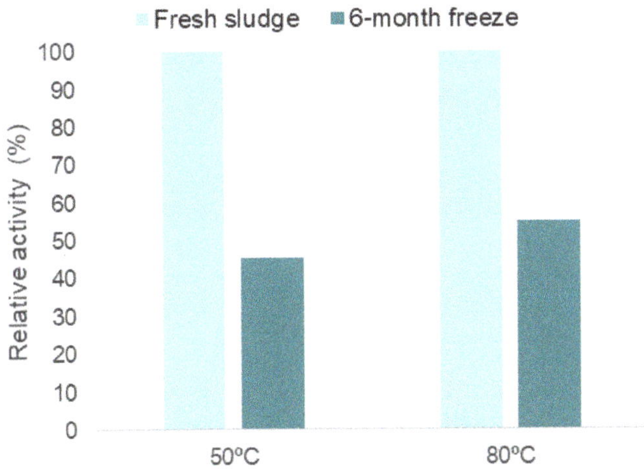

Figure 4. Effect of six-month frozen storage on specific amylase activity.

Lipase activity was measured in a single sample extracted at 50 °C, resulting in 20.8 U/g Sludge. The obtained activity is in the range of other authors' findings. The hydrolysis of complex substrates in aerobic granular sludge was studied by Toja Ortega et al [17]. The authors found that higher hydrolytic activities were found in flocculent biomass in comparison to the granular fraction. In the mixed sludge fraction the lipase activity of 34 µmol pNP/g sludge/h. Nabarlatz et al. [15] found lipase activities ranging from 2.3 to 22.9 U/g sludge, according to the extraction procedure, which included dialysis, precipitation and lyophilization. Gessesse et al. [32] showed that different extraction factors affect the lipase activity from activated sludge flocs, from 108 to 335 U/g sludge. High lipase activity was obtained using the non-ionic detergent Triton-X.

The majority of studies express enzymatic activity on a sludge mass basis. However, considering that EPS is intended to be used as a bioproduct in its liquid form, reporting activity on a volume basis becomes more appropriate. Moreover, EPS was applied in its liquid form in the bioflocculation tests. Future investigations may determine whether the enzymes embedded within the EPS matrix can withstand drying processes, such as spray drying or lyophilization, for the preparation of a dry product.

Biological macromolecules are abundant in domestic wastewater and can be found as particulates such as cellulose fibers, microbial cells, or colloidal and soluble polymers [17]. Raunkjær et al. [33] originally quantified that lipids and fats may account for up to 40% of the influent COD, while carbohydrates can contribute up to 18%. These ranges were later reiterated by Wasmund et al. [13], who emphasized the importance of these compounds as major nutrient sources in wastewater treatment plants. In this context, the work of Flemming et al. [14] provides a link in that extracellular enzymes embedded in the EPS matrix play a crucial role in hydrolyzing and degrading these macromolecules, thereby driving the biological transformation of organic matter in wastewater treatment systems.

https://doi.org/10.3390/pr14030547

In line with this enzymatic perspective, recent genomic-based investigations have begun to unravel the microbial potential behind these processes. To better understand microbial functions in WWTPs, Wasmund et al. [13] predicted the secreted proteomes of the wastewater microbiota using more than 1000 high-quality metagenome-assembled genomes (MAGs) derived from 23 Danish WWTPs with biological nutrient removal. This genomic approach enabled the identification of secreted hydrolytic enzymes. Many of the MAGs encoding predicted secreted lipases were affiliated with taxa already known for lipase activity, thereby reinforcing the functional relevance of these predictions and supporting the enzymatic mechanisms previously proposed.

3.3. Flocculation Properties of the EPS

EPS addition markedly influenced the settling dynamics of mixed liquor activated sludge. The highest settling velocity was obtained in jar 6, which received 250 mL of EPS, reaching 4.48 m/h (Table 1). This value was substantially higher than that of the control and confirmed the capacity of EPS to accelerate biomass aggregation and compaction. Correspondingly, the sludge volume index (SVI) improved progressively with EPS dosage, with the best performance also observed in jar 6 (Figure 5). These findings demonstrate that EPS promotes denser flocs and enhances sludge settleability.

Table 1. Effect of EPS addition over settling velocity and SVI.

Jar	EPS Addition (mL)	Settling Velocity (m/h)	SVI
1	0	0.86	118.6
2	50	0.34	161.1
3	100	1.63	56.0
4	150	3.62	39.6
5	200	2.58	50.0
6	250	4.48	35.5

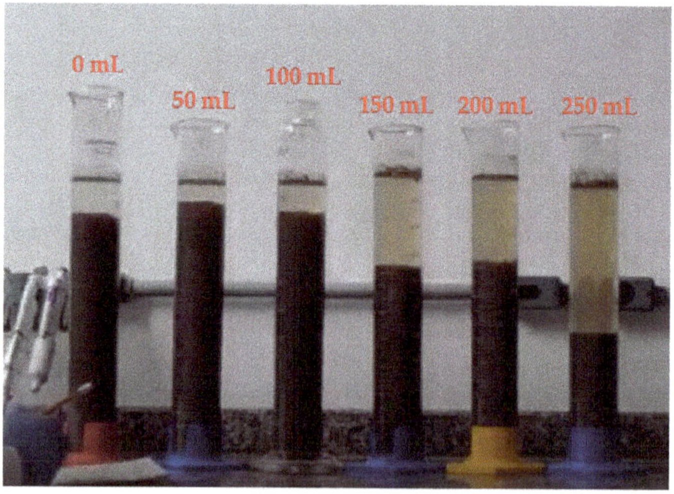

Figure 5. Sludge settling comparison with increasing EPS addition.

When applied to activated sludge mixed liquor, EPS demonstrated a bioflocculant effect, significantly improving aggregation and settling (Figure 6). The addition of EPS led to up to a fivefold increase in settling velocity compared to the control, with consistent

https://doi.org/10.3390/pr1403054

improvements in the sludge volume index (SVI), which reached values classified as "optimal" under higher dosages for activated sludge mixed liquor. These findings confirm the capacity of EPS to promote stable floc formation and accelerate clarification in biological sludge. However, some side effects were observed. The EPS application increased the turbidity in the supernatant, suggesting the release of organic matter and nutrients during the process. Together, the results highlight the dual role of EPS: while it enhances flocculation and settling performance, its application also alters effluent quality and microbial activity, aspects that must be carefully evaluated for full-scale implementation.

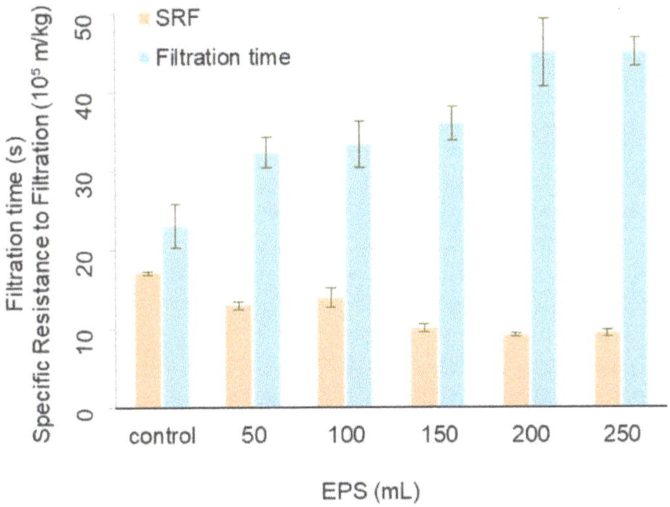

Figure 6. Specific resistance to filtration and filtration time for increasing EPS addition.

The specific resistance to filtration (SRF) allows identifying the influence that the addition of EPS has on the sludge filtration process. The SRF decreased with increasing EPS dosage, indicating improved floc cohesion and reduced passage of fine particles through the filter matrix. Conversely, the time required to filter 100 mL of mixed liquor with EPS after the jar test (filtration time) increased by nearly 50% at the highest EPS concentration compared to the control. This suggests that while EPS enhances particle retention and reduces SRF, it also tends to clog the filter pores, impairing water passage.

Overall, the results indicate that EPS improves settling and compaction of biological sludge but may worsen dewatering when filtration is the primary thickening or dewatering method. This trade-off emphasizes the importance of tailoring EPS application to treatment configurations where sedimentation rather than filtration is the key solid–liquid separation step.

Sun et al. [8] prepared a bioflocculant using residual activated sludge from a Chinese WWTP. The authors disintegrated the sludge with hydrochloric acid and used the supernatant as the bioflocculant in kaolinite clay suspensions, achieving a 99.5% flocculation rate. Zhang et al. [34] tested the use of a microbial bioflocculant produced by Proteus mirabilis TJ-1 screened out from activated sludge biomass. The bioflocculant resulted in SRF up to 27 (10^5 m/kg) and up to 8 min of time to filter during the Buchner funnel test. Compared to the control, the bioflocculant improved the sludge dewaterability, whichwas not observed in this study.

Inorganic coagulants and flocculants, such as aluminum sulfate and polyaluminum chloride (PAC), are widely applied due to their high efficiency in removing organic pollutants. However, their use is associated with important drawbacks, including potential

https://doi.org/10.3390/pr14030547

health concerns related to aluminum exposure and the generation of large volumes of sludge that require further treatment and disposal. Commercial organic flocculants also pose environmental risks, as their polymeric residues may exhibit neurotoxic or carcinogenic effects [35]. In contrast, natural bioflocculants represent a more sustainable alternative. They are typically biodegradable, non-toxic, and do not lead to secondary pollution, offering economic and environmental advantages over conventional chemical flocculation. Bioflocculants can be produced by various microorganisms, such as *Bacillus*, *Pseudomonas*, *Serratia*, and *Azotobacter*, or recovered directly from mixed and non-sterile microbial cultures like waste activated sludge [36].

Sludge management is a major challenge for wastewater treatment plants due to its high moisture content (around 80%) and the associated operational costs. Consequently, sludge dewatering represents a critical step in sludge disposal [37]. In this context, enzymatic treatment has emerged as a competitive strategy because the sludge matrix is largely composed of extracellular polymeric substances (EPS) produced by bacteria, which can be disintegrated by specific enzymes. Importantly, the enzymes naturally embedded within the EPS matrix may themselves contribute to the degradation of EPS, potentially enhancing sludge disintegration and improving dewatering performance. On the other hand, the addition of exogenous EPS—as a bioflocculant—tends to increase sludge-bound water and structural resistance, thereby hindering sludge dewatering. This trade-off represents a key bottleneck for the practical application of EPS as a bioflocculant, particularly when considering the further dewatering steps required downstream. Nevertheless, if the use of EPS is envisioned as an in situ pre-treatment for bioflocculated sludge prior to its transfer to an anaerobic digester, this approach may still offer advantages, especially by facilitating hydrolysis and enhancing subsequent anaerobic conversion.

3.4. Impact of EPS on OUR

The impact of EPS addition on microbial activity was evaluated through oxygen uptake assays (Table 2). Compared to the control, the maximum specific oxygen uptake rate (OUR) of the sludge decreased by approximately 40% after the addition of 250 mL of EPS. This reduction suggests that EPS may increase the diffusional barrier surrounding microbial cells, thickening the liquid film, and thereby limiting oxygen transfer. Reduced oxygen availability at the cell surface likely explains the observed decline in metabolic activity.

Table 2. Oxygen uptake rate of activated sludge mixed liquor before and after EPS addition.

Sample	OUR (mgO_2/L·h)	$OUR_{specific}$ (mgO_2/L·h·X)	$X_{Autotrophic}$ (gDQO/L)	$X_{Heterotrophic}$ (gDQO/L)
Sludge	15.13	147.6	15.7	38.8
Sludge + EPS	9.13	129.6		

Although the reduction in OUR was primarily attributed to an increased diffusional resistance caused by EPS accumulation around microbial cells, other mechanisms may also be involved. The addition of EPS can alter the physical and biochemical properties of sludge flocs, potentially affecting microbial accessibility to oxygen and substrates beyond simple diffusion limitations. Furthermore, EPS may induce short-term physiological stress or shifts in microbial community structure, temporarily reducing respiratory activity. Another possible contribution is the consumption of dissolved oxygen by biodegradable organic matter associated with EPS, which may compete with microbial respiration during OUR measurements. While these mechanisms were not individually quantified in the present study, their combined effects highlight the need for comprehensive OUR assessment when EPS is proposed as a multifunctional bioflocculant and catalytic additive in activated sludge systems.

https://doi.org/10.3390/pr14030547

These results highlight the importance of carefully assessing the oxygen uptake rate of activated sludge when EPS is proposed as an additive. Since EPS is intended to act simultaneously as a bioflocculant and as a catalytic agent, its interaction with microbial metabolism becomes a critical factor for process stability. In wastewater treatment plants, flocculants and catalysts are typically supplied as separate commercial products, each with distinct operational purposes. The possibility of replacing both products with a single EPS-based additive represents a promising technological advancement. However, any benefits associated with improved flocculation and catalytic activity must be balanced against potential adverse effects on microbial respiration. Therefore, OUR measurements are essential to ensure that EPS application does not compromise biological performance, particularly under aerobic conditions where oxygen transfer is a key limiting factor.

4. Conclusions

The recovery of EPS from mixed liquor in activated sludge systems represents a promising strategy for the valorization of residual streams in wastewater treatment plants. Extraction temperature influenced EPS recovery yield and physicochemical characteristics, as well as the associated enzymatic activities. However, statistical analysis indicated that variations between 50 °C and 80 °C did not result in significant differences in amylase activity, suggesting a degree of enzymatic stability within the EPS matrix rather than thermal enhancement or denaturation.

When applied to activated sludge, the recovered EPS exhibited clear bioflocculant behavior. The observed increase in sludge settling velocity and reduction in SVI confirm the potential of EPS to act as a flocculation enhancer, with possible application in aerobic reactors to improve settling performance in secondary clarifiers. In addition, the presence of active enzymes within the EPS matrix highlights its potential added value as a functional additive for sludge pre-treatment prior to anaerobic digestion or for enzymatic hydrolysis processes aimed at resource recovery.

Nonetheless, some limitations were identified. Despite reducing filtration time, EPS addition increased the specific resistance to filtration, which may negatively affect downstream dewatering processes. Moreover, the reduction in oxygen uptake rate suggests that EPS may influence oxygen transfer under bench-scale conditions. These findings indicate that operational trade-offs should be carefully considered prior to full-scale application.

Overall, the recovery of enzyme-active EPS from activated sludge constitutes a viable pathway for producing a functional bioproduct from wastewater treatment residues. This approach aligns with circular economy principles by promoting resource recovery and reintegration within WWTPs, while emphasizing the need for further studies to optimize application conditions and assess process-scale implications.

Author Contributions: Conceptualization, N.L.J.; Validation, R.d.A.M. and P.B.F.; Formal analysis, I.H.P.J., C.G. and G.U.; Investigation, S.J.A., G.P.d.S., S.K.d.S., C.G. and G.U.; Resources, R.d.A.M., P.B.F., R.H.R.d.C. and N.L.J.; Data curation, N.L.J.; Writing—original draft, G.P.d.S., I.H.P.J. and N.L.J.; Writing—review and editing, N.L.J.; Visualization, G.P.d.S., I.H.P.J. and C.G.; Supervision, N.L.J.; Project administration, R.H.R.d.C. and N.L.J.; Funding acquisition, R.d.A.M., P.B.F., R.H.R.d.C. and N.L.J. All authors have read and agreed to the published version of the manuscript.

Funding: This work was funded by the Coordenação de Aperfeiçoamento de Pessoal de Nível Superior (CAPES), Brazil, through the Move La America Program (Grant No. 88881.016894/2024-01), and by the Conselho Nacional de Desenvolvimento Científico e Tecnológico (CNPq), Brazil, under the Universal Project (Grant No. 403786/2023-1).

https://doi.org/10.3390/pr14030547

Data Availability Statement: The original contributions presented in this study are included in the article. Further inquiries can be directed to the corresponding author.

Conflicts of Interest: The authors declare no conflicts of interest.

References

1. Sancho, I.; Lopez-Palau, S.; Arespacochaga, N.; Cortina, J.L. New Concepts on Carbon Redirection in Wastewater Treatm Plants: A Review. *Sci. Total Environ.* **2019**, *647*, 1373–1384. [CrossRef]
2. Cecconet, D.; Capodaglio, A.G. Sewage Sludge Biorefinery for Circular Economy. *Sustainability* **2022**, *14*, 14841. [CrossRef]
3. Wetsus. *IWA Resource Recovery Conference Magazine 2025*; Wetsus: Leeuwarden, The Netherlands, 2025.
4. Kehrein, P.; Van Loosdrecht, M.; Osseweijer, P.; Posada, J. Exploring Resource Recovery Potentials for the Aerobic Granu Sludge Process by Mass and Energy Balances—Energy, Biopolymer and Phosphorous Recovery from Municipal Wastewa *Environ. Sci. Water Res. Technol.* **2020**, *6*, 2164–2179. [CrossRef]
5. Schambeck, C.M.; Girbal-Neuhauser, E.; Böni, L.; Fischer, P.; Bessière, Y.; Paul, E.; Da Costa, R.H.R.; Derlon, N. Chemical a Physical Properties of Alginate-like Exopolymers of Aerobic Granules and Flocs Produced from Different Wastewaters. *Biores Technol.* **2020**, *312*, 123632. [CrossRef]
6. Pronk, M.; Neu, T.R.; Van Loosdrecht, M.C.M.; Lin, Y.M. The Acid Soluble Extracellular Polymeric Substance of Aerobic Granu Sludge Dominated by *Defluviicoccus* sp. *Water Res.* **2017**, *122*, 148–158. [CrossRef]
7. Feng, C.; Lotti, T.; Canziani, R.; Lin, Y.; Tagliabue, C.; Malpei, F. Extracellular Biopolymers Recovered as Raw Biomaterials fr Waste Granular Sludge and Potential Applications: A Critical Review. *Sci. Total Environ.* **2021**, *753*, 142051. [CrossRef]
8. Sun, J.; Zhang, X.; Miao, X.; Zhou, J. Preparation and Characteristics of Bioflocculants from Excess Biological Sludge. *Biores Technol.* **2012**, *126*, 362–366. [CrossRef]
9. Zhang, X.; Sun, J.; Liu, X.; Zhou, J. Production and Flocculating Performance of Sludge Bioflocculant from Biological Slud *Bioresour. Technol.* **2013**, *146*, 51–56. [CrossRef]
10. Sheng, G.-P.; Yu, H.-Q.; Li, X.-Y. Extracellular Polymeric Substances (EPS) of Microbial Aggregates in Biological Wastewat Treatment Systems: A Review. *Biotechnol. Adv.* **2010**, *28*, 882–894. [CrossRef]
11. Frølund, B.; Palmgren, R.; Keiding, K.; Nielsen, P.H. Extraction of Extracellular Polymers from Activated Sludge Using a Cati Exchange Resin. *Water Res.* **1996**, *30*, 1749–1758. [CrossRef]
12. Yu, H.-Q. Molecular Insights into Extracellular Polymeric Substances in Activated Sludge. *Environ. Sci. Technol.* **2020**, 5 7742–7750. [CrossRef]
13. Wasmund, K.; Singleton, C.; Dahl Dueholm, M.K.; Wagner, M.; Nielsen, P.H. The Predicted Secreted Proteome of Activat Sludge Microorganisms Indicates Distinct Nutrient Niches. *mSystems* **2024**, *9*, e00301-24. [CrossRef] [PubMed]
14. Flemming, H.-C.; Van Hullebusch, E.D.; Little, B.J.; Neu, T.R.; Nielsen, P.H.; Seviour, T.; Stoodley, P.; Wingender, J.; Wuertz, Microbial Extracellular Polymeric Substances in the Environment, Technology and Medicine. *Nat. Rev. Microbiol.* **2025**, *23*, 87–1 [CrossRef] [PubMed]
15. Nabarlatz, D.; Stüber, F.; Font, J.; Fortuny, A.; Fabregat, A.; Bengoa, C. Extraction and Purification of Hydrolytic Enzymes fro Activated Sludge. *Resour. Conserv. Recycl.* **2012**, *59*, 9–13. [CrossRef]
16. Liu, Z.; Smith, S.R. Enzyme Recovery from Biological Wastewater Treatment. *Waste Biomass Valoriz.* **2021**, *12*, 4185–42 [CrossRef]
17. Toja Ortega, S.; Pronk, M.; De Kreuk, M.K. Anaerobic Hydrolysis of Complex Substrates in Full-Scale Aerobic Granular Slud Enzymatic Activity Determined in Different Sludge Fractions. *Appl. Microbiol. Biotechnol.* **2021**, *105*, 6073–6086. [CrossRef]
18. Felz, S.; Al-Zuhairy, S.; Aarstad, O.A.; Van Loosdrecht, M.C.M.; Lin, Y.M. Extraction of Structural Extracellular Polymer Substances from Aerobic Granular Sludge. *J. Vis. Exp.* **2016**, *115*, 54534. [CrossRef]
19. Pencreac'h, G.; Baratti, J.C. Hydrolysis of *p*-Nitrophenyl Palmitate in *n*-Heptane by the *Pseudomonas cepacia* Lipase: A Simple Te for the Determination of Lipase Activity in Organic Media. *Enzym. Microb. Technol.* **1996**, *18*, 417–422. [CrossRef]
20. Rondel, C.; Marcato-Romain, C.-E.; Girbal-Neuhauser, E. Development and Validation of a Colorimetric Assay for Simultaneo Quantification of Neutral and Uronic Sugars. *Water Res.* **2013**, *47*, 2901–2908. [CrossRef]
21. Felz, S.; Vermeulen, P.; Van Loosdrecht, M.C.M.; Lin, Y.M. Chemical Characterization Methods for the Analysis of Structur Extracellular Polymeric Substances (EPS). *Water Res.* **2019**, *157*, 201–208. [CrossRef]
22. Baird, R.B.; Eaton, A.D.; Rice, E.W. (Eds.) *Standard Methods for the Examination of Water and Wastewater*, 23rd ed.; America Public Health Association: Washington, DC, USA; American Water Works Association: Denver, CO, USA; Water Environmer Federation: Alexandria, VA, USA, 2017; ISBN 978-0-87553-287-5.
23. Lo, I.M.C.; Lai, K.C.K.; Chen, G.H. Salinity Effect on Mechanical Dewatering of Sludge with and without Chemical Conditionin *Environ. Sci. Technol.* **2001**, *35*, 4691–4696. [CrossRef] [PubMed]

 https://doi.org/10.3390/pr1403054

24. Andreottola, G.; Oliveira, E.L.D.; Foladori, P.; Dallago, L.; Peterlini, R.; Cadonna, M. Método respirométrico para o monitoramento de processos biológicos. *Eng. Sanit. Ambient.* **2005**, *10*, 14–23. [CrossRef]
25. Henze, M.; Grady, C.P.L.; Gujer, W.; Marais, G.V.R.; Matsuo, T. A General Model for Single-Sludge Wastewater Treatment Systems. *Water Res.* **1987**, *21*, 505–515. [CrossRef]
26. De Bruin, S.; Riisgaard-Jensen, M.; Hansen, S.H.; Van Loosdrecht, M.C.M.; Nielsen, P.H.; Lin, Y. Global Insights into Extracellular Polymeric Substances from Activated Sludge: Yield, Composition, and Microbial Communities. *Water Res.* **2026**, *289*, 124726. [CrossRef]
27. Li, J.; Hao, X.; Gan, W.; Van Loosdrecht, M.C.M.; Wu, Y. Recovery of Extracellular Biopolymers from Conventional Activated Sludge: Potential, Characteristics and Limitation. *Water Res.* **2021**, *205*, 117706. [CrossRef]
28. Frolund, B.; Griebe, T.; Nielsen, P.H. Enzymatic Activity in the Activated-Sludge Floc Matrix. *Appl. Microbiol. Biotechnol.* **1995**, *43*, 755–761. [CrossRef]
29. Liu, Z.; Smith, S.R. Enzyme Activity of Waste Activated Sludge Extracts. *Water Sci. Technol.* **2019**, *80*, 1861–1869. [CrossRef]
30. Yu, G.-H.; He, P.-J.; Shao, L.-M.; Lee, D.-J. Enzyme Activities in Activated Sludge Flocs. *Appl. Microbiol. Biotechnol.* **2007**, *77*, 605–612. [CrossRef]
31. Toja Ortega, S.; Van Den Berg, L.; Pronk, M.; De Kreuk, M.K. Hydrolysis Capacity of Different Sized Granules in a Full-Scale Aerobic Granular Sludge (AGS) Reactor. *Water Res. X* **2022**, *16*, 100151. [CrossRef]
32. Gessesse, A.; Dueholm, T.; Petersen, S.B.; Nielsen, P.H. Lipase and Protease Extraction from Activated Sludge. *Water Res.* **2003**, *37*, 3652–3657. [CrossRef]
33. Raunkjær, K.; Hvitved-Jacobsen, T.; Nielsen, P.H. Measurement of Pools of Protein, Carbohydrate and Lipid in Domestic Wastewater. *Water Res.* **1994**, *28*, 251–262. [CrossRef]
34. Zhang, Z.; Xia, S.; Zhang, J. Enhanced Dewatering of Waste Sludge with Microbial Flocculant TJ-F1 as a Novel Conditioner. *Water Res.* **2010**, *44*, 3087–3092. [CrossRef]
35. Shahadat, M.; Teng, T.T.; Rafatullah, M.; Shaikh, Z.A.; Sreekrishnan, T.R.; Ali, S.W. Bacterial Bioflocculants: A Review of Recent Advances and Perspectives. *Chem. Eng. J.* **2017**, *328*, 1139–1152. [CrossRef]
36. Paul, E.; Bessière, Y.; Dumas, C.; Girbal-Neuhauser, E. Biopolymers Production from Wastes and Wastewaters by Mixed Microbial Cultures: Strategies for Microbial Selection. *Waste Biomass Valoriz.* **2021**, *12*, 4213–4237. [CrossRef]
37. Liu, W.; Zhong, X.; Cheng, L.; Wang, J.; Sun, Y.; Deng, Y.; Zhang, Z. Cellular and Compositional Insight into the Sludge Dewatering Process Using Enzyme Treatment. *Environ. Sci. Pollut. Res.* **2018**, *25*, 28942–28953. [CrossRef]

https://doi.org/10.3390/pr14030547

processes

MDPI

Article

Circular Bioprocessing of *Chlorella* sp. Biomass via *Wickerhamomyces* sp. UFFS-CE-3.1.2 Fermentation for the Production of High-Value Enzymes, Glycerol, and Acetic Acid

Vitória Dassoler Longo [1,2], Marcelli Powzum Amorim [2,3], Nair Mirely Freire Pinheiro Silveira [1,2], Isabely Sandi Baldasso [1,2], Emanuely Fagundes da Silva [1,2], Arielle Cristina Fornari [4], Sérgio L. Alves, Jr. [5], Mateus Torres Nazari [6] and Helen Treichel [1,2,*]

1 Undergraduate Program in Environmental and Sanitary Engineering, Federal University of Fronteira Sul, Erechim 99700-000, RS, Brazil; vitorialongo22@gmail.com (V.D.L.); nairfreire460@gmail.com (N.M.F.P.S.); isabelysandibaldasso@gmail.com (I.S.B.); emanuelyfagundesdasilva@gmail.com (E.F.d.S.)
2 Laboratory of Microbiology and Bioprocess, Federal University of Fronteira Sul, Erechim 99700-000, RS, Brazil; marcellipowzum@gmail.com
3 Graduate Program in Environmental Science and Technology, Federal University of Fronteira Sul, Erechim 99700-000, RS, Brazil
4 Laboratory of Analytical Tests, Federal University of Fronteira Sul, Erechim 99700-000, RS, Brazil; arielle.fornari@uffs.edu.br
5 Laboratory of Yeast Biochemistry, Federal University of Fronteira Sul, Chapecó 89815-899, SC, Brazil; slalvesjr@uffs.edu.br
6 Graduate Program in Civil and Environmental Engineering (PPGEng), University of Passo Fundo (UPF), Passo Fundo 99052-900, RS, Brazil; nazari.eas@gmail.com
* Correspondence: helentreichel@gmail.com

Abstract

The transition to a circular economy and the pursuit of environmental sustainability are driving humanity to develop alternative technologies for producing a range of bioproducts. In this context, microbial-mediated fermentation processes have gained prominence. Although yeasts are well known for their ability to produce alcohols, they can also generate a wide range of value-added bioproducts. At the same time, microalgae emerge as an advantageous unconventional raw material, as their cultivation does not require arable land, thus avoiding competition with food production. To meet this demand, this study aimed to produce biocomposites through submerged fermentation using biomass from the microalgae *Chlorella* sp. Enzymatic hydrolysis was optimized using a 2^2 Central Composite Rotational Design (CCRD), with algal biomass and enzyme mass as independent variables. This step was followed by fermentation with the yeast *Wickerhamomyces* sp. UFFS-CE-3.1.2. The enzyme alpha amylase employed is of commercial origin, commonly used in the brewing industry, characterized by its easy accessibility and lower environmental impact compared to chemical hydrolysis methods. The results demonstrated that the combination of microalgae biomass with the enzyme preparation led to the production of several compounds of interest, such as highly active enzymes, mainly protease (560 U/mL), catalase (3381 U/mL), and peroxidase (277 U/mL), as well as other compounds, such as glycerol (32.5 g/L) and acetic acid (22.8 g/L). These products have wide industrial applications and a strong market demand, reinforcing the potential of the yeast–microalgae synergy for the sustainable production of high-value biocompounds, which represents a matrix of environmentally friendly products.

Keywords: biorefinery; catalase; circular economy; microalgae; peroxidase; protease; yeast

1. Introduction

Microalgae are a low-cost biomass with high potential for the practical production of environmentally relevant compounds. They can serve as energy sources and do not require arable land for cultivation; moreover, they grow rapidly and with relatively low water demands [1,2]. Microalgal biomass is primarily composed of carbohydrates, including polysaccharides such as glycogen, starch, and cellulose, which can be further processed in industry to produce target compounds, such as enzymes, glycerol, and organic acids, including acetic acid [1,3]. According to industry market reports and published surveys, the enzymes market size was USD 5.6 billion in 2023 and is expected to reach USD 10.7 billion by 2032, growing at a compound annual growth rate (CAGR) of 7.5% during the forecast period from 2024 to 2032. Microorganisms dominated the specific enzymes market, accounting for approximately 72%, in 2023 (http://www.globenewswire.com).

Typically, these fermentation processes are carried out using strains of *Saccharomyces cerevisiae*, characterized by rapid growth and reproduction, a short metabolic cycle with minimal byproducts, ease of cultivation and separation, and tolerance to specific concentrations of ethanol, acetic acid, and other inhibitors. However, the exclusive use of *S. cerevisiae* reduces the biochemical complexity of the process, ultimately decreasing the diversity of compounds and biocompounds [4]. Fermentations using non-*Saccharomyces* yeasts, such as *Wickerhamomyces* sp., produce a wide range of specific extracellular enzymes, including proteases, pectinases, cellulases, glycosidases, and lipolytic hydrolases, that act on relevant substrates for the production of alcohol, esters, fatty acids, terpenes, and other metabolites [5–7].

Recent research has increasingly focused on the use of microalgal biomass as a fermentation substrate, providing experimental evidence that algal-derived carbohydrates can be efficiently converted into value-added metabolites by different microorganisms. For example, microalgal hydrolysates obtained from *Chlorella* and *Scenedesmus* species have been successfully fermented by yeasts and bacteria, yielding products such as ethanol, organic acids, and polyols, with performances strongly dependent on hydrolysis efficiency and fermentation conditions. Studies using *Saccharomyces cerevisiae* demonstrated that properly conditioned microalgal hydrolysates can achieve ethanol yields comparable to those obtained from conventional lignocellulosic feedstocks, highlighting the technical feasibility of algal biomass in fermentation-based bioprocesses [8].

Beyond ethanol, microalgae-derived substrates have also been explored for the microbial production of organic acids. Chen et al. reported efficient lactic acid production from *Chlorella vulgaris* hydrolysates using immobilized *Lactobacillus plantarum*, achieving high productivities under optimized operating conditions [9]. In addition, fermentation and wet preservation of microalgal biomass have been shown to promote the formation of short-chain organic acids, with acetic acid frequently identified as a dominant metabolite, reinforcing the suitability of microalgal carbohydrates for acidogenic fermentation pathways [10]. These results demonstrate that microalgae can serve as a versatile carbon source not only for single-target products but also for integrated biorefinery schemes generating multiple biocompounds.

In parallel, increasing attention has been given to the use of non-*Saccharomyces* yeasts to modulate fermentation outcomes and expand product diversity. Several studies have shown that non-conventional yeasts can redirect carbon flux toward metabolites such as glycerol and organic acids, owing to differences in redox balancing, stress tolerance, and enzyme secretion compared with *S. cerevisiae*. For instance, *Starmerella bacillaris* has been associated with enhanced glycerol formation and altered organic acid profiles under controlled fermentation conditions, illustrating how yeast selection can be strategically employed to tailor metabolite production [11,12]. Although many of these investigations

https://doi.org/10.3390/pr14010111

are conducted in food- or beverage-related systems, the underlying metabolic principles are directly transferable to bioprocesses based on microalgal substrates.

Glycerol is a simple polyol widely used in the food and pharmaceutical industries for the production of cosmetics, paints, medicines, paper, textiles, leather, and explosives [13]. It is expected to become a key platform compound for the development of biopolymers and other high-value chemicals [14]. An alternative method for glycerol production involves microbial cells converting carbohydrates or CO_2 into glycerol. New strains of yeast, algae, and cyanobacteria, found in nature or genetically modified, can be used [15]. Under anaerobic conditions, glycerol production is consistently associated with the generation of byproducts, including ethanol, acetate, acetic acid, and acetoin, all of which have industrial value [16]. Acetic acid is an essential organic acid, widely used in the food, pharmaceutical, and chemical industries [17]. It is produced through an initial fermentation step and prepared from starchy or sugary raw materials [18]. Other compounds are generated during fermentation, such as enzymes, which can be applied in various areas, including sanitation, energy production, herbicide production, and hydrolysis [19].

Despite the growing body of literature on microalgae-based fermentation, there remains a lack of studies that systematically integrate microalgal biomass hydrolysis, fermentation with non-*Saccharomyces* yeasts, and operation in a controlled stirred-tank bioreactor (STR). In particular, limited attention has been given to how alternative enzymatic hydrolysis strategies affect downstream fermentation performance and the formation of targeted biocompounds, such as glycerol, organic acids, and enzymes, during scale-relevant bioreactor operation. Moreover, while non-*Saccharomyces* yeasts are increasingly recognized for their metabolic versatility, their application as biocatalysts in microalgae-based fermentation systems remains underexplored. The use of *Wickerhamomyces* sp., therefore, represents an additional distinguishing feature of this study, as this genus combines fermentative capacity with extracellular enzyme production and metabolic traits that may favor the formation of diverse biocompounds from complex substrates.

The integration of biotechnology with microalgal biomass has strong potential to contribute to the development of a low-carbon circular economy by enabling the conversion of renewable resources into multiple value-added products. Within this context, the novelty of the present work lies in combining an alternative enzymatic hydrolysis approach with fermentation optimization in a controlled stirred-tank bioreactor using *Wickerhamomyces* sp. as the production microorganism. Therefore, this study aimed to optimize fermentation performance for the production of targeted biocompounds from microalgae-derived substrates under STR conditions, providing insights into process behavior and metabolite formation relevant to the design and scale-up of microalgae-based bioprocesses.

2. Materials and Methods

2.1. Microalgal Biomass

Commercial microalgae of the genus *Chlorella* sp. were purchased from a commercial supplier (Brasbol, lot 10271, Sao Paulo, Brazil). They were stored at −60 °C until use. The moisture content was measured using a moisture analyzer to standardize the residual moisture in the biomass. According to the supplier, the microalgae biomass contains 2 g of carbohydrates, 5 g of protein, and 1.3 g of total fat per 10 g of biomass (https://www.zonacerealista.com.br, accessed on March, 2025).

2.2. Pretreatment and Saccharification

To optimize enzymatic saccharification, an experimental design was conducted with algal biomass mass and the volume of commercial alpha-amylase (200 U/mL) as inde-

 https://doi.org/10.3390/pr1401011

pendent variables. The experimental design was performed using a Central Composite Rotational Design (CCRD) (Table 1), with total reducing sugars as the response variable.

Table 1. CCRD for saccharification (absolute and coded values).

Assay	Mass (g)	Volume of Enzyme (mL)/Unit Concentration (U)
1	20 (−1)	2/200 (−1)
2	20 (−1)	7/1400 (1)
3	40 (1)	2/200 (−1)
4	40 (1)	7/1400 (1)
5	30 (0)	0.96/192 (−1.41)
6	30 (0)	8.04/1608 (1.41)
7	15.86 (−1.41)	4.50/900 (0)
8	44.14 (1.41)	4.50/900 (0)
9	30 (0)	4.50/900 (0)
10	30 (0)	4.50/900 (0)
11	30 (0)	4.50/900 (0)

The procedure began with a physical pretreatment to release carbohydrates from the microalgae. The experimental biomass masses (Table 1), corrected for moisture content, were diluted to 100 mL in 0.2 M sodium phosphate buffer (pH 5.5). The solution was frozen at −20 °C for 24 h, then incubated at 4 °C for 24 h, and finally placed in a thermostatic water bath at 100 °C for 10 min, as described by Rempel et al. [20].

Subsequently, saccharification was performed by adding α-amylase to the microalgal biomass (Table 1) and maintaining the mixture at 50 °C and 150 rpm in an orbital shaker. Samples were collected to determine available reducing sugars using the 3,5-dinitrosalicylic acid (DNS) method [21].

2.3. *Microorganism and Inoculum*

The yeast used in fermentation was *Wickerhamomyces* sp. UFFS-CE-3.1.2 [22]. It was maintained in YPD growth medium, composed of 1% yeast extract, 2% peptone, 2% glucose, and 2% agar. The strain was transferred to liquid YPD medium (without agar) and incubated at 30 °C for 24 h before inoculation into the wort at 10% (*v*/*v*) [23].

2.4. *Shake-Flask Fermentation*

The wort, with a volume of 250 mL and a working volume of 100 mL, was adjusted to pH 5.0. After inoculation, the experiments were maintained at 30 °C and 120 rpm for 48 h. Subsequently, the wort was subjected to fermentation with *Wickerhamomyces* sp. UFFS-CE-3.1.2 [24]. Aliquots of 2.5 mL were collected at 0, 12, 24, and 48 h for quantification of sugars, glycerol, carboxylic acids, and ethanol.

2.5. *Scale-Up Fermentation*

To scale up the process and assess the impact of volume on compound production, the experiment yielding the best results was fermented in a stirred tank reactor (STR) (BIO TEC, Tecnal, Piracicaba, Brazil) with a total volume of 7 L, as shown in Figure 1. A total of 800 g (dry biomass, corrected for moisture) of microalgae was weighed and diluted into 2 L of 0.2 M sodium phosphate buffer (pH 5.5). The wort was autoclaved at 121 °C and 1 atm to sterilize the medium and pre-treat the biomass. Due to the high temperature, the sterilization process also served as a pretreatment step, fractionating the structural polymers to enhance the accessibility of hydrolytic enzymes to carbohydrates in the subsequent step (hydrolysis/saccharification).

https://doi.org/10.3390/pr14010111

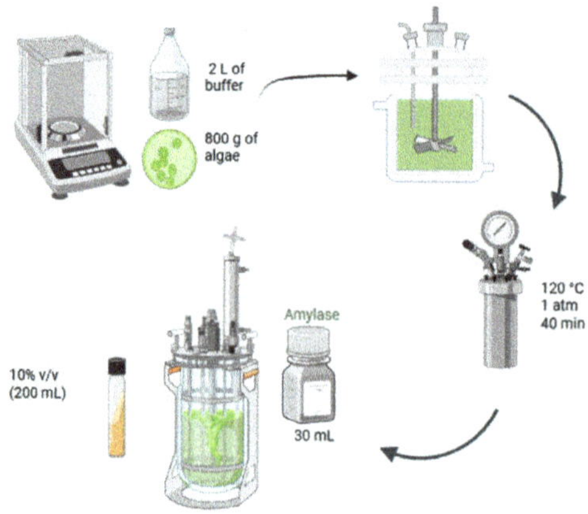

Figure 1. Scale-up of the process using an STR.

Then, 45 mL of the enzyme (activity as specified in Table 1) was added to the bioreactor to initiate saccharification. The amounts of microalgae and enzyme corresponded to the optimal conditions obtained in the shaken-flask fermentation but were scaled up to a final volume of 2 L. An additional 1 L was added, bringing the total to 3 L, to improve homogenization of the medium and facilitate subsequent steps, given the medium's viscosity. After one hour, yeast was inoculated at 10% (v/v) and transferred into the fermentation tank, as described by Bonatto et al. [24]. Fermentation was conducted for 72 h at 30 °C and 80 rpm. Samples were collected at 0, 12, 24, 48, and 72 h for further analysis.

2.6. Enzymatic Analysis

To analyze and quantify the enzymes present in the reactor fermentation, the methods described by Kubeneck et al. [19] were used. Blank assays containing reaction buffer and substrate without cell extract were included in all measurements to account for background signals. For amylase (with starch as the substrate) and cellulase (cellulose as the standard substrate), the methodology adopted was to quantify total reducing sugars, with readings taken on a spectrophotometer at 540 nm using the DNS method [21]. The enzymatic activities of amylase and cellulase were calculated from the glucose standard curve and expressed in units per milliliter (U/mL).

Peroxidase activity, using 8% hydrogen peroxide as the standard substrate, was determined by measuring absorbance at 470 nm and expressed as units per milliliter (U/mL). The substrate for the laccase enzyme reaction was 2,2′-azino-di-3-ethylbenzothiazoline-6-sulfonic acid (ABTS), and U was defined as the amount of enzyme capable of forming one µmol of ABTS+ per minute under the reaction conditions. Protease activity with casein as the substrate was determined by spectrophotometry at 660 nm, and U was defined as the amount of enzyme required to release 1 µg of tyrosine per minute under the test conditions.

Catalase activity, using 0.0125 M hydrogen peroxide as the substrate, was measured at 240 nm for 3 min, with readings taken every 30 s, to monitor the formation of oxidized products. For ascorbate peroxidase, a wavelength of 290 nm was used, with readings taken every 15 s for 1 min, using 0.008 M ascorbic acid as the substrate. One unit (U) of catalase activity was defined as the amount of enzyme catalyzing the conversion of 1 µmol of hydrogen peroxide per minute under the assay conditions. Finally, superoxide dismutase activity was measured under light exposure, using a 15 kW fluorescent lamp, except for the control, which was kept in the dark. Enzymatic activity was quantified at 560 nm every

https://doi.org/10.3390/pr14010111

1 min for 15 s. Superoxide dismutase activity is determined by the amount of enzyme required to inhibit 50% of the photoreduction of NBT (4-Nitro blue tetrazolium chloride).

2.7. Analytical Methods

Quantification of glucose, cellobiose, arabinose, and fructose, as well as ethanol, glycerol, citric acid, and acetic acid, was performed by High-Performance Liquid Chromatography (HPLC). Samples were diluted with 0.005 M sulfuric acid, vacuum-filtered using a Millipore® (Merck Millipore, Burlington, MA, USA) 0.45 μm membrane, and degassed in an ultrasonic bath for 15 min [18]. The chromatographic system consisted of a Shimadzu instrument equipped with a refractive index detector (RID-10A) and an Aminex Biorad HPX-87H column (Shimadzu do Brasil, Barueri, Brazil). Chromatographic conditions were as follows: mobile phase (H_2SO_4), flow rate 0.6 mL/min, and temperature 45 °C [22].

2.8. Statistical Analysis

Statistical analysis of the CCRD 2^2 was performed using Protimiza Experimental Design software (https://experimental-design.protimiza.com.br/, accessed in 2025), with a 95% confidence level ($p < 0.05$). The central point of the experimental design, as recommended by the tool, was used to determine the standard deviation.

3. Results and Discussion

3.1. Optimization of Enzymatic Hydrolysis

The results of the experimental trials demonstrated the high potential of commercial amylase to convert biomass polysaccharides into fermentable sugars, as shown in Table 2, thereby catalyzing the hydrolysis of starch and other α-glucans [25]. In Assay 3, with 40 g of microalgae biomass and 2 mL of enzyme, approximately 31.8 g/L of total reducing sugars (TRS) were obtained after saccharification. This condition was selected for scale-up because it was identified as the most promising for producing compounds of interest through fermentation in a bioreactor. Given the amount of sugar available, this condition underscores the importance of enzyme loading in process feasibility. Among the compounds analyzed, ethanol was produced at low concentrations under the tested conditions, whereas acetic acid reached 23 g/L after 48 h of fermentation. This concentration is technically relevant, as acetic acid is a key platform chemical in biorefinery concepts and can be integrated as an intermediate for downstream valorization routes, rather than being considered solely as a low-value end product [26,27]. In addition, acetic acid is increasingly recognized as a versatile building block for the synthesis of fuels, solvents, polymers, and esters, which supports its inclusion in integrated bioprocess schemes that generate multiple products from renewable feedstocks [26]. Reported acetic acid titers in microalgae-based or mixed-substrate fermentation systems vary widely depending on microorganism and process configuration, typically ranging from a few grams per liter to tens of grams per liter, placing the value obtained in this study within the upper range of reported concentrations for biologically derived acetic acid [27]. Compounds such as citric acid and arabinose were not detected at any time.

Assay 1 showed an attractive sugar content; however, these sugars were not consumed during fermentation, which does not indicate the formation of bioproducts of this consumption, such as sugars and acids. The optimized model was evaluated using Analysis of Variance (ANOVA), as shown in Table 3, where the calculated F-value exceeded the tabulated F-value, and the R^2 value was 86%. These results indicate that the experimental data are well explained by Equation 1, where A represents the enzyme volume, and B represents the algal biomass mass.

https://doi.org/10.3390/pr14010111

$$\text{TRS (g/L)} = 26.55 - 3.14 \times A - 8.16 \times A^2 + 0.41 \times B - 5.52 \times B^2 + 4.62 \times A \times B \quad (1)$$

where A: enzyme volume; B: microalgal biomass mass

Table 2. Total reducing sugar production from enzymatic hydrolysis.

Assay	Mass (g)	Volume of Enzyme (mL)	Total Reducing Sugars (g/L) *
1	20 (−1)	2 (−1)	29.86
2	20 (−1)	7 (1)	26.36
3	40 (1)	2 (−1)	31.83
4	40 (1)	7 (1)	30.72
5	30 (0)	0.96 (−1.41)	18.14
6	30 (0)	8.04 (1.41)	15.42
7	15.86 (−1.41)	4.50 (0)	23.62
8	44.14 (1.41)	4.50 (0)	30.01
9	30 (0)	4.50 (0)	39.82 **
10	30 (0)	4.50 (0)	34.22 **
11	30 (0)	4.50 (0)	37.46 **

* Standard deviation of each experiment was less than 5% (n = 3). ** Standard deviation of 2.81 g/L.

Table 3. Analysis of variance (ANOVA) for total reducing sugar (TRS) production.

Source of Variation	Sum of Squares	Degrees of Freedom	Mean Square	F-Test
Regression	601.7	5	120.3	6.1
Residual	98.6	5	19.7	
Lack of fit	97.7	3		
Pure error	0.9	2		
Total	700.3	10		

Regression Coefficient: $R = 0.85$; $F_{(0.95;5;5)} = 5.05$.

Between enzyme concentration and algal biomass, intermediate concentrations were favorable for the process. In this study, the enzyme used was readily available, allowing feasible concentration ranges; however, using smaller amounts of enzyme is preferable. A contour plot was constructed based on the model validation, as shown in Figure 2, highlighting the central region.

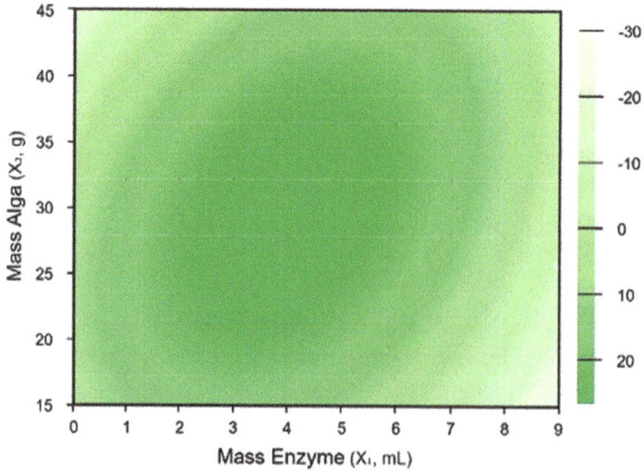

Figure 2. Reducing sugar obtained by enzymatic hydrolysis, represented by the CCRD 2^2 response surface.

https://doi.org/10.3390/pr1401011

Some assays, such as 5 and 6, demonstrated significant sugar consumption during fermentation, 80% and 84%, respectively. However, in Assay 5, the low availability of sugars released during hydrolysis suggests a potentially lower product yield. On the other hand, Assay 6, which used 30 g of biomass and 8.04 mL of enzyme, achieved considerable sugar conversion; however, its enzyme volume was 4 times that of Assay 3, making the process less economically viable.

As shown in Figure 3, Assay 3 produced 2.44 g/L of glycerol and 0.67 g/L of acetic acid in 12 h, representing the best condition for total reducing sugars (TRS), as it contained 15.84 g/L at the start of fermentation. Next, Assay 4 stands out for producing 32.5 g/L of glycerol in 24 h and 18.86 g/L of TRS, while Assay 1 produced 22.8 g/L of acetic acid in 48 h with 36 g/L of TRS.

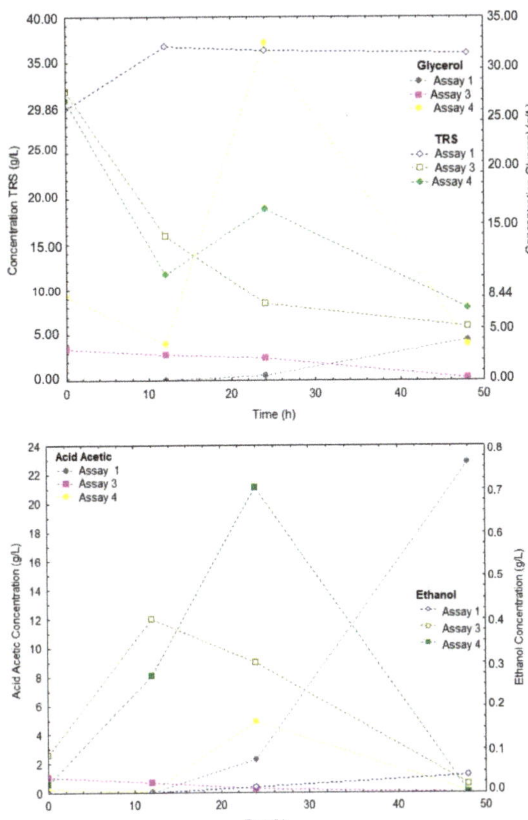

Figure 3. Sugar consumption and production of different compounds during fermentation. Standard deviation of each experiment was less than 5% ($n = 3$).

Studies demonstrate a relationship between high glycerol production and low ethanol yield, caused by the diversion of dihydroxyacetone phosphate from glycolysis toward glycerol-3-phosphate via the enzyme glycerol-3-phosphate dehydrogenase. This process consumes NADH and reduces the fermentative flux, thereby decreasing ethanol production. However, due to redox imbalance, acetic acid accumulates [28], a primary fermentation inhibitor that impairs yeast growth and metabolism [29,30]. Consequently, in experiment 1, ethanol production was hampered by the high acetic acid concentration resulting from sugar degradation [31].

https://doi.org/10.3390/pr14010111

3.2. Scale-Up

During scale-up, it was observed that 2 L of buffer was insufficient for fermentation, as the medium became dense, hindering reactor agitation and other operational parameters. Therefore, an additional 1 L of buffer was added before sterilization and fermentation. It is important to note that scale-up is not necessarily linear; bioprocess scaling typically relies on empirical and semi-empirical approaches to maintain consistency in key process variables [32].

The fermentation results are shown in the Supplementary Material (Table S1). The central values found were: 36.34 g/L of TRS at zero h, 2.10 g/L of glycerol at zero h, 1.47 g/L of ethanol at 24 h, and 0.68 g/L of acetic acid at 48 h. The ethanol concentration was lower compared to optimized fermentations with *Chlorella* sp., where values above 10 g/L were reported [33] and up to 20 g/L with efficient pretreatment and the use of *Saccharomyces cerevisiae* [34]. This difference may be related to the limited availability of fermentable sugars.

Regarding acetic acid, the accumulation of 0.68 g/L is considered moderate. In fermentations with *S. cerevisiae* or *Zymomonas mobilis*, concentrations between 5 and 10 g/L already exert strong inhibitory effects, while under extreme conditions (7.5–15 g/L), significant reductions in growth and sugar consumption occur. Thus, the value obtained in this study is below the critical threshold, suggesting it did not substantially compromise fermentation [35–37].

3.3. Evaluation of Enzymatic Activities

This study successfully documented the presence of various enzymes during fermentation in a reactor using the added microorganism. The yeast *Wickerhamomyces* sp. UFFS-CE-3.1.2 has been previously used for ethanol production; however, different studies are expanding the range of products derived from its metabolism. This study highlights its potential for producing a fermented composite rich in enzymes with diverse applications. A significant increase in the production of various enzymes was observed after 24 h of fermentation. This is because decomposition processes drive the synthesis and secretion of enzymes [38].

The results demonstrate that the enzyme composite is rich in catalase, protease, and peroxidase, as shown in Figure 4. Crucial antioxidant enzymes, such as superoxide dismutase, peroxidase, catalase, and ascorbate peroxidase, play a vital role in scavenging free radicals. Catalase is responsible for the degradation or reduction of hydrogen peroxide into water and oxygen [39,40], reaching an activity of 3381 U/mL in 48 h, highlighting that catalase activity was already elevated at the beginning of fermentation when compared to baseline levels typically reported for yeasts under non-stressed or early growth conditions [41]. Catalase is a key oxidative stress-response enzyme in yeasts, and its activity increases in response to reactive oxygen species generated during aerobic cultivation, substrate complexity, or metabolic shifts, which may explain the early activation observed in this study [41,42].

In this study, a protease production of 560.55 U/mL was achieved by the end of fermentation. Protease facilitates the hydrolysis of proteins into amino acids, making them more readily available for absorption [43]. The synergistic action of other enzymes present in the fermentation matrix can enhance protease activity. Cofactors, coenzymes, or activators derived from plant extracts and yeast strains can facilitate protease activation and enhance overall proteolytic activity [44,45]. Egbune et al. [46] reported a protease activity of 39.2 U/mL. Consequently, the biomass and microorganisms used in this fermentation produced a substantially higher protease yield than in other studies. Enzymes such as ascorbate peroxidase, cellulase, and laccase showed consistently low activities (<2 U/mL)

https://doi.org/10.3390/pr14010111

at all sampling times (Figure 5). Blank assays confirmed that these values were close to background signal levels.

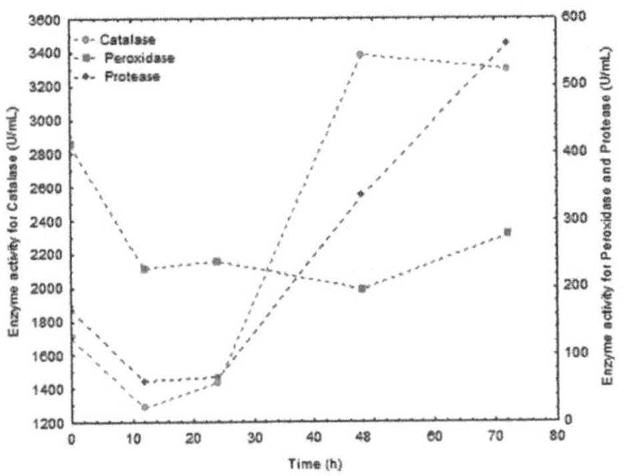

Figure 4. Enzymatic activities during fermentation. Standard deviation of each experiment was less than 5% (n = 3).

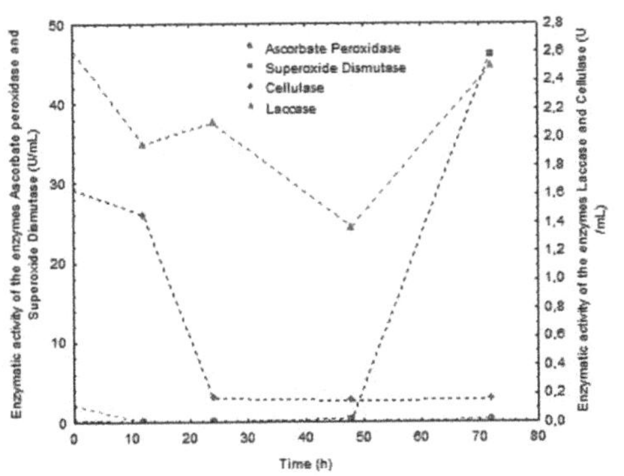

Figure 5. Other enzymes quantified in fermentation. Standard deviation of each experiment was less than 5% (n = 3) (ascorbate peroxidase and superoxide dismutase refer to the left Y-axis, and the other enzymes to the right Y-axis).

The enzyme superoxide dismutase showed a significant activity level at 72 h, with a value of 46 U/mL. Specifically, this enzyme facilitates the dismutation of the superoxide anion (O_2^-) into O_2 and H_2O_2, while peroxidase limits the accumulation of free radicals in plant cells, mitigating oxidative stress. Ascorbate peroxidase further detoxifies H_2O_2, thereby protecting plant cells from oxidative stress-induced damage [47,48]. For peroxidase, the highest activity was 277.78 U/mL at 72 h of fermentation. This value is based on the initial amount of enzyme present in the must, which was not produced by the microorganism. This enzyme requires organic hydroperoxides or H_2O_2 as co-substrates to stimulate oxidative reactions [33].

4. Conclusions

This study investigated the conversion of microalgae-derived substrates into targeted biocompounds via fermentation with *Wickerhamomyces* sp. in a stirred-tank bioreactor (STR) using an alternative enzymatic hydrolysis strategy. The results demonstrated that microalgal biomass can be effectively converted into a fermentable medium and processed under controlled bioreactor conditions, yielding organic acids, polyols, and enzyme-related activities. The observed fermentation profiles highlighted the importance of integrating

 https://doi.org/10.3390/pr14010111

upstream hydrolysis conditions with downstream fermentation performance to control metabolite distribution.

The use of a non-*Saccharomyces* yeast was a critical aspect of this work, as *Wickerhamomyces* sp. exhibited metabolic versatility when cultivated on microalgae-derived substrates, supporting the concept of diversified bioproduct generation in microalgae-based biorefineries. Moreover, the application of the STR operation enabled a more realistic assessment of process behavior, contributing to the understanding of fermentation performance under scale-relevant conditions.

From a future perspective, further development of this type of research may focus on optimizing operational parameters, such as aeration, agitation, and feeding strategies, to enhance process robustness and selectively steer metabolite formation. In addition, integrating techno-economic analysis and life cycle assessment would provide valuable insights into the feasibility and sustainability of microalgae-based fermentation routes. Exploring different microalgal species, hydrolysis strategies, and microbial systems, including co-cultivation approaches, may further expand the portfolio of value-added products and advance integrated microalgae biorefinery concepts.

Supplementary Materials: The following supporting information can be downloaded at: https://www.mdpi.com/article/10.3390/pr14010111/s1, Table S1. Compounds monitored during 72 h STR fermentation.

Author Contributions: Conceptualization: V.D.L. and H.T.; Formal analysis and investigation: V.D.L., M.P.A., N.M.F.P.S., I.S.B., E.F.d.S. and A.C.F.; Writing—original draft preparation: V.D.L., M.P.A., N.M.F.P.S., I.S.B., E.F.d.S. and A.C.F.; Writing—review and editing: M.T.N., S.L.A.J. and H.T.; Supervision: H.T. All authors have read and agreed to the published version of the manuscript.

Funding: This study was supported by the following Brazilian Funding Agencies: the National Council for Scientific and Technological Development (CNPq—302484/2022-1) and the Coordination for the Improvement of Higher Education Personnel (CAPES – 001). The support of the Bioprocess and Biotechnology for Food Research Center (Biofood), which is funded through the Research Support Foundation of Rio Grande do Sul (FAPERGS-22/2551-0000397-4) and PqGaúcho FAPERGS (24/2551-0001209-5), and the Federal University of Fronteira Sul (UFFS) for the financial support.

Data Availability Statement: The original contributions presented in this study are included in the article/Supplementary Material. Further inquiries can be directed to the corresponding author.

Conflicts of Interest: The authors declare no conflicts of interest.

References

1. Samoylova, Y.V.; Sorokina, K.N.; Parmon, V.N. Use of microalgae biomass to synthesize marketable products: 4. Production biofuels from microalgae using bioengineering approaches. *Catal. Ind.* **2024**, *16*, 89–101. [CrossRef]
2. Konwar, G.; Banik, R.; Geed, S.R. Bioprocess strategies for bioethanol production from algae-derived carbohydrates: Scalab solutions and industry prospects in a circular bioeconomy. *Chem. Eng. J.* **2025**, *515*, 163456. [CrossRef]
3. Farkas, C.; Rezessy-Szabó, J.M.; Gupta, V.K.; Truong, D.H.; Friedrich, L.; Felföldi, J.; Nguyen, Q.D. Microbial saccharification wheat bran for bioethanol fermentation. *J. Clean. Prod.* **2019**, *240*, 118269. [CrossRef]
4. Padilla, B.; Gil, J.V.; Manzanares, P. Challenges of the non-conventional yeast *Wickerhamomyces anomalus* in winemakin *Fermentation* **2018**, *4*, 68. [CrossRef]
5. Chen, L.; Li, D.; Ren, L.; Song, S.; Ma, X.; Rong, Y. Effects of Simultaneous and Sequential Co-Fermentation on Microbi Interactions and Aroma of Rice Wine. *Food Sci. Nutr.* **2021**, *9*, 71–86. [CrossRef]
6. Sun, N.; Gao, Z.; Li, S.; Chen, X.; Guo, J. Assessment of chemical constitution and aroma properties of kiwi wines obtained fro pure and mixed fermentation with *Wickerhamomyces anomalus* and *Saccharomyces cerevisiae*. *J. Sci. Food Agric.* **2022**, *102*, 175–18 [CrossRef]
7. Lai, Y.-T.; Chen, C.-H.; Lo, Y.-C.; Hsieh, C.-W.; Hsu, F.-C.; Cheng, K.-C. Application of aroma-producing yeasts and agein technology in Kyoho-fortified wine. *Eur. Food Res. Technol.* **2023**, *249*, 2849–2860. [CrossRef]

https://doi.org/10.3390/pr140101

8. Seon, G.; Kim, H.S.; Cho, J.M.; Kim, M.; Park, W.-K.; Chang, Y.K. Effect of post-treatment process of microalgal hydrolysate on bioethanol production. *Sci. Rep.* **2020**, *10*, 16698. [CrossRef]
9. Chen, P.-T.; Hong, Z.-S.; Cheng, C.-L.; Ng, I.-S.; Lo, Y.-C.; Nagarajan, D.; Chang, J.-S. Exploring fermentation strategies for enhanced lactic acid production with polyvinyl alcohol-immobilized *Lactobacillus plantarum* 23 using microalgae as feedstock. *Bioresour. Technol.* **2020**, *308*, 123266. [CrossRef]
10. Verspreet, J.; Kuchendorf, C.M.; Ackermann, B.; Bastiaens, L. The Impact of Nutrient Limitation and Harvest Method on the Wet Preservation of *Chlorella vulgaris* Biomass. *Bioengineering* **2023**, *10*, 600. [CrossRef]
11. Nadai, C.; Duarte, V.d.S.; Sica, J.; Vincenzi, S.; Carlot, M.; Giacomini, A.; Corich, V. *Starmerella bacillaris* Released in Vineyards at Different Concentrations Influences Wine Glycerol Content Depending on the Vinification Protocols. *Foods* **2022**, *12*, 3. [CrossRef] [PubMed]
12. Rossetti, A.P.; Perpetuini, G.; Tofalo, R. Sniffing the wine differences: The role of Starmerella bacillaris biofilm-detached cells. *Heliyon* **2024**, *10*, e35692. [CrossRef] [PubMed]
13. Semkiv, M.; Dmytruk, K.; Abbas, C.; Sibirny, A. Biotechnology of glycerol production and conversion in yeasts. In *Biotechnology of Yeasts and Filamentous Fungi*; Springer: Cham, Switzerland, 2017; pp. 117–148. [CrossRef]
14. Pagliaro, M. Glycerol. In *Green Chemicals and Processes*; Elsevier: Amsterdam, The Netherlands, 2017; pp. 109–132. [CrossRef]
15. Zhao, X.; Procopio, S.; Becker, T. Flavor impacts of glycerol in the processing of yeast fermented beverages: A review. *J. Food Sci. Technol.* **2015**, *52*, 7588–7598. [CrossRef] [PubMed]
16. Semkiv, M.V.; Ruchala, J.; Dmytruk, K.V.; Sibirny, A.A. 100 Years Later, What Is New in Glycerol Bioproduction? *Trends Biotechnol.* **2020**, *38*, 907–916. [CrossRef]
17. Solieri, L.; Giudici, P. *Vinegars of the World*; Springer: Milan, Italy, 2009; pp. 1–16.
18. Saichana, N.; Matsushita, K.; Adachi, O.; Frébort, I.; Frebortova, J. Acetic acid bacteria: A group of bacteria with versatile biotechnological applications. *Biotechnol. Adv.* **2015**, *33*, 1260–1271. [CrossRef]
19. Kubeneck, S.; Camargo, A.F.; Longo, V.D.; Romani, L.C.; Nerling, J.P.; Bazoti, S.F.; Pagno, C.H.; Rodrigues, E.; Treichel, H. Characterization of enzymatic and metabolic properties of a biocomposite based on *Trichoderma koningiopsis* and *Chlorella* biomass. *Biocatal. Agric. Biotechnol.* **2025**, *65*, 103542. [CrossRef]
20. Rempel, A.; Machado, T.; Treichel, H.; Colla, E.; Margarites, A.C.; Colla, L.M. Saccharification of *Spirulina platensis* biomass using free and immobilized amylolytic enzymes. *Bioresour. Technol.* **2018**, *263*, 163–171. [CrossRef]
21. Miller, G.L. Use of dinitrosalicylic acid reagent for the determination of reducing sugar. *Anal. Chem.* **1959**, *31*, 426–428. [CrossRef]
22. Bazoti, S.F.; Golunski, S.; Pereira Siqueira, D.; Scapini, T.; Barrilli, É.T.; Alex Mayer, D.; Barros, K.O.; Rosa, C.A.; Stambuk, B.U.; Alves, S.L.; et al. Second-generation ethanol from non-detoxified sugarcane hydrolysate by a rotting wood isolated yeast strain. *Bioresour. Technol.* **2017**, *244*, 582–587. [CrossRef]
23. Zanivan, J.; Bonatto, C.; Scapini, T.; Dalastra, C.; Bazoti, S.F.; Alves, S.L., Jr.; Fongaro, G.; Treichel, H. Evaluation of bioethanol production from mixed fruit waste by *Wickerhamomyces* sp. UFFS-CE-3.1.2. *BioEnergy Res.* **2021**, *15*, 175–182. [CrossRef]
24. Bonatto, C.; Scapini, T.; Zanivan, J.; Dalastra, C.; Bazoti, S.F.; Alves, S.L., Jr.; Fongaro, G.; Oliveira, D.; Treichel, H. Utilization of seawater and wastewater from shrimp production in the fermentation of papaya residues to ethanol. *Bioresour. Technol.* **2021**, *321*, 124501. [CrossRef]
25. Siqueira, J.G.W.; Rodrigues, C.; Vandenberghe, L.P.S.; Woiciechowski, A.L.; Soccol, C.R. Current advances in on-site cellulase production and application on lignocellulosic biomass conversion to biofuels: A review. *Biomass Bioenergy* **2020**, *132*, 105419. [CrossRef]
26. Straathof, A.J.J. Transformation of biomass into commodity chemicals using enzymes or cells. *Chem. Rev.* **2014**, *114*, 1871–1908. [CrossRef]
27. Blöbaum, L.; Haringa, C.; Grünberger, A. Microbial Lifelines in Bioprocesses: From Concept to Application. *Biotechnol. Adv.* **2023**, *62*, 108071. [CrossRef] [PubMed]
28. Remize, F.; Roustan, J.-L.; Sablayrolles, J.-M.; Barre, P.; Dequin, S. Glycerol overproduction by engineered *Saccharomyces cerevisiae* wine yeast strains leads to substantial changes in byproduct formation and to a stimulation of fermentation rate in stationary phase. *Appl. Environ. Microbiol.* **1999**, *65*, 143–149. [CrossRef] [PubMed]
29. Guaragnella, N.; Bettiga, M. Acetic acid stress in budding yeast: From molecular mechanisms to applications. *Yeast* **2021**, *38*, 391–400. [CrossRef]
30. Li, Y.-C.; Du, W.; Meng, F.-B.; Rao, J.-W.; Liu, D.-Y.; Peng, L.-X. Tartary buckwheat protein hydrolysates enhance the salt tolerance of the soy sauce fermentation yeast *Zygosaccharomyces rouxii*. *Food Chem.* **2021**, *342*, 128382. [CrossRef]
31. Han, J.; Li, D.; Han, F.; Huang, K.; Yang, F.; Xu, Y. A practical regeneration approach and model simulation for poisoned-resin recycle to selectively detoxify acetic acid-like bio-inhibitors in acidic lignocellulose hydrolysate. *Sep. Purif. Technol.* **2024**, *328*, 125110. [CrossRef]
32. Garcia-Ochoa, F.; Gomez, E. Bioreactor scale-up and oxygen transfer rate in microbial processes: An overview. *Biotechnol. Adv.* **2009**, *27*, 153–176. [CrossRef]

 https://doi.org/10.3390/pr14010111

33. Ngamsirisomsakul, M.; Reungsang, A.; Liao, Q.; Kongkeitkajorn, M.B. Enhanced bioethanol production from *Chlorella* sp. bioma by hydrothermal pretreatment and enzymatic hydrolysis. *Renew. Energy* **2019**, *141*, 482–492. [CrossRef]
34. Condor, B.E.; de Luna, M.D.G.; Chang, Y.-H.; Chen, J.-H.; Leong, Y.-K.; Chen, P.-T.; Chen, C.-Y.; Lee, D.-J.; Chang, J.-S. Bioethan production from microalgae biomass at high-solids loadings. *Bioresour. Technol.* **2022**, *363*, 128002. [CrossRef] [PubMed]
35. Samakkarn, W.; Vandecruys, P.; Moreno, M.R.F.; Thevelein, J.M.; Ratanakhanokchai, K.; Soontorngun, N. New biomarke underlying acetic acid tolerance in the probiotic yeast *Saccharomyces cerevisiae* var. *boulardii*. *Appl. Microbiol. Biotechnol.* **202** *108*, 153. [CrossRef] [PubMed]
36. Chen, Y.; Stabryla, L.; Wei, N. Improved acetic acid resistance in *Saccharomyces cerevisiae* by overexpression of the *WHI2* ger identified through inverse metabolic engineering. *Appl. Environ. Microbiol.* **2016**, *82*, 2156–2166. [CrossRef] [PubMed]
37. Zhao, J.; Wang, Z.; Wang, M.; He, Q.; Zhang, H. The inhibition of *Saccharomyces cerevisiae* cells by acetic acid quantified b electrochemistry and fluorescence. *Bioelectrochemistry* **2008**, *72*, 117–121. [CrossRef]
38. Yang, L.; Cheng, J.; Zhao, Y.; Guo, F. Quality control and law exploration of microbial oil production from spent grains fermente by *Wickerhamomyces anomalus* CY2. *J. Environ. Manag.* **2025**, *380*, 124854. [CrossRef]
39. Gauthier, M.R.; Senhorinho, G.N.A.; Scott, J.A. Microalgae under environmental stress as a source of antioxidants. *Algal Res.* **202** *52*, 102104. [CrossRef]
40. Ighodaro, O.M.; Akinloye, O.A. First Line Defence Antioxidants—Superoxide Dismutase (SOD), Catalase (CAT) and Glutathion Peroxidase (GPx): Their Fundamental Role in the Entire Antioxidant Defence Grid. *Alex. J. Med.* **2018**, *54*, 287–293. [CrossRef]
41. Jamieson, D.J. Oxidative stress responses of the yeast *Saccharomyces cerevisiae*. *Yeast* **1998**, *14*, 1511–1527. [CrossRef]
42. Morano, K.A.; Grant, C.M.; Moye-Rowley, W.S. The response to heat shock and oxidative stress in *Saccharomyces cerevisiae*. *Genetic* **2012**, *190*, 1157–1195. [CrossRef]
43. Egbune, E.O.; Avwioroko, O.J.; Orororo, O.C.; Egbune, O.U.; Aganbi, E.; Anigboro, A.A.; Tonukari, N.J. *Rhizopus oligosporu* alkaline protease in cassava fermentation: Characterization and detergent potential. *Biocatal. Agric. Biotechnol.* **2023**, *47*, 10295 [CrossRef]
44. Rai, K.K.; Rai, N.; Pandey-Rai, S. Unlocking pharmacological and therapeutic potential of hyacinth bean (*Lablab purpureus* L. Role of omics-based biology, biotic and abiotic elicitors. In *Legumes*; IntechOpen: London, UK, 2021. [CrossRef]
45. Abu-Khudir, S.M.; Salem, M.M.; Allam, N.G.; Ali, E.M. Production, partial purification, and biochemical characterization of thermotolerant alkaline metalloprotease from *Staphylococcus sciuri*. *Appl. Biochem. Biotechnol.* **2019**, *189*, 87–102. [CrossRef]
46. Egbune, E.O.; Egbune, O.U.; Ezedom, T.; Dennis-Eboh, U.; Eraga, L.I.; Ichipi-Ifukor, P.C.; Orororo, O.C.; Adoh, N.G.; Adongo D.L.; Afure, C.A.; et al. Enhancement of Biochemical Parameters and Enzyme Activity in Solid-State Fermented and Biofortifie Maize Cobs Utilizing Yeasts and Plant Extracts. *Bioresour. Technol. Rep.* **2024**, *25*, 101874. [CrossRef]
47. Egbune, E.O.; Avwioroko, O.J.; Anigboro, A.A.; Aganbi, E.; Amata, A.I.; Tonukari, N.J. Characterization of a surfactant-stabl α-amylase produced by solid-state fermentation of cassava (*Manihot esculenta* Crantz) tubers using *Rhizopus oligosporus*: Kinetics thermal inactivation, thermodynamics, and potential application in laundry industries. *Biocatal. Agric. Biotechnol.* **2022**, *39* 102290. [CrossRef]
48. Zhang, K.; Zhang, T.-T.; Guo, R.-R.; Ye, Q.; Zhao, H.-L.; Huang, X.-H. The regulation of Key Flavors in Traditional Fermented Foods by Microbial Metabolism: A Review. *Food Chem. X* **2023**, *19*, 100871. [CrossRef]

https://doi.org/10.3390/pr14010111

processes

MDPI

ticle

alorization of Green Arabica Coffee Coproducts for Iannanase Production and Carbohydrate Recovery

quel Coldibelli Ribeiro [1,2,†], Leonardo João Bicalho de Moraes de Barros [1,†], Laura Braga de Menezes [1], audia Moraes de Rezende [2], Ayla Sant'Ana da Silva [3], Elba Pinto da Silva Bon [1]
d Ricardo Sposina Sobral Teixeira [1,*]

1 Laboratório Bioetanol (LB), Instituto de Química, Universidade Federal do Rio de Janeiro, Cidade Universitária, Rio de Janeiro 21941-630, Brazil; raquel.coldibelli@pos.iq.ufrj.br (R.C.R.); leonardojbmb@gmail.com (L.J.B.d.M.d.B.); lauramenezes@eq.ufrj.br (L.B.d.M.); elba1996@gmail.com (E.P.d.S.B.)
2 Laboratório de Análise de Aroma (LAROMA), Instituto de Química, Universidade Federal do Rio de Janeiro, Cidade Universitária, Rio de Janeiro 21941-630, Brazil; claudia.rezendeufrj@gmail.com
3 Laboratório de Biocatálise, Bioprocessos e Bioprodutos, Divisão de Catálise, Biocatálise e Processos Químicos, Instituto Nacional de Tecnologia, Ministério da Ciência, Tecnologia, Inovações, Rio de Janeiro 70067-900, Brazil; ayla.santana@int.gov.br
* Correspondence: ricardot@iq.ufrj.br; Tel.: +55-21-987524829
† These authors contributed equally to this work.

Abstract

Agro-industrial residues rich in carbohydrates represent low-cost and sustainable feedstock for enzyme production. This study demonstrates that green Arabica coffee press cake, a mannan-rich coproduct of oil extraction, is an efficient carbon source for *Aspergillus niger* (CFAM 1234) cultivation and for inducing mannanase production. Furthermore, the enzymes obtained were tested for mannose recovery in the enzymatic hydrolysis of healthy and defective coffee beans to investigate their hydrolytic potential. Mannanase production was investigated using various carbon sources—including ground coffee beans; coffee press cake; different particle sizes of coffee press cake; aqueous coffee cake extract (prepared at 30 g·L^{-1} under constant stirring (300 rpm) at 80 °C for 2 h, followed by filtration.); and a commercial galactomannan, locust bean gum (LBG). CNHSO analysis was performed in the best carbon source (coffee press cake) and LBG. Statistical optimization (Plackett–Burman and Central Composite Rotatable Design) simplified the culture medium composition to coffee press cake (48.78 g·L^{-1}), yeast extract (4 g·L^{-1}), and potassium phosphate (0.25 g·L^{-1}, pH 5.5) and increased mannanases productivity to 22.4 ± 0.6 U·mL^{-1} within only 3 days (a 42.9% improvement compared to non-optimized conditions, which were 30 g·L^{-1}, carbon source, 4 g·L^{-1} yeast extract, 1 g·L^{-1} Al_2O_3, 0.5 g·L^{-1} potassium phosphate buffer (pH 5.5), 0.5 g·L^{-1} of $MgSO_4{\cdot}7H_2O$, and 0.05 g·L^{-1} of $CaCl_2{\cdot}2H_2O$, which resulted in a maximum of ~20 U·mL^{-1} in 7 days). The crude extract also exhibited β-mannosidase activity (1.39 ± 0.06 U·mL^{-1}). When applied to the hydrolysis of untreated healthy and defective coffee beans, the enzyme preparation enabled ~25% mannose recovery (considering the value obtained through acid hydrolysis as 100%), highlighting its potential as a mannose resource. The results demonstrate that coproducts from the coffee production chain can be used as an efficient carbon source (coffee cake) for mannanase production, as well as sugar recovery (defective coffee beans), offering an integrated strategy to strengthen the circular bioeconomy and generate carbohydrates with potential industrial and nutritional applications.

 https://doi.org/10.3390/pr13123874

Keywords: mannanase; β-mannosidase; *Aspergillus niger*; coffee cake; agro-industrial coproducts; submerged cultivation; enzymatic hydrolysis; mannose

1. Introduction

The inappropriate disposal of agro-industrial waste from agriculture and food processing constitutes a significant environmental problem. However, these residues hold remarkable potential for biotechnology applications, since they are sources of cellulose, hemicellulose, and lignin [1]. Their application in bioprocesses, being used as a carbon source for microbial enzyme production, can simultaneously reduce environmental impacts while adding value to by-products that would otherwise be discarded [2–4]. Moreover, the conversion of agro-industrial residues into high-value-added products is aligned with the concept of the circular bioeconomy, a growing trend in global sustainable development [5], and contributes directly to the United Nations' Sustainable Development Goals (SDGs) 9 (Industry, Innovation and Infrastructure) and 12 (Responsible Consumption and Production) [6].

Among agro-industrial residues, those generated by the coffee industry are particularly noteworthy, given that, according to the International Coffee Organization (2023) [7], only 5% of the coffee pulp remains in the final beverage for consumers. Waste from the coffee sector accounts for approximately 40% of the total production volume, consisting of coffee husks, pulp, mucilage, parchment, silverskin, and coffee grounds [8–11]. In addition, other residues can be considered, such as coffee press cake (which represents approximately 90% of the residual biomass from green coffee oil extraction [12]) and defective beans, which represent up to 20% of green coffee production [13]. Such biomass is often disposed of in landfills or incinerated, which can pose a significant risk to the environment, or incorporated into fodder and animal feed [14].

Brazil, as the world's largest producer and exporter of coffee, generated 55.1 million processed 60 kg bags in 2023 [15], leading to a substantial volume of residues. Arabica coffee (*Coffea arabica* L.), the most widely cultivated species [16], contains about 50% polysaccharides in its dry matter (mainly mannans, galactomannans, and type II arabinogalactans) [17] and 7–17% lipids [16]. Approximately 70% of these lipids are triglycerides, which are widely exploited for coffee oil production [18–20]. Oil extraction by mechanical pressing yields a solid by-product known as coffee press cake [21]. This by-product is rich in the polysaccharide fraction of green coffee, mainly composed of cellulose, type II arabinogalactans, and galactomannans [22]. Due to its high mannan content (making up about 50%) [17,22], a hemicellulose composed of mannose chains linked by β-1,4 glycosidic bonds, this residue represents an attractive carbon source for microorganisms capable of producing mannan-degrading enzymes, such as mannanases (EC 3.2.1.78 and EC 3.2.1.25) [23].

Mannanases constitute a group of enzymes with diverse catalytic action. Endo-β-mannanases cleave internal (1,4-β-D-mannosidic) glycosidic bonds in the main chain of mannans, while β-mannosidases hydrolyze terminal mannose residues, releasing monosaccharides. Additionally, there are other accessory enzymes, including α-galactosidase, which catalyze the hydrolysis of galactose groups from galactomannans, as well as acetyl esterases and feruloyl esterases, which catalyze the hydrolysis of acetyl and ferulic groups, depending on the type of mannan present [23,24]. These enzymes have wide-ranging industrial applications, including juice clarification, wastewater treatment, papermaking, and improving oil and sugar extraction from plant matrices [25]. Furthermore, β-mannanases can perform partial hydrolysis of plant mannans, generating β-mannan-oligosaccharides (β-MOS), which exhibit prebiotic activity that stimulates the growth of beneficial gut bacteria in vitro [26–28]. Owing to these properties, mannanases have attracted significant interest from the food and pharmaceutical industries [29].

The production of mannanases can be carried out by different microorganisms, with fungi such as *Aspergillus niger* being among the most efficient producers due to their ability to secrete large amounts of extracellular enzymes [25,30]. This fungus is widely employed in fermentation processes due to its capacity to grow on a wide range of carbon sources [24,31]. Moreover, *A. niger* exhibits high resistance to pH and temperature variations, making it suitable for large-scale industrial applications [3,24], particularly in the production of enzyme cocktails for the degradation of plant polysaccharides into oligosaccharides and monosaccharides [30,32,33].

Submerged fermentation (SmF) is suitable for fungi growth, offering precise control of environmental parameters and nutrient availability, which ensures uniform and efficient microbial growth [3]. Even though SmF is a cultivation in liquid medium, there is the possibility of using solid components. In this context, the use of agro-industrial residues rich in mannan as carbon and energy sources in SmF represents an effective strategy to boost mannanase production. When optimized, SmF can yield significantly higher enzyme levels, requiring studies to define optimal cultivation conditions such as nutrient concentrations, pH, and incubation time [25,34]. Statistical approaches, including Plackett–Burman (PB) design and the Response Surface Methodology (RSM), are particularly useful, as they enable the identification of critical variables and fine-tuning of fermentation parameters to maximize enzyme production [29,35].

There are few studies reporting the production of mannanases using coffee grounds or husks [3,36–38], while green coffee press cake, the solid residue generated after oil extraction, remains largely underexplored for enzyme production, even though it is particularly rich in mannans. Thus, this is the first study to report the use of Arabica coffee press cake as a carbon source for the submerged fermentation of *Aspergillus niger* aimed at mannanase production. Furthermore, few studies address the production of β-mannosidase, which is essential for the complete hydrolysis of mannans into fermentable sugars such as mannose. The use of such low-cost substrates not only reduces enzyme production costs but also provides an environmentally sustainable route for agro-industrial waste valorization [29].

In this context, the present study investigates coffee press cake as a mannan-rich carbon source for submerged fermentation with *Aspergillus niger*, aiming at the induction of endo-β-mannanase and β-mannosidase production. Statistical optimization approaches were employed to enhance enzymatic yield, while the enzymes obtained were further evaluated in the hydrolysis of healthy and defective coffee beans to examine their hydrolytic potential, thus integrating waste valorization, process optimization, and circular bioeconomy opportunities.

2. Materials and Methods

2.1. Materials

2.1.1. Sample Preparation

The green Arabica coffees of the Catuaí Amarelo variety were obtained by semi-mechanized harvesting and post-harvesting by dry processing on a terrace. The coffee beans were obtained from the 2018 harvest from a farm located in São José do Vale do Rio Preto, Rio de Janeiro, Brazil (22°11′35.2″ S, 42°59′8.6″ W).

The coffee beans were ground using a Pulverisette 19 knife mill (Fritsch, Pittsboro, NC, USA) equipped with a 1 mm sieve, followed by lipid extraction through pressing (CA59O, IBG Monforts, Mönchengladbach, Germany) without heating, at 18 rpm, and with a 5 mm outlet diameter, according to a previously reported method for optimizing lipids extraction from green Arabica coffee beans [39]. The solid residue from pressing (coffee press cake) was reground and subjected to granulometry adjustment using a sieving system (Analysette 3 Spartan, Fritsch, Pittsboro, NC, USA) with 80- and 20-mesh sieves, amplitude of 2 mm, for 15 min.

Ground coffee beans, coffee cake, and commercial galactomannan (locust bean gum, LBG, Sigma-Aldrich, St. Louis, Missouri, USA) were tested as carbon to evaluate their effect as a carbon source for fungal mannanase production under submerged cultivation. The influence of particle size was also investigated by using two coffee cake fractions (80/20 and 20 mesh). In addition, an aqueous extract of coffee cake was also tested as a carbon source, prepared at 30 $g \cdot L^{-1}$ under constant stirring (300 rpm) at 80 °C for 2 h, followed by filtration.

For enzymatic hydrolysis, the coffee beans were ground using a Pulverisette 19 knife mill (Fritsch, Pittsboro, NC, USA) equipped with a 1 mm sieve.

2.1.2. Elementary Organic Analysis (CHNSO) in the Best Carbon Source

Elemental analyses were carried out on the selected carbon source (coffee cake) and on commercial mannan (LBG) for comparison, using an Unicube organic elemental analyzer (Elementar, Germany) equipped with a thermal conductivity detector and using helium as carrier gas. The analysis determined the mass percentage of carbon (C), nitrogen (N), hydrogen (H), sulfur (S), and oxygen (O) and allowed for the calculation of the C/N ratio in the culture media.

2.1.3. Microorganism

The microorganism used was a wild strain of *Aspergillus niger* from the Amazon Cultivation Collection (CFAM—Fiocruz), code 1234, isolated from drinking water in the community of Serra Baixa, Iranduba, Amazônia, Brazil. This strain was selected due to its high potential for mannanase production compared to other *Aspergillus* strains [40]. It was propagated on potato agar dextrose agar (PDA, Sigma-Aldrich) at 27 °C for 7 days in an incubator (Incucell 111, MMM Group, Planegg/München Germany). Spores were suspended in 0.9% NaCl solution and centrifuged at 9000 rpm for 15 min. The supernatant was discarded, and the conidia were resuspended in 20% glycerol to achieve 10^8 spores.mL^{-1}, and stored in cryogenic vials at −18 °C (for later use in inoculation).

2.2. *Enzyme Production*

2.2.1. Preliminary Growth Medium Composition and Cultivation

The initial medium for mannanase production (Table 1) was formulated based on previous reports [41–45]. Potassium phosphate buffer was prepared by mixing 9.55 g of KH_2PO_4 with 0.24 g of K_2HPO_4, dissolving it in 800 mL of distilled water, and adjusting the pH to 5.5 with KOH or HCl. The final solution was brought to a volume of 1 L using a volumetric flask. Aluminum oxide (Al_2O_3) was used to prevent excessive growth of filamentous fungi, acting to reduce the size of fungal pellets and, consequently, helping to control hyphal development and minimize cell leakage [44]. Submerged cultivations were carried out in 1000 mL Erlenmeyer flasks containing 250 mL of medium, incubated in a shaker (Innova 44R, New Brunswick, NJ, USA) at 200 rpm and 30 °C. The cultivation time varied according to the purpose of each test. The pre-inoculum was prepared by inoculating 1% (v/v) of the spore suspension into the medium and incubating under the same conditions for 48 h. Each cultivation was then inoculated with 10% (v/v) of the pre-inoculum.

Table 1. Initial cultivation media formulated based on scientific prospecting [41–45].

Compound	Concentration ($g \cdot L^{-1}$)
Carbon Source *	30.0
Yeast extract	4.0
Potassium phosphate buffer (pH 5.5)	0.5
$CaCl_2 \cdot 2H_2O$	0.05
$MgSO_4 \cdot 7H_2O$	0.5
Al_2O_3	1.0

* ground coffee bean, coffee cake, coffee cake 80/20 mesh, coffee cake 20 mesh, coffee cake extracts, or LBG.

2.2.2. Determination of Mannanase Activity

Mannanase activity was performed using LBG as substrate, prepared at 0.5% (*w*/*v*) in 50 mM sodium citrate buffer (pH 4.8) [46]. The reaction mixture, which consisted of 0.25 mL of enzyme extract and 0.25 mL of substrate solution, was incubated at 50 °C for 10 min. The reaction was stopped by adding dinitrosalicylic acid (DNS), followed by heating at 100 °C for 5 min. The released reducing sugars were quantified according to Teixeira and coauthors [47]. One unit of enzymatic activity (U) was defined as the amount of enzyme required to release 1 μmol of reducing sugar (D-mannose-based) per minute at 50 °C.

2.2.3. Statistical Experimental Design for Mannanase Production

Plackett–Burman Design (PB)

The PB was carried out to evaluate the significance of six independent factors, tested at levels from −1 to +1, as shown in Table 2. Data analysis was performed in the Statistica 12.0 software, considering a 10% error level.

Table 2. Coded levels and corresponding values of the independent factors in the Plackett–Burman design.

ID	Independent Factor ($g \cdot L^{-1}$)	Level		
		−1	0	1
X_1	Coffee cake	20	30	40
X_2	Yeast extract	2	4	6
X_3	Phosphate buffer (pH 5.5)	0.25	0.5	0.75
X_4	$CaCl_2 \cdot 2H_2O$	0	0.005	0.1
X_5	$MgSO_4 \cdot 7H_2O$	0	0.5	1
X_6	Al_2O_3	0	1	2

Central Composite Rotatable Design (CCRD)

The factors identified as significant in PB design were further evaluated using CCRD, tested at levels from −1.41 to +1.41, as shown in Table 3. Data analysis was carried out in the Statistica 12.0 software, considering a 10% error level.

Table 3. Coded (−1.41, −1, 0, +1, +1.41) and decoded values of central composite rotatable design factors.

ID	Independent Factor ($g \cdot L^{-1}$)	Level				
		−1.41	−1	0	+1	+1.41
Z_1	Coffee cake	25	30.82	45	59.18	65
Z_2	Yeast extract	4	5.16	8	10.84	12

This approach generated a predictive model equation for mannanase production, which was validated by comparing theoretical values (calculated by substituting the optimal conditions into the model equation) with the experimental results.

2.2.4. Determination of β-mannosidase Activity

The specific production of β-mannosidases was evaluated in the culture medium optimized for mannanase production after 3, 5, and 7 days of cultivation. β-mannosidase activity was carried out according to an adapted method from Gottschalk and coauthor [48], using 4-nitrophenyl-β-D-mannopyranoside (PNP-m) as substrate. The reaction mixture contained 0.1 mL of enzyme (diluted in 50 mM sodium acetate buffer, pH 5.0), 0.6 mL of ultrapure water, 0.2 mL of 500 mM sodium acetate buffer (pH 5.0), and 0.1 mL of substrate solution (10 mM). Reactions were incubated at 50 °C for 10 min in a water bath and stopped by adding 0.5 mL of 100 mM sodium carbonate solution. Absorbance was measured at 405 nm in a UV-1800 spectrophotometer (Shimadzu, Kyoto, Japan). An analytical curve of *p*-nitrophenol (0.02 to 0.20 mM) was used for quantification. One unit of β-mannosidase activity (U) was defined as the amount of enzyme required to release 1 μmol of PNP per minute under the assay conditions.

2.3. *Hydrolysis Experiments of Coffee Beans*

2.3.1. Enzymatic Hydrolysis

A crude mannanase preparation (culture supernatant) was used for the enzymatic hydrolysis of healthy and defective milled Arabica coffee beans to recover their monomeric sugars. Enzymatic hydrolysis was performed with 12% (w/v) dry biomass, enzymatic activity of 15 U·g^{-1} of dry biomass, and 100 mM sodium citrate buffer (pH 4.8) to complete 10 mL medium. Reactions were carried out at 50 °C and 200 rpm in a shaker incubator (Innova 44R, New Brunswick, NJ, USA). Aliquots were withdrawn in 0, 6, 24, and 48 h, heated at 100 °C for 5 min to stop the enzymatic reaction, and centrifuged at 8000 rpm for 10 min.

Monosaccharides were analyzed by HPLC-RI, using a Dionex Ultimate 3000 system (Thermo Fischer Scientific, Germany) equipped with a RefractoMax 521 refractive index detector (Thermo Fischer Scientific, Germany), and an Aminex HPX-87P column (300 mm × 7.8 mm, 9 μm, Bio-Rad, Hercules, CA, USA). The mobile phase was Milli-Q water at a flow rate of 0.6 mL·min^{-1}, with a total run time of 25 min. Quantification was carried out using an external analytical curve with a mixture of sugar standards such as: D-glucose (6.2 mg·mL^{-1}), D-xylose (2.98 mg·mL^{-1}), D-galactose (2.12 mg·mL^{-1}), L-arabinose (2.95 mg·mL^{-1}), and D-mannose (4.91 mg·mL^{-1}). Mannose and fructose content were reported together due to co-elution.

2.3.2. Acid Hydrolysis

To determine the yield of enzymatic hydrolysis (Equation (1)), acid hydrolysis was carried out on healthy and defective coffee beans according to the NREL Protocol [44], including extractives determination and hydrolysis with sulfuric acid. Monosaccharides were quantified as described for enzymatic hydrolysis.

$$Yield\ (\%) = 100\% \times \frac{manose\ content\ (enzymatic\ hydrolysis)}{manose\ content\ (acid\ hydrolysis)} \quad (1)$$

2.4. *Statistical Analyses*

Statistical analyses were performed using Statistica 12 (StatSoft) and Microsoft Excel. All experiments were carried out in triplicate. Data were analyzed by one-way ANOVA, followed by Student's *t*-test (for comparisons between two variables) and Tukey's test (for comparisons with more than two variables), and differences were considered not significant for $p \leq 0.05$.

3. Results

3.1. Enzyme Production

3.1.1. Influence of Carbon Source Arrangement

Ground coffee bean, coffee cake, coffee cake fractions (80/20 and 20 mesh), coffee cake extracts, and LBG were tested as carbon sources to evaluate their effect on mannanase production. Cultivations were conducted at 30 °C and 200 rpm, conditions commonly reported as optimal for *Aspergillus* [43,48–50]. The pH was adjusted to 4.8, based on previous studies on mannanase production from *Aspergillus* [41–45].

Figure 1 shows the mannanase production profile under these conditions with different carbon sources. The highest mannanase production was observed on day 7 of cultivation, consistent with the results reported by Saleh and coauthors [29], who obtained 20.92 U·mL^{-1} using *A. niger* MSSFW in submerged fermentation of coffee powder waste over 7 days.

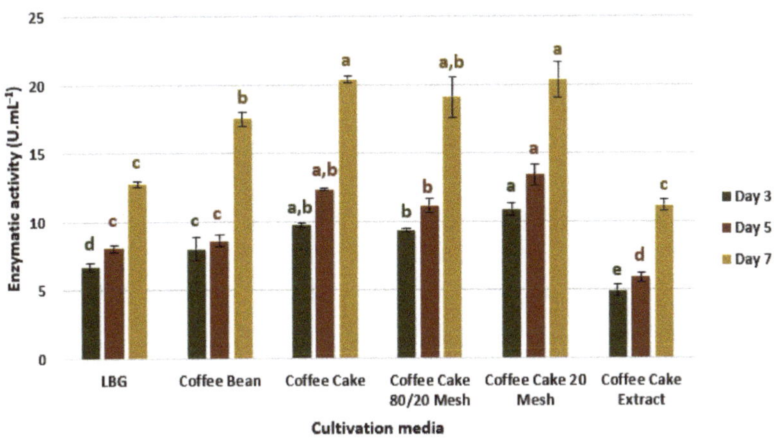

Figure 1. Mannanase production profile measured on days 3, 5, and 7 of cultivation using the initial medium described in Table 1 and different carbon sources, incubated in a shaker at 30 °C and 200 rpm. The comparison of mannanase activity between cultivation days was performed using a one-way ANOVA. Identical letters, for the same day, indicate no significant difference ($p \leq 0.05$) between carbon sources for mannanase production, according to Tukey's test.

The medium containing only LBG, a commercially available galactomannan, resulted in lower mannanase activity compared to media containing coffee cake or green coffee beans. These results indicate that coffee beans are an excellent substrate for mannanase production. Furthermore, since coffee cake is an industrial waste product, its use in the enzyme production process could be highly cost-effective.

The lowest mannanase activities were observed in media containing coffee cake extracts, indicating that the nutrient extraction process from the coffee cake was inefficient. The presence of lipids in green coffee beans negatively affects enzymatic activity compared to coffee cake. A hypothesis for this is that the fungus may be using the lipids present in the substrate as a source of carbon, redirecting its metabolism toward the production of enzymes related to lipid degradation, such as lipases, to the detriment of mannanases. Lin et al. (2004) [51] indicate that the presence of oil in copra (a fat-rich matrix) may depress mannanase production.

The highest activities were obtained in media containing coffee cake of different particle sizes, with no significant differences among them ($p \leq 0.05$). Therefore, subsequent experiments were conducted using unprocessed coffee cake (20.39 ± 1.50 U·mL^{-1}), as this simplifies the procedure and avoids a 3% mass loss.

3.1.2. Influence of Cultivation Time

Mannanase production using coffee cake and LBG was evaluated over several days, as shown in Figure 2. On all sampling days, LBG showed significantly lower activity compared to coffee cake ($p \geq 0.05$).

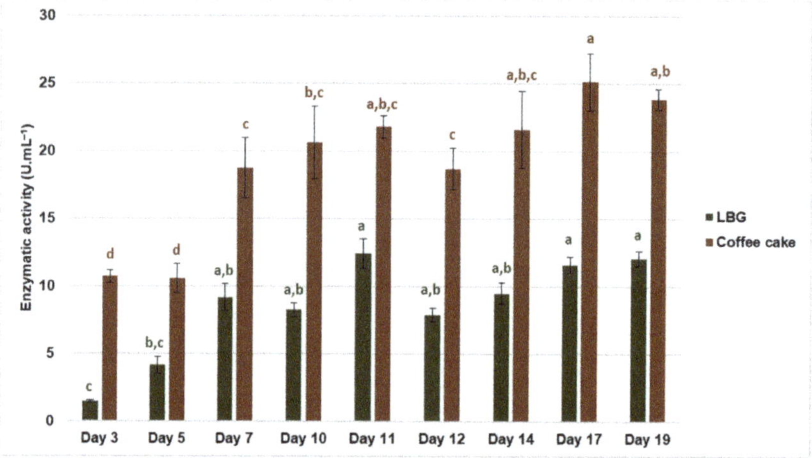

Figure 2. Mannanase production profile over 19 days of cultivation using coffee cake and LBG as carbon sources, in the columns, with the initial medium described in Table 1, incubated in a shaker at 30 °C and 200 rpm. The comparison of mannanase activity between cultivation days was performed using a one-way ANOVA. Identical letters, in the same carbon source, indicate no significant difference ($p \leq 0.05$) between cultivation days for mannanase production, according to Tukey's test.

Peak mannanase production in the LBG-based medium occurred on day 11 (12.44 U·mL^{-1}), followed by stabilization or a slight decline, suggesting substrate depletion. In contrast, the coffee cake medium maintained high activity for longer periods, peaking on day 17 (25.15 U·mL^{-1}), which may be related to the greater structural complexity of the substrate and the gradual release of nutrients. In short, a notable discrepancy was observed between the maximum activity levels: the coffee cake medium reached an average of 25.15 ± 2.08 U·mL^{-1}, while the LBG medium reached only 12.44 ± 1.09 U·mL^{-1}, consistent with the preliminary tests. Considering productivity, the optimal cultivation day was day 7, which may reflect a characteristic of *Aspergillus niger,* as this trend was observed in both media.

One possible explanation for this activity difference between media is that coffee cake provides more favorable and sustained conditions for mannanase production, possibly because it contains components that act as inducers or because it offers a richer and more diverse nutritional environment. Coffee cake exhibited higher carbon, nitrogen, and sulfur content compared to LBG (Table 4), highlighting its potential as a low-cost source of mannan, compared to the commercial galactomannan extracted from *Ceratonia siliqua* seeds (LBG).

The availability of carbon and nitrogen in the culture medium is fundamental for the growth and metabolite production of *Aspergillus niger*. According to Chauhan and coauthors [52], carbon serves as both an energy source and an essential structural element. It can also influence the production of specific enzymes, such as mannanases, depending on the type and concentration present in the medium.

Table 4. Elementary organic analysis (CHNSO) of the coffee cake and locust bean gum (LBG).

Carbon Source	%C	%H	%N	%S	%O
LBG	38.85 ± 0.12 [a]	6.64 ± 0.04 [a]	0.87 ± 0.01 [b]	0.15 ± 0.03 [a]	53.49 ± 0.17 [a]
Coffee cake	43.42 ± 0.05 [a]	6.36 ± 0.00 [b]	2.61 ± 0.00 [a]	0.23 ± 0.01 [a]	47.38 ± 0.04 [a]

The comparison of elementary organic analysis between LBG and coffee cake was performed using one-way ANOVA. Identical letters, in the same element, indicate no significant difference ($p \leq 0.05$) between the carbon sources, according to Student's *t*-test.

Although nitrogen is supplied to the medium through yeast extract, the nitrogen content in the biomass also contributes to fungal growth and enzyme synthesis. Different nitrogen sources may enhance the yield of specific enzymes. Moreover, the carbon-to-nitrogen (C/N) ratio plays a key role in regulating fungal growth and metabolite production [53]. Considering that the yeast extract used in the medium has 38.15 ± 0.07% carbon (%C) and 10.85 ± 0.24% nitrogen (%N), the C/N ratio was calculated for the medium containing coffee cake and LBG, resulting in 11.96 and 18.96, respectively. These results indicate that the C/N ratio of the coffee bean medium favors mannanase production, in agreement with findings reported by Gottschalk and coauthors [48] for *Aspergillus awamori* 2B.361 U2/1 cultivated on wheat bran and yeast extract (C/N equal to 10.3).

3.1.3. Validation of Preliminary Tests

Once the best arrangement of the carbon source had been determined, a new test was carried out, in a shorter time, to validate the results obtained, as shown in Figure 3.

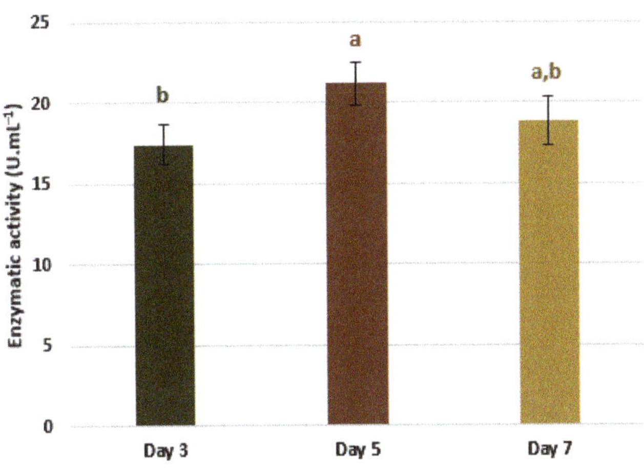

Figure 3. Mannanase production profile over 7 days of cultivation using coffee cake as a carbon source, with the initial medium described in Table 1, incubated in a shaker at 30 °C and 200 rpm. The comparison of mannanase activity between cultivation days was performed using a one-way ANOVA. Identical letters indicate no significant difference ($p \leq 0.05$) between cultivation days for mannanase production, according to Tukey's test.

In this experiment, the peak enzymatic activity of mannanases did not differ significantly ($p \leq 0.05$) between the 5th and 7th days. It is common for biotechnological processes such as this to vary in terms of the ideal time, as everything depends on the development of the strain under the cultivation conditions [54]. As the peak of mannanase enzyme activity occurred on the fifth day of cultivation, this was considered the ideal day for enzyme production in subsequent studies.

3.1.4. Statistical Experimental Design

Data from the preliminary tests supported the application of statistical experimental designs to optimize mannanase production by modifying the nutritional composition of the culture medium. A Plackett–Burman (PB) design was employed to evaluate the influence of six independent variables and identify those with significant effects on mannanase production. Subsequently, a Central Composite Rotatable Design (CCRD) was applied to optimize the significant variables, enabling a more detailed evaluation of their individual and interactive effects through a full factorial approach. The statistical analyses were performed using response surface methodology (RSM) and analysis of variance (ANOVA), following established procedures for bioprocess optimization [54,55]. Results were expressed as means ± standard deviations, and variance analysis was performed using Tukey's test at the 5% significance level.

Table 5 presents the characteristics of each test (12 experimental points and 4 central points), along with the results of the dependent variable under study. The results showed very close mannanase activities from 19 to 21 U·mL^{-1}, which may indicate that the concentrations studied had no effect on the production of mannanases. Only assays 8 and 12 presented values below 15 U·mL^{-1}.

Table 5. Results of the Plackett–Burman design, represented in codified variables, for mannanase production on the fifth day of cultivation.

ID	X_1	X_2	X_3	X_4	X_5	X_6	VI_1	VI_2	VI_3	VI_4	VI_5	Mannanase Activity (U·mL^{-1})
1	1	−1	1	−1	−1	−1	1	1	1	−1	1	21.87 ± 1.64
2	1	1	−1	1	−1	−1	−1	1	1	1	−1	21.49 ± 0.24
3	−1	1	1	−1	1	−1	−1	−1	1	1	1	19.42 ± 0.61
4	1	−1	1	1	−1	1	−1	−1	−1	1	1	20.44 ± 0.41
5	1	1	−1	1	1	−1	1	−1	−1	−1	1	21.67 ± 0.77
6	1	1	1	−1	1	1	−1	1	−1	−1	−1	20.77 ± 0.93
7	−1	1	1	1	−1	1	1	−1	1	−1	−1	19.96 ± 0.81
8	−1	−1	1	1	1	−1	1	1	−1	1	−1	13.56 ± 0.83
9	−1	−1	−1	1	1	1	−1	1	1	−1	1	19.53 ± 1.34
10	1	−1	−1	−1	1	1	1	−1	1	1	−1	20.79 ± 0.43
11	−1	1	−1	−1	−1	1	1	1	−1	1	1	20.65 ± 0.30
12	−1	−1	−1	−1	−1	−1	−1	−1	−1	−1	−1	14.52 ± 0.22
13	0	0	0	0	0	0	0	0	0	0	0	20.74 ± 0.14
14	0	0	0	0	0	0	0	0	0	0	0	20.57 ± 0.14
15	0	0	0	0	0	0	0	0	0	0	0	20.20 ± 0.17
16	0	0	0	0	0	0	0	0	0	0	0	20.52 ± 0.07

ID—identification assay number; X_1—Coffee cake; X_2—Yeast extract; X_3—Phosphate buffer (pH 5.5); X_4—$CaCl_2·2H_2O$; X_5—$MgSO_4·7H_2O$; X_6—Al_2O_3; $IV_{1–5}$—dummy variables, included to complete the design matrix, estimate the experimental error, and allow identification of the real factors that have a significant effect on mannanase production.

After analyzing the results with Statistica 12 software, the information from each assay was consolidated to generate the Pareto chart (Figure 4), which enabled the statistical interpretation of the studied variables. Pareto chart analysis revealed that only two variables were statistically significant: coffee cake (carbon source) and yeast extract (nitrogen source). Consequently, all independent factors with statistically insignificant effects—except for phosphate buffer—were excluded from the medium in the subsequent CCRD. The buffer was retained due to its essential role in adjusting the initial pH to levels suitable for *Aspergillus niger* growth. Since the phosphate buffer exhibited a negative effect, it was maintained at the minimum concentration tested (level −1, corresponding to 0.25 g·L^{-1}, expressed as phosphate).

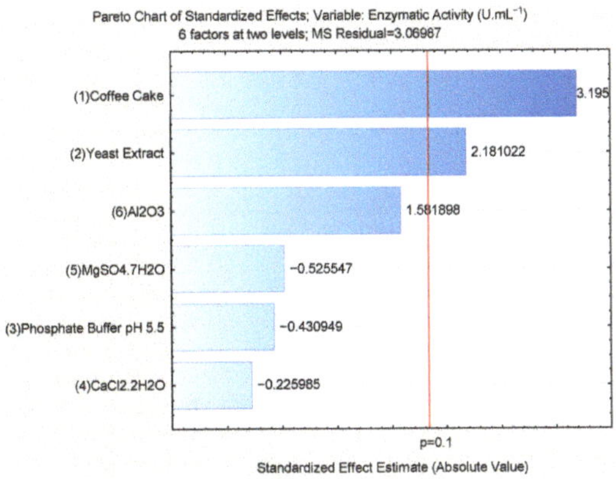

Figure 4. Pareto chart of effects for mannanase production ($U{\cdot}mL^{-1}$).

The CCRD was conducted with eight factorial points and four central points to improve the reliability of the results, as shown in Table 6. The highest mannanase activities were obtained in assays 8, 9, and 10, of which two tests correspond to the central points of the design.

Table 6. Results of the Central Composite Rotatable Design for mannanase production, on the fifth day of cultivation, where Z_1 is the coffee cake concentration, and Z_2 is the yeast extract concentration, represented in codified variables.

ID	Z_1	Z_2	Mannanase Activity ($U{\cdot}mL^{-1}$)
1	−1	−1	21.01 ± 0.27
2	1	−1	22.97 ± 0.45
3	−1	1	21.30 ± 0.18
4	1	1	22.65 ± 0.27
5	−1.41	0	21.07 ± 0.59
6	1.41	0	23.07 ± 0.43
7	0	−1.41	22.02 ± 0.61
8	0	1.41	25.43 ± 0.84
9	0	0	25.63 ± 0.48
10	0	0	25.33 ± 0.30
11	0	0	23.64 ± 0.29
12	0	0	24.50 ± 0.52

Based on the results processed in Statistica 12, a Pareto chart was generated (Figure 5a) to interpret the significance of the studied variables, along with a response surface plot predicting the tested conditions and their corresponding responses (Figure 5b). Both the linear and quadratic terms for coffee cake were statistically significant, whereas neither term for yeast extract showed significance, leading to its exclusion from the model.

The mathematical model (Equation (2)), obtained for the Pareto chart, was used even though the variables corresponding to yeast extract (L and Q) were not statistically significant, due to the necessity of a nitrogen source to support fungal growth. Although yeast extract did not have a significant effect on the evaluated response, it is well known to be an essential nutrient source. Therefore, since the central composite rotatable design (CCRD) did not include experiments with zero concentration of this component, the minimum studied value was adopted. The model predicted a mannanase production (Man_{prod}) of 24.32 U·mL^{-1}.

$$Man_{prod}\ (U \cdot mL^{-1}) = -1.58866{Z_1}^2 - 0.75652{Z_2}^2 + 0.76809Z_1 + 0.59818Z_2 + 24.77747 \quad (2)$$

The validation assay of the statistical experimental design was performed using the yeast extract at the lowest level studied (4 g·L^{-1}), since it had no significant effect. After five days of cultivation, the experimental activity was 21.85 ± 0.73 U·mL^{-1}, close to the theoretical value of 24.32 U·mL^{-1} predicted by the CCRD model, with an error of approximately 10%. This confirmed the validity of the statistical model. It is important to emphasize that the equation enables the calculation of mannanase activity under varying cultivation conditions, allowing for the prediction of potential outcomes based on different concentration levels.

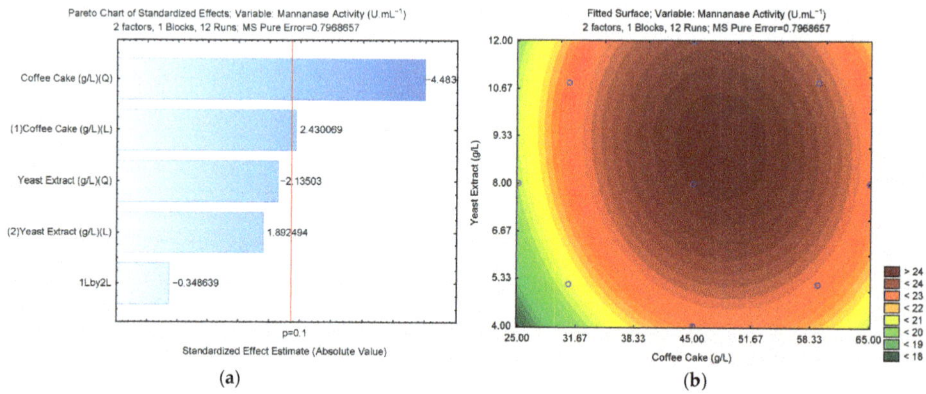

Figure 5. (**a**) Pareto chart of effects and (**b**) contour curves graph obtained through the two-factor CCRD conditions (coffee cake and yeast extract content) from culture medium for mannanase production (U·mL^{-1}).

Additional assays under the optimized condition showed activities of 22.43 ± 0.59 U·mL^{-1} at three days and 17.26 ± 0.56 U·mL^{-1} at seven days of cultivation. The activities on days three and five were not significantly different ($p \leq 0.05$), indicating that the peak of enzymatic activity shifted to the third day of cultivation.

The maximum activity obtained in the present was higher than that reported by Agu and coauthors [56], who used wild-type *Aspergillus* strains and agro-industrial residues as carbon sources. In that study, three species (*A. niger*, *A. flavus*, and *A. tamari*) were isolated from decomposing palm kernel cake and cultivated under submerged fermentation with coconut yam powder as the sole carbon source. *A. niger* produced the highest mannanase activity (0.35 U·mL^{-1}), followed by *A. flavus* (0.18 U·mL^{-1}) and *A. tamari* (0.15 U·mL^{-1}).

The medium composition optimization allowed an increase in mannanase production of approximately 10% and a 42.9% increase in productivity, going from 20.39 ± 1.50 U·mL^{-1} (at seven days) to 22.44 ± 0.61 U·mL^{-1} (at three days). The reduction in cultivation time from seven to three days is particularly relevant for industrial applications, since shorter fermentations reduce energy consumption, contamination risks, and downstream processing costs. Moreover, the elimination of inorganic salts ($CaCl_2$, $MgSO_4$, Al_2O_3) from the medium highlights the robustness of the process, enabling a simplified and cost-effective formulation that relies almost exclusively on the coffee coproduct. Thus, the optimized cultivation medium consisted only of 48.78 g·L^{-1} of coffee cake, 4 g·L^{-1} of yeast extract, and 0.25 g·L^{-1} of potassium phosphate buffer (pH 5.5).

3.1.5. Determination of β-mannosidase Enzyme Activity

In addition to the high production of mannanases, the specific production of β-mannosidases was evaluated under the optimized culture medium using coffee cake. Enzyme activity was assessed after 3, 5, and 7 days of cultivation, resulting in 0.52 ± 0.01 U·mL^{-1}, 0.88 ± 0.06 U·mL^{-1}, and 1.39 ± 0.06 U·mL^{-1}, respectively. The maximum β-mannosidase activity was observed on the seventh day, differing from β-mannanase production, which peaked on the third day. This value was 5.6-fold higher than that previously reported for *A. niger* (0.25 U·mL^{-1}) cultivated with soya flour [57].

These results suggest that the strain used in this study has considerable potential for β-mannosidase production, even in a culture medium that has not been optimized for its production. β-Mannosidase catalyzes the hydrolysis of β-1,4-mannosidic bonds in mannose-containing polysaccharides such as galactomannan, playing a key role in converting complex carbohydrates into simpler sugars. Its applications extend to the food industry, where it improves ingredient digestibility and produces prebiotics, as well as to biotechnology, biofuel production, and animal feed, where it enhances nutritional efficiency and supports sustainable bioconversion processes [58–60]. A noteworthy aspect of the present study is the concomitant production of β-mannosidase, which broadens the applicability of the crude enzymatic cocktail. While most reports focus exclusively on β-mannanases, the simultaneous presence of β-mannosidase increases hydrolytic efficiency, particularly in generating fermentable mannose. Although this is a very positive result, the addition of an external β-mannosidase (either commercial or laboratory-concentrated) to balance the β-mannosidase/β-mannanase ratio could enhance the enzymatic hydrolysis of this material, enabling the complete conversion of polysaccharides into monosaccharides.

Using coffee press cake as a carbon source for β-mannosidase production also aligns with the principles of the circular economy and agro-industrial residue valorization. By-products of the coffee industry contain galactomannan and have been shown to support enzyme production by fungi of the *Aspergillus* species [61,62]. Leveraging coffee cake reduces production costs, promotes environmental sustainability, and repurposes waste that would otherwise be discarded, reinforcing its potential as an efficient and sustainable carbon source for enzyme production.

To expand this study, the enzymes produced were applied to the enzymatic hydrolysis of defective coffee beans, aiming to release fermentable sugars that could potentially be used for the generation of higher-value-added products.

3.2. Hydrolysis Experiments of Coffee Beans

It is estimated that approximately 20% of global coffee production consists of defective beans, which, due to their poor sensory quality, are unsuitable for consumption [8]. These beans, therefore, represent a potential worldwide residue, rich in mannan, whose processing faces significant challenges. To explore alternative uses, this study investigated the potential of the produced enzyme for mannose recovery from defective beans through enzymatic hydrolysis, with comparisons to the hydrolysis of healthy beans. Valorizing defective beans as a substrate is particularly relevant, as mannose can serve as a precursor for diverse bioproducts, such as immunostimulants [63], anti-tumor agents [64], vitamins [65], and D-mannitol [66].

Polysaccharides, which account for 50–70% of the dry weight of green coffee beans, are mainly composed of galactomannans, arabinogalactans, and cellulose [17]. During hydrolysis, these polysaccharides are depolymerized into monosaccharides, mainly mannose, whose release was monitored at 0, 6, 24, and 48 h, as shown in Figure 6. Since the chromatographic column used did not separate mannose and fructose, their contents were quantified together. The reactions were conducted at 50 °C and 200 rpm in buffer at pH 4.8—conditions commonly reported as suitable for enzymatic hydrolysis—while agitation enhanced enzyme–substrate contact and activity [67–71].

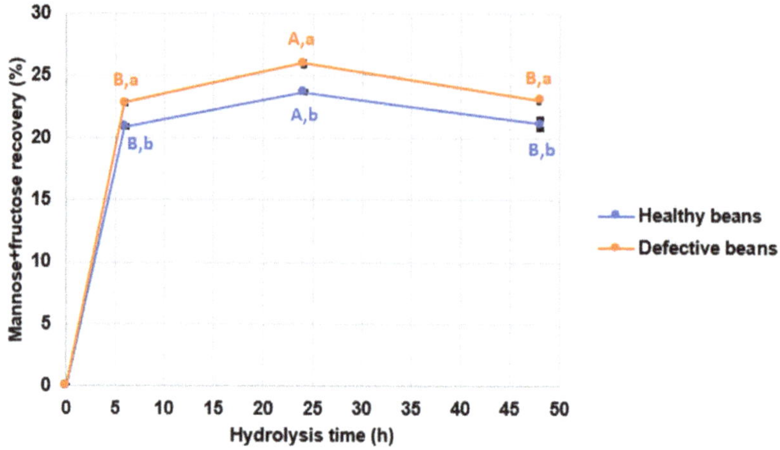

Figure 6. Mannose plus fructose recovery (%) obtained from the enzymatic hydrolysis of healthy and defective coffee beans at 50 °C and 250 rpm, using the optimized enzyme productized. The mannose value obtained by acid hydrolysis was considered 100%. The comparison of mannose + fructose recovery between cultivation days and between biomass was performed using a one-way ANOVA. Identical uppercase letters indicate no significant difference ($p \leq 0.05$) between hydrolysis time, in the same biomass, for mannose recovery, according to Tukey's test. Identical lowercase letters indicate no significant difference ($p \leq 0.05$) between biomass, in the same hydrolysis time, for mannose recovery, according to Student's *t* test.

The best mannose yield was obtained after 24 h, as shown in Figure 6. The mannose value obtained by acid hydrolysis was considered 100%. The efficiency of mannose recovery by enzymatic hydrolysis was 23.68 ± 0.03% for healthy beans and 25.98 ± 0.10% for defective beans, in 24 h of reaction. Although relatively low, these values demonstrate the enzyme's potential, achieving ~25% mannose recovery directly from untreated biomass. Limited yields are attributed to the recalcitrant structure of coffee beans, where crystalline mannans hinder enzymatic access. To improve recovery, pretreatments—physical, chemical, or combined—are required to disrupt the cell wall, solubilize hemicelluloses and lignin, and increase surface area for enzymatic action [32,33,71–73]. Examples include extrusion, hydrothermal processing, acid or alkaline hydrolysis, and treatments with organic solvents [74]. Although only monosaccharides were quantified, presented in Table 7, mannanoligosaccharides (MOS) may also have been formed and remained in the reaction medium without being converted to mannose, due to the imbalance between β-mannosidase and β-mannanase activities.

In a related study [75], coffee grounds were used as a mannose-rich biomass (19.3 g 100 g^{-1}). After enzymatic hydrolysis carried out with 50 mM sodium citrate buffer (pH 4.8), 10% dry matter, and an enzyme cocktail (cellulase—17.74 mg·g^{-1} of dry biomass; pectinase—16 mg·g^{-1} of dry biomass) for 24 h, a mannose recovery of approximately 47% was achieved. The higher yield observed in roasted beans was likely due to the previous processing, such as roasting, grinding, and hot-water extraction, which may remove enzyme inhibitors and promote biomass deconstruction, facilitating enzymatic access.

Table 7. Monosaccharides from the acid and enzymatic hydrolysis of healthy and defective coffee beans. Enzymatic hydrolysis was performed at 50 °C and 200 rpm.

Samples	Monosaccharides (g·100 g^{-1})			
	Glucose	Galactose	Arabinose	Mannose + Fructose
Acid hydrolysis				
Healthy beans	6.56 ± 0.21	13.53 ± 0.70	1.91 ± 0.38	19.69 ± 4.06
Defective beans	5.52 ± 0.53	12.59 ± 0.76	1.68 ± 0.13	18.50 ± 2.07
Enzymatic hydrolysis (24 h)				
Healthy beans	5.01 ± 0.33	0.18 ± 0.00	0.00	4.66 ± 0.01
Defective beans	3.96 ± 0.39	0.17 ± 0.01	0.00	4.81 ± 0.02

Xylose was not detected for any sample.

The enzyme produced in this study also demonstrated good potential for recovery of glucose (76% in healthy beans and 72% in defective beans) but limited recovery of galactose and arabinose. To maximize sugar release, integrated strategies should be adopted, including appropriate pretreatments, optimization of hydrolysis parameters (enzyme loading, pH, and temperature), and the use of tailored enzymatic cocktails containing accessory enzymes (e.g., β-galactosidase and β-glucosidase) to enhance the conversion of complex polysaccharides into fermentable sugars [74].

Furthermore, optimizing enzymatic hydrolysis conditions is essential, considering adjustments in solid matter concentration, enzyme proportion, and precise control of operational parameters such as pH and temperature. Another critical aspect is the use of tailored enzymatic cocktails containing accessory enzymes such as β-galactosidase and β-glucosidase, which work synergistically to enhance the conversion of structural biomass components into fermentable sugars, like mannose and glucose. These integrated approaches can significantly improve the efficiency of biotechnological processes.

4. Conclusions

This study demonstrated that green Arabica coffee press cake is an efficient and sustainable substrate for β-mannanase and β-mannosidase production by *Aspergillus niger*. The comparison of enzyme productivity was performed using the same carbon source (coffee press cake). After statistical optimization, the medium composition was simplified to 48.78 g·L^{-1} coffee cake, 4 g·L^{-1} yeast extract, and 0.25 g·L^{-1} potassium phosphate buffer (pH 5.5), which increased mannanase productivity to 22.4 ± 0.6 U·mL^{-1} within 3 days, representing a 42.9% improvement. The simplified medium composition—based solely on coffee press cake, yeast extract, and phosphate buffer—further enhances economic feasibility by eliminating the need for additional supplements (Al_2O_3, $MgSO_4{\cdot}7H_2O$, and $CaCl_2{\cdot}2H_2O$). Although mannose recovery from untreated coffee beans reached only ~25% (using the acid hydrolysis value at 100%), the results demonstrate the enzyme's capacity to act on recalcitrant biomass, with higher efficiencies expected through pretreatment strategies and tailored enzymatic cocktails.

From an industrial and sustainability perspective, these findings align with circular bioeconomy principles. A low-value by-product (coffee press cake) was used as a carbon source for *A. niger* cultivation and production of a high-value enzymatic mixture, capable of valorizing another waste stream (defective beans), enabling the recovery of functional monosaccharides for food, nutritional, and pharmaceutical applications.

Author Contributions: Conceptualization, R.C.R., L.J.B.d.M.d.B., A.S.d.S. and R.S.S.T.; methodology, R.C.R. and L.J.B.d.M.d.B.; validation, R.C.R. and L.J.B.d.M.d.B.; formal analysis, R.C.R., L.J.B.d.M.d.B. and L.B.d.M.; investigation, L.J.B.d.M.d.B.; data curation, R.C.R., L.J.B.d.M.d.B. and L.B.d.M.; writing—original draft preparation, R.C.R. and L.J.B.d.M.d.B.; writing—review and editing, R.C.R., C.M.d.R., A.S.d.S., E.P.d.S.B. and R.S.S.T.; supervision, C.M.d.R. and R.S.S.T.; project administration, R.S.S.T.; funding acquisition, C.M.d.R., E.P.d.S.B. and R.S.S.T. All authors have read and agreed to the published version of the manuscript.

Funding: This research was funded by Fundação Carlos Chagas Filho de Amparo à Pesquisa do Estado do Rio de Janeiro, grant number E-26/010.002491/2019, the Financiadora de Estudos e Projetos, number 2621/22, the Coordenação de Aperfeicoamento de Pessoal de Nível Superior (CAPES), and the Institutional Scholarship Program for Scientific Initiation from the National Council for Scientific and Technological Development (CNPq) for the scholarships.

Data Availability Statement: The raw data supporting the conclusions of this article will be made available by the authors on request.

Acknowledgments: The authors express their thanks to the National Council for Scientific and Technological Development (CNPq), the Research Support Foundation for the State of Rio de Janeiro (FAPERJ), the Funding Authority of Studies and Projects (FINEP), and the Coordination for higher Education Staff Development (CAPES) for the resources granted for the development of this project. The authors also thank the partner laboratory, Laboratório de Análises Térmicas e Reologia (IQ/UFRJ), for their part in the analyses.

Conflicts of Interest: The authors declare no conflicts of interest.

References

1. Ferreira-Leitão, V.; Gottschalk, L.M.F.; Ferrara, M.A.; Nepomuceno, A.L.; Molinari, H.B.C.; Bon, E.P.d.S. Biomass Residues in Brazil: Availability and Potential Uses. *Waste Biomass Valoriz.* **2010**, *1*, 65–76. [CrossRef]
2. Castro, A.M.; Pereira, N. Produção, propriedades e aplicação de celulases na hidrólise de resíduos agroindustriais. *Quim. Nova* **2010**, *33*, 181–188. [CrossRef]
3. Basmak, S.; Turhan, I. Production of β-Mannanase, Inulinase, and Oligosaccharides from Coffee Wastes and Extracts. *Int. J. Biol. Macromol.* **2024**, *261*, 129798. [CrossRef]
4. Alencar, V.d.N.e.S.; Batista, J.M.d.S.; Nascimento, T.P.; da Cunha, M.N.C.; Leite, A.C.L. Resíduos Agroindustriais: Uma Alternativa Promissora e Sustentável Na Produção de Enzimas Por Microrganismos. In *Ciência, Tecnologia e Inovação: Do Campo a Mesa. Proceedings of the Congresso Internacional da Agroindústria, Virtual Event, 25 September 2020*; Editora IIDV: Recife, Brazil; pp. 1–16.
5. Berto, P.J.; Ferraz, D.; Rebelatto, D.A.d.N. The Circular Economy, Bioeconomy, and Green Investments: A Systematic Review of the Literature. *Rev. Gestão Produção Operações Sist.* **2022**, *17*, 46–63. [CrossRef]
6. United Nations. The 17 Goals. Available online: https://sdgs.un.org/goals (accessed on 7 September 2024).
7. ICO. *Beyond Coffee: Towards a Circular Coffee Economy*; International Coffee Organization: London, UK, 2023.
8. Kalschne, D.L.; Viegas, M.C.; De Conti, A.J.; Corso, M.P.; Benassi, M.d.T. Steam Pressure Treatment of Defective Coffea Canephora Beans Improves the Volatile Profile and Sensory Acceptance of Roasted Coffee Blends. *Food Res. Int.* **2018**, *105*, 393–402. [CrossRef]
9. Klingel, T.; Kremer, J.I.; Gottstein, V.; De Rezende, T.R.; Schwarz, S.; Lachenmeier, D.W. A Review of Coffee By-Products Including Leaf, Flower, Cherry, Husk, Silver Skin, and Spent Grounds as Novel Foods within the European Union. *Foods* **2020**, *9*, 665. [CrossRef]
10. Ribeiro, R.C.; Teixeira, R.S.S.; de Rezende, C.M. Extrusion Pretreatment of Green Arabica Coffee Beans for Lipid Enhanced Extraction. *Ind. Crops Prod.* **2024**, *221*, 119318. [CrossRef]
11. Pongsiriyakul, K.; Wongsurakul, P.; Kiatkittipong, W.; Premashthira, A.; Kuldilok, K.; Najdanovic-Visak, V.; Adhikari, S.; Cognet, P.; Kida, T.; Assabumrungrat, S. Upcycling Coffee Waste: Key Industrial Activities for Advancing Circular Economy and Overcoming Commercialization Challenges. *Processes* **2024**, *12*, 2851. [CrossRef]
12. Vidal, O.L.; Tsukui, A.; Garrett, R.; Miguez Rocha-Leão, M.H.; Piler Carvalho, C.W.; Pereira Freitas, S.; Moraes de Rezende, C.; Simões Larraz Ferreira, M. Production of Bioactive Films of Carboxymethyl Cellulose Enriched with Green Coffee Oil and Its Residues. *Int. J. Biol. Macromol.* **2020**, *146*, 730–738. [CrossRef] [PubMed]
13. Franca, A.S.; Oliveira, L.S.; Mendonça, J.C.F.; Silva, X.A. Physical and Chemical Attributes of Defective Crude and Roasted Coffee Beans. *Food Chem.* **2005**, *90*, 89–94. [CrossRef]

Getachew, A.T.; Chun, B.S. Influence of Pretreatment and Modifiers on Subcritical Water Liquefaction of Spent Coffee Grounds: A Green Waste Valorization Approach. *J. Clean. Prod.* **2017**, *142*, 3719–3727. [CrossRef]

Companhia Nacional de Abastecimento. Produção de Café Cresce 8,2% Em 2023 e Chega a 55,1 Milhões De. Available online: https://www.conab.gov.br/ultimas-noticias/5323-producao-de-cafe-cresce-8-2-em-2023-e-chega-a-55-1-milhoes-de-sacas (accessed on 7 September 2024).

Silva, A.C.R.; da Silva, C.C.; Garrett, R.; de Rezende, C.M. Comprehensive Lipid Analysis of Green Arabica Coffee Beans by LC-HRMS/MS. *Food Res. Int.* **2020**, *137*, 109727. [CrossRef] [PubMed]

Redgwell, R.; Fischer, M. Coffee Carbohydrates. *Braz. J. Plant Physiol.* **2006**, *18*, 165–174. [CrossRef]

Dong, W.; Chen, Q.; Wei, C.; Hu, R.; Long, Y.; Zong, Y.; Chu, Z. Comparison of the Effect of Extraction Methods on the Quality of Green Coffee Oil from Arabica Coffee Beans: Lipid Yield, Fatty Acid Composition, Bioactive Components, and Antioxidant Activity. *Ultrason. Sonochem.* **2021**, *74*, 105578. [CrossRef] [PubMed]

Farah, A. Coffee Constituents. In *Coffee: Emerging Health Effects and Disease Prevention*; Chu, Y.-F., Ed.; Blackwell Publishing Ltd.: Oxford, UK, 2012.

Franca, A.S.; Oliveira, L.S. Chemistry of defective coffee beans. In *Food Chemistry Research Developments*; Nova Science Publishers: Hauppauge, NY, USA, 2008; p. 234. ISBN 9781604563030.

Ramadan, M.F. *Cold Pressed Oils: Green Technology, Bioactive Compounds, Functionality, and Applications*; Elsevier: Amsterdam, The Netherlands, 2020; Volume 1.

Arya, M.; Rao, L.J.M. An Impression of Coffee Carbohydrates. *Crit. Rev. Food Sci. Nutr.* **2007**, *47*, 51–67. [CrossRef]

Singh, S.; Singh, G.; Arya, S.K. Mannans: An Overview of Properties and Application in Food Products. *Int. J. Biol. Macromol.* **2018**, *119*, 79–95. [CrossRef]

Takahashi, J.A.; Lima, G.D.S.; Dos Santos, G.F.; Lyra, F.H.; Da Silva-Hughes, A.F.; Gonçalves, F.A.G. Filamentous Fungi and Chemistry: Old Friends, New Allies. *Rev. Virtual Quim.* **2017**, *9*, 2351–2382. [CrossRef]

Srivastava, P.K.; Kapoor, M. Production, Properties, and Applications of Endo-β-Mannanases. *Biotechnol. Adv.* **2017**, *35*, 1–19. [CrossRef]

Li, Y.; Liu, H.; Shi, Y.; Yan, Q.; You, X.; Jiang, Z. Preparation, Characterization, and Prebiotic Activity of Manno-Oligosaccharides Produced from Cassia Gum by a Glycoside Hydrolase Family 134 β-Mannanase. *Food Chem.* **2020**, *309*, 125709. [CrossRef]

Jana, U.K.; Kango, N. Characteristics and Bioactive Properties of Mannooligosaccharides Derived from Agro-Waste Mannans. *Int. J. Biol. Macromol.* **2020**, *149*, 931–940. [CrossRef]

Mary, P.R.; Prashanth, K.V.H.; Vasu, P.; Kapoor, M. Structural Diversity and Prebiotic Potential of Short Chain β-Manno-Oligosaccharides Generated from Guar Gum by Endo-β-Mannanase (ManB-1601). *Carbohydr. Res.* **2019**, *486*, 107822. [CrossRef]

Saleh, S.A.A.; Mostafa, F.A.; Ahmed, S.A.; Zaki, E.R.; Salama, W.H.; Abdel Wahab, W.A. Date Nawah Powder as a Promising Waste for β-Mannanase Production from a New Isolate *Aspergillus niger* MSSFW, Statistically Improving Production and Enzymatic Characterization. *Int. J. Biol. Macromol.* **2024**, *277*, 134447. [CrossRef] [PubMed]

Cairns, T.C.; Nai, C.; Meyer, V. How a Fungus Shapes Biotechnology: 100 Years of *Aspergillus niger* Research. *Fungal Biol. Biotechnol.* **2018**, *5*, 13. [CrossRef] [PubMed]

Ntana, F.; Mortensen, U.H.; Sarazin, C.; Figge, R. Aspergillus: A Powerful Protein Production Platform. *Catalysts* **2020**, *10*, 1064. [CrossRef]

Moro, M.K.; Teixeira, R.S.S.; da Silva, A.S.; Fujimoto, M.D.; Melo, P.A.; Secchi, A.R.; Bon, E.P.d.S. Continuous Pretreatment of Sugarcane Biomass Using a Twin-Screw Extruder. *Ind. Crops Prod.* **2017**, *97*, 509–517. [CrossRef]

Fasheun, D.O.; de Oliveira, R.A.; Bon, E.P.S.; da Silva, A.S.A.; Teixeira, R.S.S.; Ferreira-Leitão, V.S. Dry Extrusion Pretreatment of Cassava Starch Aided by Sugarcane Bagasse for Improved Starch Saccharification. *Carbohydr. Polym.* **2022**, *285*, 119256. [CrossRef]

Ganguly, A.; Mandal, A. Production and Optimization of Xylanase Enzyme from Bacillus Cereus BSA1 by Submerged Fermentation. *Int. Res. J. Basic Appl. Sci.* **2024**, *9*. Available online: https://www.researchgate.net/publication/385899118_Production_and_Optimization_of_Xylanase_Enzyme_from_Bacillus_cereus_BSA1_by_Submerged_Fermentation (accessed on 7 September 2024).

5. Blibech, M.; Chaari, F.; Bhiri, F.; Dammak, I.; Ghorbel, R.E.; Chaabouni, S.E. Production of Manno-Oligosaccharides from Locust Bean Gum Using Immobilized Penicillium Occitanis Mannanase. *J. Mol. Catal. B Enzym.* **2011**, *73*, 111–115. [CrossRef]

Cilmeli, S.; Doruk, T.; Könen-Adıgüzel, S.; Adıgüzel, A.O. A Thermostable and Acidophilic Mannanase from Bacillus Mojavensis: Its Sustainable Production Using Spent Coffee Grounds, Characterization, and Application in Grape Juice Processing. *Biomass Convers. Biorefin.* **2022**, *14*, 3811–3825. [CrossRef]

7. Favaro, C.P.; Baraldi, I.J.; Casciatori, F.P.; Farinas, C.S. β-Mannanase Production Using Coffee Industry Waste for Application in Soluble Coffee Processing. *Biomolecules* **2020**, *10*, 227. [CrossRef]

8. Ismail, S.A.; Kalthoum Khattab, O.H.; Nour, S.A.; Awad, G.E.A.; Abo-Elnasr, A.A.; Hashem, A.M. A Thermodynamic Study of Partially-Purified Penicillium Humicola β-Mannanase Produced by Statistical Optimization. *Jordan J. Biol. Sci.* **2019**, *12*, 209–217.

39. Silva, R.; Brand, A.L.; Tinoco, N.; Freitas, S.; Rezende, C. Bioactive Diterpenes and Serotonin Amides in Cold-Pressed Gre Coffee Oil (*Coffea arabica* L.). *J. Braz. Chem. Soc.* **2023**, *35*, 20230131. [CrossRef]
40. Nunes, O.C.; Tupi, L.P.C.; Teixeira, R.S.S. *Prospecção de Fungos Do Gênero Aspergillus Produtores de Mananases*; Final Course W Universidade do Grande Rio: Rio de Janeiro, Brazil, 2019.
41. Karahalil, E.; Germeç, M.; Turhan, I. β-Mannanase Production and Kinetic Modeling from Carob Extract by Using Recombin *Aspergillus sojae*. *Biotechnol. Prog.* **2019**, *35*, e2885. [CrossRef]
42. Mohamad, S.N.; Ramanan, R.N.; Mohamad, R.; Ariff, A.B. Improved Mannan-Degrading Enzymes' Production by *Aspergi niger* through Medium Optimization. *New Biotechnol.* **2011**, *28*, 146–152. [CrossRef] [PubMed]
43. Ozturk, B.; Cekmecelioglu, D.; Ogel, Z.B. Optimal Conditions for Enhanced β-Mannanase Production by Recombinant *Aspergi sojae*. *J. Mol. Catal. B Enzym.* **2010**, *64*, 135–139. [CrossRef]
44. Yatmaz, E.; Germec, M.; Karahalil, E.; Turhan, I. Enhancing β-Mannanase Production by Controlling Fungal Morphology in Bioreactor with Microparticle Addition. *Food Bioprod. Process.* **2020**, *121*, 123–130. [CrossRef]
45. Yilmazer, C.; Gürler, H.N.; Erkan, S.B.; Ozcan, A.; Hosta Yavuz, G.; Germec, M.; Yatmaz, E.; Turhan, I. Optimization Mannooligosaccharides Production from Different Hydrocolloids via Response Surface Methodology Using a Recombin *Aspergillus sojae* β-Mannanase Produced in the Microparticle-Enhanced Large-Scale Stirred Tank Bioreactor. *J. Food Process. Pres* **2021**, *45*, e14916. [CrossRef]
46. Stalbrand, H.; Siika-Aho, M.; Tenkanen, M.; Viikari, L. Purification and Characterization of Two B-Mannanases from Trichoder Reesei. *J. Biotechnol.* **1993**, *29*, 229–242. [CrossRef]
47. Teixeira, R.S.S.; Da Silva, A.S.; Ferreira-Leitão, V.S.; Bon, E.P.d.S. Amino Acids Interference on the Quantification of Reduci Sugars by the 3,5-Dinitrosalicylic Acid Assay Mislead Carbohydrase Activity Measurements. *Carbohydr. Res.* **2012**, *363*, 33– [CrossRef]
48. Gottschalk, L.M.F.; Paredes, R.D.S.; Teixeira, R.S.S.; Da Silva, A.S.; Bon, E.P.D.S. Efficient Production of Lignocellulolytic Enzym Xylanase, b-Xylosidase, Ferulic Acid Esterase and b-Glucosidase by the Mutant Strain *Aspergillus awamori* 2B.361 U2/1. *Braz Microbiol.* **2013**, *44*, 569–576. [CrossRef]
49. Piza, F.A.T.; Siloto, A.P.; Carvalho, C.V.; Franco, T.T. Production, Characterization and purification of chitosanase from Bacill Cereus. *Braz. J. Chem. Eng.* **1999**, *16*, 185–192. [CrossRef]
50. Abd-Aziz, S.; Ong, L.G.A.; Hassan, M.A.; Karim, M.I.A. Process Parameters Optimisation of Mannanase Production fro *Aspergillus niger* FTCC 5003 Using Palm Kernel Cake as Carbon Source. *Asian J. Biochem.* **2008**, *3*, 297–307. [CrossRef]
51. Lin, T.C.; Chen, C. Enhanced Mannanase Production by Submerged Culture of *Aspergillus niger* NCH-189 Using Defatted Cop Based Media. *Process Biochem.* **2004**, *39*, 1103–1109. [CrossRef]
52. Chauhan, P.S.; Puri, N.; Sharma, P.; Gupta, N. Mannanases: Microbial Sources, Production, Properties and Potential Biotechnolo ical Applications. *Appl. Microbiol. Biotechnol.* **2012**, *93*, 1817–1830. [CrossRef]
53. Brandl, J.; Aguilar-Pontes, M.V.; Schäpe, P.; Noerregaard, A.; Arvas, M.; Ram, A.F.J.; Meyer, V.; Tsang, A.; de Vries, R.P.; Anderse M.R. A Community-Driven Reconstruction of the *Aspergillus niger* Metabolic Network. *Fungal Biol. Biotechnol.* **2018**, *5*, 16– [CrossRef]
54. Lee, K.-M.; Gilmore, D.F. Statistical Experimental Design for Bioprocess Modeling and Optimization Analysis. *Appl. Bioche Biotechnol.* **2006**, *135*, 101–116. [CrossRef]
55. Rodrigues, M.I.; Iemma, A.F. *Planejamento de Experimentos e Otimização de Processos: Uma Estratégia Sequencial de Planejamentos*, 3 ed.; Cárita Editora: Campinas, Brazil, 2014.
56. Agu, K.C.; Okafor, F.C.; Amadi, O.C.; Mbachu, A.E.; Awah, N.S.; Odili, L.C. Production of Mannanase Enzyme Using *Aspergill* Spp. Isolated from Decaying Palm Press Cake. *Sch. Acad. J. Biosci.* **2014**, *2*, 863–870.
57. Fliedrová, B.; Gerstorferová, D.; Křen, V.; Weignerová, L. Production of *Aspergillus niger* β-Mannosidase in Pichia Pastoris. *Prote Expr. Purif.* **2012**, *85*, 159–164. [CrossRef]
58. Moreira, L.R.S.; Filho, E.X.F. An Overview of Mannan Structure and Mannan-Degrading Enzyme Systems. *Appl. Microbi Biotechnol.* **2008**, *79*, 165–178. [CrossRef] [PubMed]
59. Subramaniyan, S.; Prema, P. Cellulase-Free Xylanases from Bacillus and Other Microorganisms. *FEMS Microbiol. Lett.* **2000**, *18* 1–7. [CrossRef] [PubMed]
60. Srivastava, N.; Srivastava, M.; Mishra, P.K.; Gupta, V.K.; Molina, G.; Rodriguez-Couto, S.; Manikanta, A.; Ramteke, P.V Applications of Fungal Cellulases in Biofuel Production: Advances and Limitations. *Renew. Sustain. Energy Rev.* **2018**, *8* 2379–2386. [CrossRef]
61. Murthy, P.S.; Madhava Naidu, M. Sustainable Management of Coffee Industry By-Products and Value Addition—A Revie *Resour. Conserv. Recycl.* **2012**, *66*, 45–58. [CrossRef]
62. Panagiotou, G.; Kekos, D.; Macris, B.J.; Christakopoulos, P. Production of Cellulolytic and Xylanolytic Enzymes by Fusariu Oxysporum Grown on Corn Stover in Solid State Fermentation. *Ind. Crops Prod.* **2003**, *18*, 37–45. [CrossRef]

63. Ranta, K.; Nieminen, K.; Ekholm, F.S.; Poláková, M.; Roslund, M.U.; Saloranta, T.; Leino, R.; Savolainen, J. Evaluation of Immunostimulatory Activities of Synthetic Mannose-Containing Structures Mimicking the β-(1→2)-Linked Cell Wall Mannans of Candida Albicans. *Clin. Vaccine Immunol.* **2012**, *19*, 1889–1893. [CrossRef]
64. Kamel, M.M.; Ali, H.I.; Anwar, M.M.; Mohamed, N.A.; Soliman, A.M. Synthesis, Antitumor Activity and Molecular Docking Study of Novel Sulfonamide-Schiff's Bases, Thiazolidinones, Benzothiazinones and Their C-Nucleoside Derivatives. *Eur. J. Med. Chem.* **2010**, *45*, 572–580. [CrossRef]
65. Chen, F.-E.; Zhao, J.-F.; Xiong, F.-J.; Xie, B.; Zhang, P. An Improved Synthesis of a Key Intermediate for (+)-Biotin from D-Mannose. *Carbohydr. Res.* **2007**, *342*, 2461–2464. [CrossRef]
66. Mishra, D.K.; Hwang, J.S. Selective Hydrogenation of D-Mannose to d-Mannitol Using NiO-Modified TiO2 (NiO-TiO2) Supported Ruthenium Catalyst. *Appl. Catal. A Gen.* **2013**, *453*, 13–19. [CrossRef]
67. Filipigh, A.A.; Rojo, E.M.; Pila, A.N.; Bolado, S. Fractional Recovery of Proteins and Carbohydrates from Secondary Sludge from Urban Wastewater Treatment Plants. *Chem. Eng. J. Adv.* **2024**, *20*, 100686. [CrossRef]
68. Baraldi, I.J.; Giordano, R.L.C.; Zangirolami, T.C. Enzymatic Hydrolysis as an Environmentally Friendly Process Compared to Thermal Hydrolysis for Instant Coffee Production. *Braz. J. Chem. Eng.* **2016**, *33*, 763–771. [CrossRef]
69. Carvalho, M.L.; Sousa, R., Jr.; Rodríguez-Zúñiga, U.F.; Suarez, C.A.G.; Rodrigues, D.S.; Giordano, R.C.; Giordano, R.L.C. Kinetic Study of the Enzymatic Hydrolysis of Sugarcane Bagasse. *Braz. J. Chem. Eng.* **2013**, *30*, 437–447. [CrossRef]
70. Eugenio, M.E.; Domínguez, G.; Molina-Guijarro, J.M.; Hernández, M.; Arias, M.E.; Ibarra, D. Boosting Enzymatic Hydrolysis of Steam-Pretreated Softwood by Laccase and Endo-β-Mannanase Enzymes from Streptomyces Ipomoeae CECT 3341. *Wood Sci Technol* **2023**, *57*, 965–987. [CrossRef]
71. Fasheun, D.O.; da Silva, A.S.; Teixeira, R.S.S.; Ferreira-Leitão, V.S. Enhancing Methane Production from Cassava Starch: The Potential of Extrusion Pretreatment in Single-Stage and Two-Stage Anaerobic Digestion. *Fuel* **2023**, *366*, 131406. [CrossRef]
72. Jiao, T.; Liang, F.; Fang, G.; Jiao, J.; Huang, C.; Tian, Q.; Zhu, B.; Deng, Y.; Han, S.; Zhou, X. An Integrated Pretreatment Strategy for Enhancing Enzymatic Hydrolysis Efficiency of Poplar: Hydrothermal Treatment Followed by a Twin-Screw Extrusion. *Ind. Crops Prod.* **2024**, *211*, 118169. [CrossRef]
73. Monteiro, A.F.; Miguez, I.S.; Silva, J.P.R.B.; da Silva, A.S.A. High Concentration and Yield Production of Mannose from Açaí (Euterpe Oleracea Mart.) Seeds via Mannanase-Catalyzed Hydrolysis. *Sci. Rep.* **2019**, *9*, 10939. [CrossRef]
74. Galbe, M.; Wallberg, O. Pretreatment for Biorefineries: A Review of Common Methods for Efficient Utilisation of Lignocellulosic Materials. *Biotechnol. Biofuels* **2019**, *12*, 294. [CrossRef] [PubMed]
75. Nguyen, Q.A.; Cho, E.; Trinh, L.T.P.; Jeong, J.; Bae, H.-J. Development of an Integrated Process to Produce D-Mannose and Bioethanol from Coffee Residue Waste. *Bioresour. Technol.* **2017**, *244*, 1039–1048. [CrossRef] [PubMed]

processes

Article

Bioconversion of Ferulic Acid to 4-Vinylguaiacol by Ferulic Acid Decarboxylase from *Brucella intermedia* TG 3.48

Sylvia Patricia de Carvalho, Mohammed Anas Zaiter, Karine Sousa Dantas, Érike Jhonnathan Pereira, Ronivaldo Rodrigues da Silva, Maurício Boscolo, Roberto da Silva, Maitê Bernardo Correia dos Santos and Eleni Gomes *

Laboratory of Unesp's Bioenegy Institute IPBEN, São Paulo State University, UNESP, São José do Rio Preto 15054-000, SP, Brazil; sylvia.patricia@unesp.br (S.P.d.C.); anas.zaiter@unesp.br (M.A.Z.); karine.dantas@unesp.br (K.S.D.); jhonnathan.pereira@unesp.br (É.J.P.); ronivaldo.r.silva@unesp.br (R.R.d.S.); mauricio.boscolo@unesp.br (M.B.); roberto.silva@unesp.br (R.d.S.); maite.bernardo@unesp.br (M.B.C.d.S.)

* Correspondence: eleni.gomes@unesp.br; Tel.: +55-17-3221-2393

Abstract

4-vinylguaiacol (4-VG) is a commercially important compound due to its characteristic clove-like aroma and its use as a flavoring in the food, beverage, and cosmetics industries. However, its extraction from natural sources or by a chemical method is expensive. The bioconversion of ferulic acid (FA) to 4-VG via microorganisms is an alternative, considering the market trend toward biotechnological and environmentally friendly processes and products. This study aimed to evaluate the tolerance of the bacterial strain *Brucella intermedia* (basonym *Ochrobactrum intermedium*) TG 3.48 to FA, its bioconversion to 4-VG, and the activity of the FA decarboxylase enzyme (FADase), which is key to the 4-VG production process. The strain tolerated FA concentrations up to 700 mg L^{-1}. When the microorganism grew at 300 mg L^{-1} FA in Mineral Liquid Medium (MLM), it converted 99.5% of FA to 4-VG within 12 h. The FADase activity was cell-associated with 5.17 U mL-1 in the whole cell, 4.40 U mL^{-1} in the intracellular extract, and 3.54 U mL^{-1} in the cell wall fragments, while the specific activity was 778.90 U mg^{-1}.

Keywords: ferulic acid; 4-vinylguaiacol; decarboxylase; *Brucella intermedia* TG 3.48; *Ochrobactrum intermedium* TG 3.48

1. Introduction

Several processes that use lignocellulosic raw material result in an excessive amount of lignin that is not optimally utilized. This polymer and its derivatives with high content of aromatic compounds have potential applications in the biosynthesis of various products [1]. Ferulic acid (FA) is present in high concentrations in hydrolyzed lignocellulosic biomass and serves as a substrate for the synthesis of flavor compounds such as vanillic acid (VA), vanillin, and 4-vinylguaiacol (4-VG) [2,3].

4-VG is a phenolic volatile substance with a spicy clove-like aroma, which makes it a key aroma compound in the beverages and beer industries [4], and as an additive in flavors and fragrances industries [5]. On the other hand, 4-VG is a well-documented volatile phenolic compound that occurs in roasted coffee beans during roasting process by thermal decarboxylation of FA [6,7], while in citrus, research reports 4-VG among identified aroma compounds in citrus peels and dried citrus products, especially when peel is processed (drying, extraction) or when bound precursor is hydrolyzed, as well as in cold-pressed grapefruit oil [8,9]. In addition, its antioxidant activity makes it a potential pharmaceutical agent [10,11]. 4-VG can be extracted from plants, yet the low concentration of this compound makes the process economically unfeasible. Chemical synthesis is an alternative representing around 80% of total 4-VG production [12,13].

The biological synthesis of 4-VG by fungi and bacteria using FA as a substrate has been reported [2,5,13,14]. These biocatalytic routes use low-cost renewable FA, operate under mild aqueous conditions with high chemo-selectivity and reduced by-product formation, simplifying downstream processing [15]. In contrast, classical chemical routes such as Wittig-type alkene formation produce stoichiometric phosphine-oxide waste, typically require harsher conditions and organic solvents, and exhibit poor green chemistry metrics [16].

The biotransformation of FA to 4-VG is catalyzed by FA decarboxylase enzyme (FADase, EC 4.1.1.102) via non-oxidative decarboxylation of FA to 4-VG with release of CO_2 from the substrate's terminal carboxyl carbon [12] (Figure 1). FADas has been reported in various microorganisms such as *Aspergillus luchuensis*, *Candida guilliermondii*, *Bacillus* sp., and *Klebsiella pneumoniae*, where it generally involves in culture media detoxification processes and, in some species, forms part of the metabolic pathway for assimilating xenobiotic compounds [2,11].

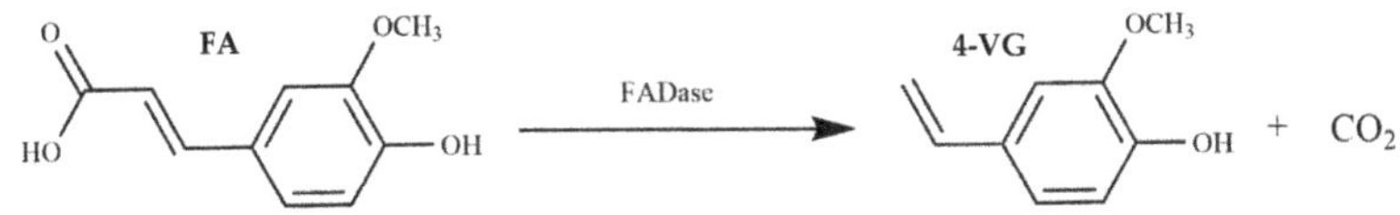

Figure 1. FADase non-oxidative decarboxylation of FA to 4-VG with release of CO_2.

The bacterium *Brucella intermedia* TG 3.48 demonstrates tolerance to compounds that typically inhibit microbial growth, such as lead and chromium VI, and can degrade xenobiotic substances including diuron and piracetam (2-(2-oxopyrrolidin-1-yl) acetamide) [17–22]. A 16S rRNA gene partial sequence (1329 bp) of *B. intermedia* TG 3.48 is available in GenBank under accession number MG214517, as reported by Egea et al. [21].

Previous studies report large inter- and intra-species variation in FA tolerance, *Klebsiella pneumoniae* TD4.7 showed growth and activity only at 0.3–0.5 g L^{-1} [2], as for *Bacillus subtilis* B7-S lost growth and bioconversion at levels around 1.3 g L^{-1} [23], while adaptive laboratory evolution (ALE) of *Pseudomonas putida* KT2440 markedly increased tolerance up to the 30 g L^{-1} range, showing that baseline tolerance is strain- and condition-dependent and can be substantially improved by ALE [24].

Unlike many fungal and yeast ferulic acid decarboxylases that require the prenylated-FMN (prFMN) cofactor and its biosynthetic partner (UbiX/PAD1) for activity [25], the enzyme described here is cofactor independent, which simplifies heterologous expression and process design, avoiding the co-expression or supplementation of accessory cofactor pathways, and thereby facilitates robust single step bioconversion of FA from lignocellulosic hydrolysates to 4-VG [5,26].

The objective of this work is to assess the FA tolerance, study the potential of *B. intermedia* TG 3.48 to produce 4-VG via decarboxylation of the FA and evaluate the expression and characterization of the FADase enzyme.

2. Materials and Methods

2.1. Microorganism

The bacterium *Brucella intermedia* (basonym *Ochrobactrum intermedium*) TG 3.48 [27], previously isolated [21], is part of the working collection of the Biochemical and Applied

Microbiology laboratory, Unesp Bioenergy Research Institute, São José do Rio Preto, SP, Brazil. The strain has been maintained at −80 °C in a 15% glycerol solution. Identification was carried out by DNA extraction using the commercial AxyPrep Bacterial Genomic DNA Miniprep Kit (Axygen, Union City, CA, USA) from a colony obtained after cultivation on Luria-Bertani agar medium (LB) for 12 h at 30 °C. The partial sequence of the 16S rRNA gene is available on NCBI website https://www.ncbi.nlm.nih.gov/nuccore/MG214517.1/, accessed on 20 August 2025.

2.2. Culture Medium

The Liquid Nutrient Medium (LNM) [28] consisted of 0.2% glucose, 0.1% sodium chloride, 1% tryptone, and 0.5% yeast extract. An adaptation of the Mineral Liquid Medium (MLM) proposed by Bushnell and Haas [29], composed of 11% $(NH_4)_2SO_4$, 0.02% $MgSO_4$, 0.002% $CaCl_2$, 0.1% $KHPO_4$, and 0.1% KH_2PO_4 was also used. The solid medium contained the same nutrients as LNM, with the addition of 1.5% agar.

2.3. Bacterial Tolerance to FA and Potential Biotransformatio of FA to 4-VG

For all cultivation procedures, the pre-inoculum was prepared by suspending bacterial cells in a liquid nutrient medium at pH 6.0. Pre-inoculum cultures were incubated in an orbital shaker at 28 °C and 150 rpm. The optical density (O.D) of the culture was measured at 600nm using a spectrophotometer until an O.D of 0.8 was reached.

Bacterial tolerance to FA was assessed in 96-well microtiter plates containing 196.0 μL of LNM, with FA concentrations ranging from 100 up to 700 mg L^{-1}, and after addition of ferulic acid the medium pH was readjusted to pH 6.0 with 1 M NaOH (or HCl where required) prior to inoculation to avoid pH-driven effects on bacterial growth, incubated at 28 °C and 190 rpm.

For the decarboxylation of FA to 4-VG, the methods described above were followed, with 250 mL of LB medium containing 300 mg L^{-1} of FA in a 500 mL Erlenmeyer flask, which was inoculated with one mL of inoculum obtained as previously described and left for 48 h. During the first 24 h of cultivation, samples were collected every two hours, and subsequently every eight hours, for the microbial growth evaluation by O.D at 600 nm. The concentrations of glucose, FA, 4-VG, and other metabolites were determined. The initial FA concentration was used to calculate product yields (%).

FA, 4-VG, VA, catechol and vanillin, metabolites commonly reported in the FA bioconversion pathways, were assayed by HPLC. The formation of 4-VG during cultivation was verified by mass spectrometry (MS) analysis.

Two controls were employed in this work, an abiotic control (medium supplemented with FA but not inoculated); and a biotic control (medium inoculated with the microorganism but without FA addition).

Unless indicated otherwise, all reagents were obtained from Sigma-Aldrich (St. Louis, MO, USA).

2.4. Analytical Methods

Metabolites potentially derived from FA including catechol (benzene-1,2-diol), guaiacol (2-methoxyphenol), 4-VG (2-Methoxy-4-vinylphenol), VA (4-hydroxy-3-methoxybenzoic acid) and vanillin (4-Hydroxy-3-methoxybenzaldehyde) were screened and analyzed by HPLC and LC-MS. Filtered samples were prepared using a 0.22 μm syringe filter (analitica 2202213 300 Cw syringe filter, hydrophilic PTFE membrane, filter diameter 13 mm, pore size 0.22 μm, pre-cleaned, with polypropylene (PP) pre-filter.), and 20 μL aliquots were injected into a 1220 Infinity liquid chromatograph (LC) (Agilent Technologies, Santa Clara, CA, USA) equipped with a binary pump, autosampler, column oven, and a UV-VIS detector. Chromatographic separation was achieved on a ZORBAX Eclipse Plus C18 column (4.6 × 250 mm) (Agilent Technologies, Santa Clara, CA, USA), and preserved at 25 °C.

Chromatographic separation was performed using solvent A (methanol:acetic acid:water, 10:2:88 *v*/*v*) and solvent B (methanol:acetic acid:water, 90:2:8 *v*/*v*). [30]. Retention times were determined using analytical standards, and calibration curves of FA and its metabolites were plotted at concentrations between 2.5 and 300 mg L^{-1}. The correlation coefficient was 0.999 for analyzed compounds, and the peak areas were quantified according to the calibration curves.

Sugars were quantified by ion-exchange chromatography using a Dionex ICS-5000 HPAEC-PAD (Thermo Scientific, Hampton, NH, USA) equipped with a CarboPac® PA-1 anion exchange column at a temperature of 25 °C. Eluents were prepared with ultrapure deionized water (18 MΩ) and degassed with N_2. The flow rate was set to one mL min^{-1} with solvent A (ultrapure water) and solvent B (500 mM NaOH), under isocratic condition of 96% A and 4% B for 25 min. The lint sample was centrifuged at 15,000× *g* for 15 min, and the supernatant was filtered through same previously mentioned 0.22 µm syringe filter, diluted 50-fold, and injected into the chromatograph.

2.5. FA Decarboxylase Activity (FADase)

FADase activity was evaluated in three different crude enzyme fractions: extracellular crude enzyme (culture medium), intracellular extract, and cell wall-associated enzymes (fragments). To obtain the biomass needed, 2 L of medium MLM (as described previously) with the supplemented with 0.05% of glucose (*w*/*v*) and 300 mg L^{-1} of commercial FA was inoculated and incubated at 28 °C and 150 rpm. Cell growth was monitored until OD600 reached 0.80. The entire culture volume was used to obtain the crude enzyme fractions previously mentioned as follows.

- Extracellular crude enzyme: Culture medium was centrifuged at 15,000× *g* for 15 min at 4 °C and the supernatant was filtered through a 0.22 µm filter and retained as the extracellular enzyme fracture.
- Intracellular crude enzyme: Cell biomass was washed twice with 50 mM sodium phosphate buffer (pH 6.0), the supernatant was discarded, and the pellet was resuspended in the same buffer at a concentration of 0.2 g mL^{-1} wet biomass (0.2 g wet cell per mL buffer). The resulting cell suspension was sonicated 4 times for 30 s at 20 kHz with 15 s cooling intervals in an ice bath. The lysate was centrifuged at 15,000× *g* for 15 min at 4 °C, and the supernatant was collected and used as the intracellular enzyme fraction.
- Cell wall-associated enzyme: The pellet obtained from the previous centrifugation step was resuspended in 50 mM sodium phosphate buffer (pH 6.0) and centrifuged at 15,000× *g* and 4 °C for 15 min. The supernatant was discarded, and the pellet resuspended in the same buffer at a concentration of 0.2 g mL^{-1} (wet weight), the method was described by dos Santos et al. [2].

The reactional mixture consisted of 1:9 ratio of enzyme solution to substrate, one mmol L^{-1} of dithiothreitol, and a FA (0.5 g L^{-1}) prepared in sodium phosphate buffer 50 mM (pH 6.0). Reaction was maintained at 30.0 °C for five minutes, and the enzymatic activity was then halted by adding ethanol 96 °GL in a 1:4 ratio (reaction mixture: ethanol).

FA decarboxylase activity was determined by FA reduction and 4-VG formation (µmol). One unit (U) of enzyme activity was defined as the amount of enzyme required to produce one µmol of 4-VG per minute under the assay conditions. Specific activity was calculated by relation of total enzyme unit (U) to the total proteins (mg) of the intracellular fraction used in the reaction. The total protein content was determined using the Bradford method, with bovine serum albumin (BSA) as the standard.

2.6. FA Decarboxylase Characterization

2.6.1. Effect of pH and Temperature on Enzyme Activity and Stability

During the cell wall-associated crude enzyme characterization, the enzyme activity was evaluated across a pH range of 4.0 to 9.0, using 0.1 M sodium acetate (pH 4.0–5.0); MES (pH 5.5–6.5); HEPES (pH 7.0–8.0); BICINE (pH 8.5–9.0) at 30 °C. The temperature effect on the enzyme activity was determined in the range of 20 and 60 °C, at pH 5.5, following the previously described enzyme reaction. Enzyme stability was assessed by incubating the enzyme without substrate, while for pH stability, samples were incubated in buffers ranging from pH 4.0 to 9.0 at 4 and 25 °C for 60 min. Thermal stability was determined by incubating the crude enzyme solution at a temperature range from 20 to 50 °C for 60 min. The remaining decarboxylase activity was determined under standard assay conditions described above at 40 °C and pH 5.0.

2.6.2. Stability of Enzyme on Storage at Different Temperatures

The enzyme was stored at 4 °C and −20 °C for 30, 90, and 180 days, and the remaining activities were determined as described in the previous section after filtration in a 0.22 μm syringe filter.

2.7. Data Analysis

At least three independent replicates were included for each measurement, with a control experiment performed under the same conditions. Results are expressed as the mean of replicate values with their corresponding standard deviations (mean ± SD).

Statistical analyses were conducted through one-way ANOVA and followed by Tukey's post hoc test for multiple comparisons in GraphPad Prism 10.6.0, with significance defined at $p < 0.05$.

3. Results and Discussion

3.1. Studies on Bacterial Tolerance to FA and Its Transformation to 4-VG

There was no significant difference in bacterium growth at FA concentrations between 100 and 700 mg L^{-1}. (Figure 2A), although a slight decrease was observed at concentrations above 500 mg L^{-1}. For more details check Figure S9 in Supplementary material.

Figure 2B shows that during cultivation with 300 mg L^{-1} of FA, there was a rapid decrease in FA concentration within the first 6 h, during which no bacterial growth was observed. Once the FA level reached its minimum, glucose was rapidly consumed, which marked the onset of growth. Glucose concentration continued to decrease until 12 h of cultivation when the maximum biomass and the highest 4-VG concentration (236.8 ± 76.3 mg L^{-1}) were achieved. The 4-VG concentration remained stable for up to 24 h of cultivation. See Figure S10.

LC-MS chromatography revealed a proton ion peak at 151.1 m/z (Figure S2), consistent with the mass of 4-VG (150.17 g mol^{-1}). A yield of 99.5% was achieved for the bioconversion of FA to 4-VG, starting with an initial concentration of 258.7 ± 4.0 mg L^{-1} (1.71 mmol L^{-1}).

HPLC did not detect any FA-derived metabolites, except in samples collected between 12 and 14 h of cultivation when VA was observed (Figure 3).

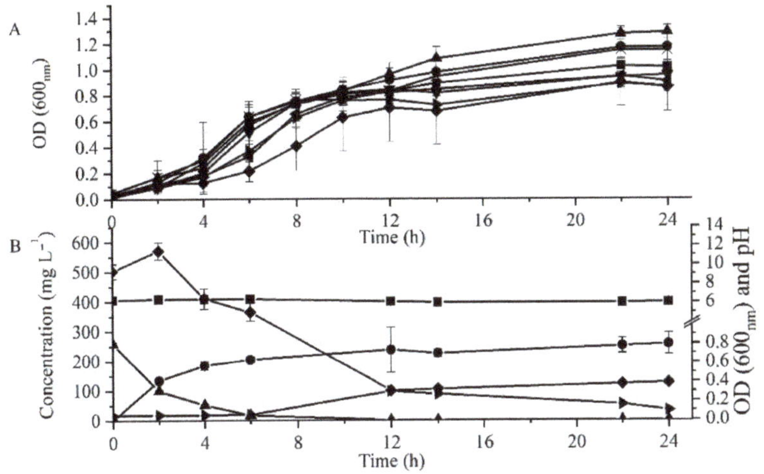

Figure 2. (**A**) Growth of *B. intermedia* TG 3.48 in nutrient medium containing 100 to 700 mg L^{-1} of FA. ■ 100 mg L^{-1}; • 200 mg L^{-1}; ▲ 300 mg L^{-1}; ▼ 400 mg L^{-1}; ▸ 500 mg L^{-1} and ◂ 600 mg L^{-1}; ♦ 700 mg L^{-1} of FA. × = biotic control; and (**B**) *B. intermedia* TG 3.48 growth in a medium with 300 mg L^{-1} of FA. Left y-axis (concentration mg L^{-1}): ▲ = FA; ♦ = Glucose; • = 4-VG. Right y-axis (pH up/OD down): ■ = pH; ▸ = microbial biomass. Data are mean ± SD of three replicates (n = 3).

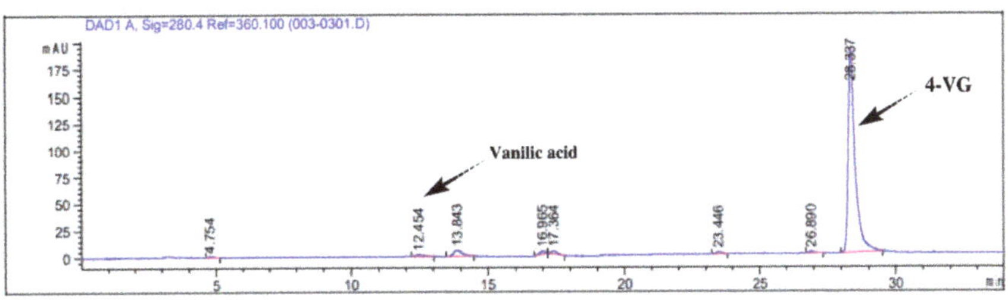

Figure 3. Chromatogram using a sample from 12 h of cultivation of *B. intermedia* TG 3.48 in a medium with 300 mg L^{-1} of FA, only showed the presence of VA as a FA derivative. The compounds were confirmed by LC-MS.

B. intermedia TG 3.48 has been shown to be capable of degrading xenobiotic compounds [21,31,32]. FA has been characterized as an antimicrobial agent with bacteriostatic effect, impacting cell mobility, biofilm formation, and energy metabolism. On the other hand, the microbial transformation of this compound could be seen as a detoxification action [33,34].

A concentration of FA around 500 mg L^{-1} inhibited the growth of *Pseudomonas aeruginosa* ATCC 10145 and *Escherichia coli* CECT4342, while *Staphylococcus aureus* CECT 976 was only inhibited at 5000 mg L^{-1} of FA [35]. *B. intermedia* TG 3.48 tolerated FA concentrations up to 700 mg L^{-1} without a significant decrease in biomass production (Figure 2A). The simultaneous consumption of glucose and FA suggests that the bacteria utilize the sugar as an energy and carbon source, while FA is biotransformed into 4-VG as a detoxification mechanism.

For the bioconversion of FA to 4-VG, 300 mg L^{-1} of FA was used to avoid inhibition in bacterial growth and to optimize the process. The concurrent decrease in FA concentration and formation of 4-VG (Figure S3) confirms the use of decarboxylation as a detoxification mechanism. Similar results have been reported for *Enterobacter* sp. Px6-4 [36] and *K. pneumoniae* [2].

3.2. FA Decarboxylase Activity (FADase)

FADase activity was examined in the intracellular extract (lysed cell) using the whole cell, the cell wall fragments, and the culture medium. It was considered an extracellular enzyme in all the samples, except the intracellular extract. When the whole cell was used, an activity of 5.17 U mL^{-1} was determined. With the intracellular extract and the cell wall fragments, the activity was 4.40 U mL^{-1} and 3.54 U mL^{-1}, respectively (Figure 4 FADase Activity, B and C), while the specific activity was 778.90 U mg^{-1}. These findings indicate that the enzyme is associated with the cell. A small amount of 4-VG detected in the culture medium (0.35 U mL^{-1}) could be the result of cell disruption during cultivation.

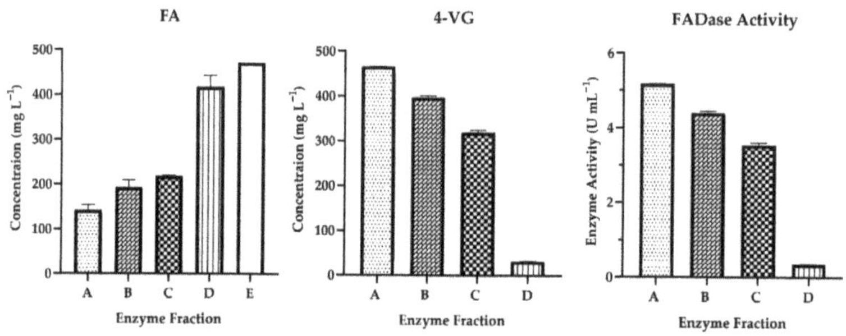

Figure 4. Residual ferulic acid (FA), 4-vinylguaiacol production (4-VG), and FADase activity. A: whole cell; B: intracellular extract; C: cell wall fragments; D: culture medium; E: control. Data are mean ± SD of three replicates (n = 3) and statistical significance (ANOVA/Tukey's post hoc test) was set at $p < 0.05$.

A one-way ANOVA confirmed the highly significant difference among the enzyme fractions for all tested parameters, including FADase activity, 4-VG production, and FA consumption (all $p < 0.0001$). Post hoc analysis with Tukey's test showed that the whole-cell fraction (A) had significantly higher FADase activity and produced significantly more 4-VG product compared to the culture medium (D) ($p < 0.0001$ for both comparisons). The negligible activity and product formation in the culture medium confirm that the FADase enzyme is cell-associated and is secreted into the medium only at low concentrations.

Our results confirm that the conversion of FA to 4-VG occurs via decarboxylation. The detection of cell-associated FADase activity supports this hypothesis. Data indicates that FADase is associated with the whole cell and cell wall fragments, suggesting it is an extracellular enzyme, but it was not released into the medium. This profile is consistent with enzymes involved in medium detoxification [37]. Similar findings were reported by Li et al. [36], where the intracellular activity of FADase was directly associated with an increase in 4-VG concentration in *Enterobacter* sp. Px6-4.

3.3. Enzyme Characterization

FADase exhibited maximum activity at pH 5.5 (Figure 5A) and at 50 °C, with activity in temperature range between 40 and 55 °C (Figure 5B). In the absence of any substrate, FADase remained stable within a pH range of 4.5 to 6.5 (Figure 5C), while remaining stable between 30 and 45 °C, it lost 40% of its initial activity at 50 °C and was inactivated at 55 °C (Figure 5D).

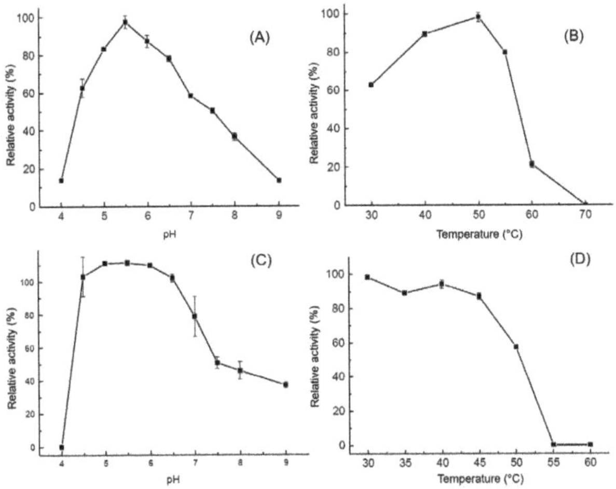

Figure 5. Effect of pH (**A**) and temperature (**B**) on enzyme activity. Effect of pH (**C**) and temperature (**D**) on the enzyme stability in absence of substrate. The maximal activity among the data was considered as 100%. Data are mean ± SD of three replicates (n = 3).

The enzyme remained stable for 180 days when stored at −20 °C. At 4 °C, it retained 60% of its initial activity after 90 days and 40% after 180 days (Figure 6).

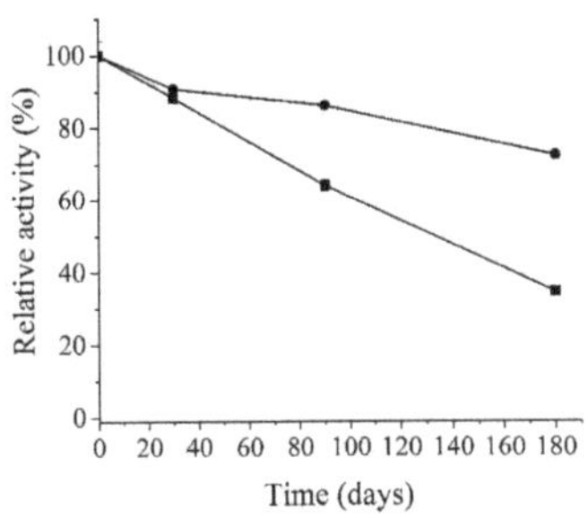

Figure 6. Effect of temperature on enzyme storage. ■ = 4 °C; • = −20 °C. 100% of activity was considered based on the unincubated enzyme.

The physicochemical properties of FADase, including maximum activity at pH 5.0 and 6.0, are consistent with other FADases, such as that described by Santos et al. [2] from *K. pneumoniae* TD 4.7 and by Maeda et al. [38] from *Bacillus* sp. BP-7. However, the highest activity observed at 40 and 55 °C indicates that these enzymes are more thermostable than those from *Candida guilliermondii*, which has an optimal temperature at 25 °C, *P. fluorescens* UI 670 at 27 to 30 °C, *B. pumilus* PS213 at 37 °C, and *K. pneumoniae* TD 4.7 at 40 °C [2,37,39,40].

3.4. Products of FADase Activity

The degradation of FA via 4-VG is a pathway commonly employed by bacteria, filamentous fungi, and yeasts, but with differences in efficiencies and resulting metabolites. In many studies, 4-VG is reported as an intermediate metabolite resulting from the decarboxylation of FA. This intermediate can be further biotransformed into acetovanillone or vanillin. Oxidation of vanillin produces VA, which can be subsequently bioconverted into protocatechuic acid or catechol [2,13,41,42].

In this study, only trace amounts of VA were detected, indicating that *B. intermedia* TG 3.48 can convert 4-VG to vanillin and subsequently to VA, as suggested in the literature [43]. The non-detection of vanillin may be due to its rapid conversion to VA. The maintenance of 4-VG concentration after the maximum production peak at 12 h of cultivation suggests that this metabolite was not used as a carbon source and was minimally converted to other metabolites (vanillin, VA, and catechol) [11]. However, it is possible that, with cultivation exceeding 24 h, further metabolization of 4-VG to vanillin and VA may occur, as observed in *Streptomyces setonii* by Salgado et al. [44]. These findings are interesting from a biotechnological perspective, indicating the potential use of this bacterium for single step production of 4-VG at high yield.

4. Conclusions

To our knowledge, this study is the first report that *B. intermedia* TG 3.48 biotransforms FA to 4-VG via a cell-wall-associated FADase. The strain tolerates high FA concentrations and achieves a high conversion yield, while the enzyme is stable between 30 and 40 °C and operates without added cofactors, features that simplify reactor design and reduce operating costs. Although vanillin was not detected in the culture, likely due to rapid conversion, the strain can further convert 4-VG into downstream derivatives such as vanillic acid, indicating useful substrate scope for valorizing lignocellulosic FA into value-added aroma and chemical intermediates. When compared with conventional biotransformation routes that require cofactor supplementation or regeneration, or to free enzyme approaches, which typically demand purification, can be less stable, and suffer greater sensitivity to substrate and product toxicity, *B. intermedia* TG 3.48 stands as a practical and competitive biocatalyst for valorizing FA from lignocellulosic biomass, because of the combination of species-level novelty, cell-wall-associated localization, cofactor independence, thermal stability in a mesophilic range, high substrate tolerance, and elevated bioconversion rates.

Supplementary Materials: The following supporting information can be downloaded at: https://www.mdpi.com/article/10.3390/pr13103367/s1, Figure S1. Chromatogram obtained from a sample of medium after 24 h of cultivation of the bacterium *B. intermedia* TG 3.48, where the peak at 28.6 min represents 4-VG. Figure S2. Chromatogram (A) and mass spectrum (B) for 4-VG, determined by LC-MS. Figure S3. FA consumption profile and 4-VG formation at different incubation times. Figure S4. Chromatogram corresponding to the retention time of the FA standard. Figure S5. Chromatogram corresponding to the retention time of the 4-VG standard. Figure S6. Chromatogram corresponding to the retention time of the catechol standard. Figure S7. Chromatogram corresponding to the retention time of the vanillic acid standard. Figure S8. Chromatogram corresponding to the retention time of the vanillin standard. Figure S9. Growth profiles of the bacterium *Brucella intermedia* TG 3.48 at concentrations of (A) 100 to 500 mg L^{-1} FA and (B) between 500 and 700 mg L^{-1} FA. Figure S10. *B. intermedia* TG 3.48 growth in a medium with 300 mg L^{-1} of FA. Left y-axis (concentration mg L^{-1}): ▲ = FA; ♦ = Glucose; • = 4-VG. Right y-axis (pH up/OD down): ■ = pH; ■ = microbial biomass.

Author Contributions: Conceptualization: E.G.; methodology: E.G., M.B.C.d.S., M.A.Z., É.J.P. and M.B.; investigation: S.P.d.C. and K.S.D.; data curation: E.G., M.B.C.d.S., M.B. and R.d.S.; formal analysis: E.G. and M.B.C.d.S.; writing—original draft preparation: S.P.d.C., E.G. and M.A.Z.; writing—review and editing: E.G., M.A.Z. and É.J.P.; visualization, R.R.d.S.; supervision: E.G. and M.B.C.d.S.; project administration: E.G., M.B. and R.d.S.; funding acquisition: E.G., M.B. and R.d.S. All authors have read and agreed to the published version of the manuscript.

Funding: The authors gratefully acknowledge the financial support from the São Paulo Research Foundation (FAPESP-Process n. 2018/21030-9 and 2021/01317-4) and National Council for Scientific and Technological Development—CNPq.

Data Availability Statement: Data is contained within the article.

Conflicts of Interest: The authors declare no conflicts of interest.

eferences

Eugenio, M.E.; Martín-Sampedro, R.; Santos, J.I.; Wicklein, B.; Martín, J.A.; Ibarra, D. Properties versus application requirements of solubilized lignins from an elm clone during different pre-treatments. *Int. J. Biol. Macromol.* **2021**, *181*, 99–111. [CrossRef]

dos Santos, M.B.C.; Scarpassa, J.A.; Monteiro, D.A.; Ladino-Orjuela, G.; Da Silva, R.; Boscolo, M.; Gomes, E. Evaluation of the tolerance and biotransformation of ferulic acid by *Klebsiella pneumoniae* TD 4.7. *Braz. J. Microbiol.* **2021**, *52*, 1181–1190. [CrossRef] [PubMed]

Pang, T.; Wang, G.; Sun, H.; Sui, W.; Si, C. Lignin fractionation: Effective strategy to reduce molecule weight dependent heterogeneity for upgraded lignin valorization. *Ind. Crops Prod.* **2021**, *165*, 113442. [CrossRef]

Lentz, M. The Impact of Simple Phenolic Compounds on Beer Aroma and Flavor. *Fermentation* **2018**, *4*, 20. [CrossRef]

Li, L.; Long, L.; Ding, S. Bioproduction of high-concentration 4-vinylguaiacol using whole-cell catalysis harboring an organic solvent-tolerant phenolic acid decarboxylase from *Bacillus atrophaeus*. *Front. Microbiol.* **2019**, *10*, 1798. [CrossRef]

Dorfner, R.; Ferge, T.; Kettrup, A.; Zimmermann, R.; Yeretzian, C. Real-Time Monitoring of 4-Vinylguaiacol, Guaiacol, and Phenol during Coffee Roasting by Resonant Laser Ionization Time-of-Flight Mass Spectrometry. *J. Agric. Food Chem.* **2003**, *51*, 5768–5773. [CrossRef]

Moon, J.-K.; Shibamoto, T. Role of Roasting Conditions in the Profile of Volatile Flavor Chemicals Formed from Coffee Beans. *J. Agric. Food Chem.* **2009**, *57*, 5823–5831. [CrossRef]

Lin, J.; Rouseff, R.L. Characterization of Aroma-Impact Compounds in Cold-Pressed Grapefruit Oil Using Time–Intensity GC–Olfactometry and GC–MS. *Flavour Fragr. J.* **2001**, *16*, 457–463. [CrossRef]

Yu, X.; Chen, X.; Li, Y.; Li, L. Effect of Drying Methods on Volatile Compounds of Citrus Reticulata Ponkan and Chachi Peels as Characterized by GC-MS and GC-IMS. *Foods* **2022**, *11*, 2662. [CrossRef]

Khan, M.R.; Fadlallah, S.; Gallos, A.; Flourat, A.L.; Torrieri, E.; Allais, F. Effect of ferulic acid derivative concentration on the release kinetics, antioxidant capacity, and thermal behaviour of different polymeric films. *Food Chem.* **2023**, *410*, 135395. [CrossRef] [PubMed]

Lubbers, R.J.M.; Dilokpimol, A.; Visser, J.; Mäkelä, M.R.; Hildén, K.S.; de Vries, R.P. A comparison between the homocyclic aromatic metabolic pathways from plant-derived compounds by bacteria and fungi. *Biotechnol. Adv.* **2019**, *37*, 107396. [CrossRef]

Detering, T.; Mundry, K.; Berger, R.G. Generation of 4-vinylguaiacol through a novel high-affinity ferulic acid decarboxylase to obtain smoke flavours without carcinogenic contaminants. *PLoS ONE* **2020**, *15*, e0244290. [CrossRef]

Sun, L.-H.; Lv, S.-W.; Yu, F.; Li, S.-N.; He, L.-Y. Biosynthesis of 4-vinylguaiacol from crude ferulic acid by *Bacillus licheniformis* DLF-17056. *J. Biotechnol.* **2018**, *281*, 144–149. [CrossRef]

Tramontina, R.; Ciancaglini, I.; Roman, E.K.B.; Chacón, M.G.; Corrêa, T.L.R.; Dixon, N.; Bugg, T.D.H.; Squina, F.M. Sustainable biosynthetic pathways to value-added bioproducts from hydroxycinnamic acids. *Appl. Microbiol. Biotechnol.* **2023**, *107*, 4165–4185. [CrossRef]

Bell, E.L.; Finnigan, W.; France, S.P.; Green, A.P.; Hayes, M.A.; Hepworth, L.J.; Lovelock, S.L.; Niikura, H.; Osuna, S.; Romero, E.; et al. Biocatalysis. *Nat. Rev. Methods Primers* **2021**, *1*, 46. [CrossRef]

Byrne, P.A.; Gilheany, D.G. The Modern Interpretation of the Wittig Reaction Mechanism. *Chem. Soc. Rev.* **2013**, *42*, 6670–6696. [CrossRef]

Woźniak-Karczewska, M.; Čvančarová, M.; Chrzanowski, Ł.; Kolvenbach, B.; Corvini, P.F.-X.; Cichocka, D. Isolation of two *Ochrobactrum* sp. strains capable of degrading the nootropic drug—Piracetam. *New Biotechnol.* **2018**, *43*, 37–43. [CrossRef] [PubMed]

Katsivela, E.; Moore, E.R.B.; Kalogerakis, N. Biodegradation of aliphatic and aromatic hydrocarbons: Specificity among bacteria isolated from refinery waste sludge. *Water Air Soil Pollut. Focus* **2003**, *3*, 103–115. [CrossRef]

Sultan, S.; Hasnain, S. Reduction of toxic hexavalent chromium by *Ochrobactrum intermedium* strain SDCr-5 stimulated by heavy metals. *Bioresour. Technol.* **2007**, *98*, 340–344. [CrossRef] [PubMed]

Waranusantigul, P.; Lee, H.; Kruatrachue, M.; Pokethitiyook, P.; Auesukaree, C. Isolation and characterization of lead-tolerant *Ochrobactrum intermedium* and its role in enhancing lead accumulation by *Eucalyptus camaldulensis*. *Chemosphere* **2011**, *85*, 584–590. [CrossRef] [PubMed]

Egea, T.C.; Da Silva, R.; Boscolo, M.; Rigonato, J.; Monteiro, D.A.; Grünig, D.; Da Silva, H.; Van Der Wielen, F.; Helmus, R.; Parsons, J.R. Diuron degradation by bacteria from soil of sugarcane crops. *Heliyon* **2017**, *3*, e00471. [CrossRef] [PubMed]

Ferhat, S.; Alouaoui, R.; Badis, A.; Moulai-Mostefa, N. Production and characterization of biosurfactant by free and immobilized cells from *Ochrobactrum intermedium* isolated from the soil of southern Algeria with a view to environmental application. *Biotechnol. Biotechnol. Equip.* **2017**, *31*, 733–742. [CrossRef]

23. Chen, P.; Yan, L.; Wu, Z.; Li, S.; Bai, Z.; Yan, X.; Wang, N.; Liang, N.; Li, H. A Microbial Transformation Using *Bacillus subtilis* B to Produce Natural Vanillin from Ferulic Acid. *Sci. Rep.* **2016**, *6*, 20400. [CrossRef]
24. Mohamed, E.T.; Werner, A.Z.; Salvachúa, D.; Singer, C.A.; Szostkiewicz, K.; Rafael Jiménez-Díaz, M.; Eng, T.; Radi, M.S.; Simmo B.A.; Mukhopadhyay, A.; et al. Adaptive Laboratory Evolution of *Pseudomonas Putida* KT2440 Improves *p*-Coumaric and Feru Acid Catabolism and Tolerance. *Metab. Eng. Commun.* **2020**, *11*, e00143. [CrossRef]
25. Lin, F.; Ferguson, K.L.; Boyer, D.R.; Lin, X.N.; Marsh, E.N.G. Isofunctional Enzymes PAD1 and UbiX Catalyze Formation c Novel Cofactor Required by Ferulic Acid Decarboxylase and 4-Hydroxy-3-Polyprenylbenzoic Acid Decarboxylase. *ACS Ch. Biol.* **2015**, *10*, 1137–1144. [CrossRef]
26. Landete, J.M.; Rodríguez, H.; Curiel, J.A.; De Las Rivas, B.; Mancheño, J.M.; Muñoz, R. Gene Cloning, Expression, a Characterization of Phenolic Acid Decarboxylase from Lactobacillus Brevis RM84. *J. Ind. Microbiol. Biotechnol.* **2010**, *37*, 617–6 [CrossRef]
27. Hördt, A.; López, M.G.; Meier-Kolthoff, J.P.; Schleuning, M.; Weinhold, L.-M.; Tindall, B.J.; Gronow, S.; Kyrpides, N.C.; Woyke, Göker, M. Analysis of 1,000+ Type-Strain Genomes Substantially Improves Taxonomic Classification of *Alphaproteobacteria*. *Frc Microbiol.* **2020**, *11*, 468. [CrossRef]
28. Bertani, G. Studies on lysogenesis I. *J. Bacteriol.* **1951**, *62*, 293–300. [CrossRef]
29. Bushnell, L.D.; Haas, H.F. The utilization of certain hydrocarbons by microorganisms. *J. Bacteriol.* **1941**, *41*, 653–673. [CrossRe
30. Rodríguez-Delgado, M.A.; Malovaná, S.; Pérez, J.P.; Borges, T.; García Montelongo, F.J. Separation of phenolic compoun by high-performance liquid chromatography with absorbance and fluorimetric detection. *J. Chromatogr. A* **2001**, *912*, 249–2 [CrossRef] [PubMed]
31. Mahendhran, K.; Arthanari, A.; Dheenadayalan, B.; Ramanathan, M. Bioconversion of oily bilge waste to polyhydroxybutyra (PHB) by marine *Ochrobactrum intermedium*. *Bioresour. Technol. Rep.* **2018**, *4*, 66–73. [CrossRef]
32. Shukla, A.; Parmar, P.; Goswami, D.; Patel, B.; Saraf, M. Characterization of novel thorium tolerant *Ochrobactrum intermedit* AM7 in consort with assessing its EPS-Thorium binding. *J. Hazard. Mater.* **2020**, *388*, 122047. [CrossRef]
33. Lemos, M.; Borges, A.; Teodósio, J.; Araújo, P.; Mergulhão, F.; Melo, L.; Simões, M. The effects of ferulic and salicylic acids *Bacillus cereus* and *Pseudomonas fluorescens* single- and dual-species biofilms. *Int. Biodeterior. Biodegrad.* **2014**, *86*, 42–51. [CrossR
34. Hu, B.-B.; Wang, J.-L.; Wang, Y.-T.; Zhu, M.-J. Specify the individual and synergistic effects of lignocellulose-derived inhibitors biohydrogen production and inhibitory mechanism research. *Renew. Energy* **2019**, *140*, 397–406. [CrossRef]
35. Borges, A.; Saavedra, M.J.; Simões, M. The activity of ferulic and gallic acids in biofilm prevention and control of pathoger bacteria. *Biofouling* **2012**, *28*, 755–767. [CrossRef]
36. Li, X.; Yang, J.; Li, X.; Gu, W.; Huang, J.; Zhang, K.-Q. The metabolism of ferulic acid via 4-vinylguaiacol to vanillin by *Enterobac* sp. Px6-4 isolated from *Vanilla* root. *Process Biochem.* **2008**, *43*, 1132–1137. [CrossRef]
37. Degrassi, G.; Polverino De Laureto, P.; Bruschi, C.V. Purification and characterization of ferulate and *p*-coumarate decarboxyla from *Bacillus pumilus*. *Appl. Environ. Microbiol.* **1995**, *61*, 326–332. [CrossRef] [PubMed]
38. Maeda, M.; Tokashiki, M.; Tokashiki, M.; Uechi, K.; Ito, S.; Taira, T. Characterization and induction of phenolic acid decarboxyla from *Aspergillus luchuensis*. *J. Biosci. Bioeng.* **2018**, *126*, 162–168. [CrossRef] [PubMed]
39. Huang, Z.; Dostal, L.; Rosazza, J.P. Purification and characterization of a ferulic acid decarboxylase from *Pseudomonas fluoresce* *J. Bacteriol.* **1994**, *176*, 5912–5918. [CrossRef]
40. Huang, H.-K.; Tokashiki, M.; Maeno, S.; Onaga, S.; Taira, T.; Ito, S. Purification and properties of phenolic acid decarboxyla from *Candida guilliermondii*. *J. Ind. Microbiol. Biotechnol.* **2012**, *39*, 55–62. [CrossRef]
41. Baqueiro-Peña, I.; Rodríguez-Serrano, G.; González-Zamora, E.; Augur, C.; Loera, O.; Saucedo-Castañeda, G. Biotransformatic of ferulic acid to 4-vinylguaiacol by a wild and a diploid strain of *Aspergillus niger*. *Bioresour. Technol.* **2010**, *101*, 4721–47 [CrossRef] [PubMed]
42. Xie, X.-G.; Dai, C.-C. Degradation of a model pollutant ferulic acid by the endophytic fungus *Phomopsis liquidambari*. *Biores Technol.* **2015**, *179*, 35–42. [CrossRef] [PubMed]
43. Girawale, S.D.; Meena, S.N.; Nandre, V.S.; Waghmode, S.B.; Kodam, K.M. Biosynthesis of Vanillic Acid by Ochrobactru Anthropi and Its Applications. *Bioorg. Med. Chem.* **2022**, *72*, 117000. [CrossRef] [PubMed]
44. Salgado, J.M.; Max, B.; Rodríguez-Solana, R.; Domínguez, J.M. Purification of ferulic acid solubilized from agroindustrial wast and further conversion into 4-vinyl guaiacol by *Streptomyces setonii* using solid state fermentation. *Ind. Crops Prod.* **2012**, *39*, 52–6 [CrossRef]

processes

MDPI

eview

'rom Waste to Wonder: Valorization of Colombian Plant 3y-Products for Peroxidase Production and 3iotechnological Innovation

ohn J. Castillo

Escuela de Química, Universidad Industrial de Santander, Bucaramanga 680002, Colombia; jcasleon@uis.edu.co; Tel.: +57-76344000 (ext. 2893)

Abstract

The valorization of agricultural by-products represents a sustainable strategy to reduce waste and create high-value biotechnological products. This review highlights Colombian plant-derived peroxidases (PODs) obtained from Guinea grass, royal palm, African oil palm, lemongrass, sleepy plant, and sweet potato. These enzymes catalyze oxidative reactions and show potential in biosensing, polymer synthesis, environmental remediation, and health monitoring. We summarize extraction and purification strategies while addressing current challenges such as operational stability, scalability, and cost. Special emphasis is given to applications like cross-linked enzymatic aggregates (CLEAs) and electrochemical biosensors, where Colombian PODs demonstrate superior stability and sensitivity compared to horseradish peroxidase (HRP). This review frames these advances within the circular bioeconomy, presenting insights into waste reduction and CO_2 savings. By integrating local biodiversity into innovative processes, Colombian PODs can drive sustainable technologies and provide industrial and environmental solutions.

Keywords: agricultural by-products; peroxidases; biotechnological applications

1. Introduction

The global shift toward sustainability has intensified interest in innovative strategies to repurpose agricultural residues [1–3]. These by-products, including crop residues, peels, leaves, and stems, are often discarded or burned, contributing to pollution and greenhouse gas emissions [3–7]. However, this organic waste contains valuable biomolecules such as enzymes, proteins, and fibers that can be repurposed for high-value applications. The concept of waste valorization, particularly in the context of the circular bioeconomy, involves transforming these by-products into new products that can be reintegrated into the economy, thus extending the lifecycle of the original resource [5,8,9]. The circular bioeconomy is a model that emphasizes the sustainable management of biological resources through the reuse, recycling, and regeneration of materials [8,10]. In the context of agriculture, this means finding innovative ways to utilize by-products that are often discarded, thereby reducing the environmental footprint of agricultural activities while adding value to waste materials [2,3,11]. Agricultural by-products, which are often rich in bioactive compounds, represent a promising source of raw materials for the production of enzymes, biopolymers, and other high-value chemicals [5,12].

Colombia, recognized for its biodiversity and strong agricultural economy, generates large volumes of plant-based residues that remain underutilized. Extracting peroxidases

(PODs) from these materials represents a dual opportunity: reducing waste and developing sustainable enzymes for industry [13]. In recent years, PODs have garnered significant attention for their role in various industrial and environmental processes [14]. These enzymes have been employed in biosensing technologies, where they facilitate the detection of H_2O_2, a critical marker in many biochemical reactions. Additionally, as is shown in Figure 1, PODs have shown promise in the synthesis of advanced materials, such as conducting polymers like polyaniline (PANI) [15], further extending their utility in material science. Their capacity to form cross-linked enzymatic aggregates (CLEAs) [16] also makes them valuable tools for bioremediation, particularly in the removal of industrial pollutants such as dyes, as well as their use in chemiluminescence assays. The biotechnological potential of PODs extracted from Colombian plant by-products represents a convergence of waste valorization and innovation. Plants such as Guinea grass (*Panicum maximum*), royal palm (*Roystonea regia*), African oil palm (*Eleais guineensis*), lemongrass (*Cymbpogon citratus*), sleepy plant (*Mimosa pudica*), and sweet potato (*Ipomea batatas*) produce significant amounts of agricultural waste [17–20]. By extracting and purifying PODs from these plants, researchers can harness their enzymatic properties for a variety of applications, contributing to both a reduction in waste and the development of sustainable technologies.

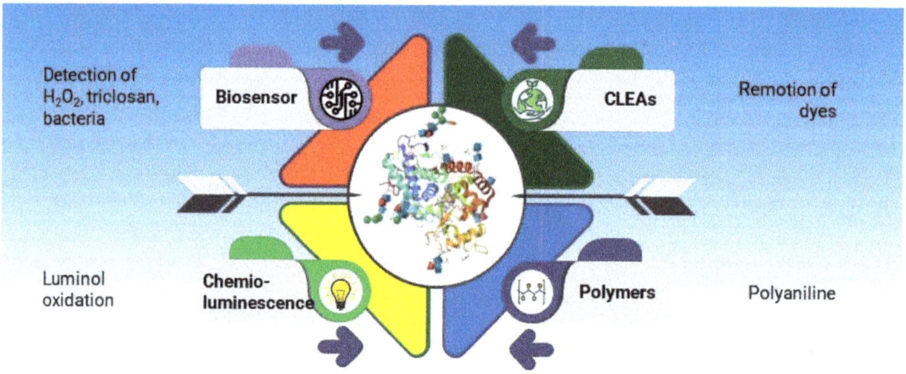

Figure 1. Novel biotechnological applications of Colombian plant-derived PODs from agricultural by-products, emphasizing their use in biosensing, advanced materials, and environmental remediation.

In Colombia, where agriculture plays a vital role in the national economy, the potential for waste valorization is particularly high. The country's diverse ecosystems and wide variety of crops generate substantial amounts of plant-based by-products that could be repurposed for biotechnological applications. By leveraging the biochemical properties of enzymes like POD, Colombia can contribute to global efforts in sustainability while also fostering innovation in sectors such as environmental remediation and health monitoring [1,21].

PODs are a class of enzymes that catalyze the oxidation of various substrates in the presence of H_2O_2. These enzymes are widely distributed in plants and play an important role in defense mechanisms against environmental stress [22,23]. In biotechnological contexts, PODs are valued for their ability to facilitate oxidative reactions, making them useful in a range of applications including biosensors, polymer synthesis, and bioremediation [24,25].

As is shown in Figure 2, Colombian plants such as Guinea grass (*Panicum maximum*), Royal palm (*Roystonea regia*), African palm (*Elaeis guineensis*), lemongrass (*Cymbopogon citratus*), sleepy plant (*Mimosa pudica*), and sweet potato (*Ipomoea batatas*) are rich sources of PODs.

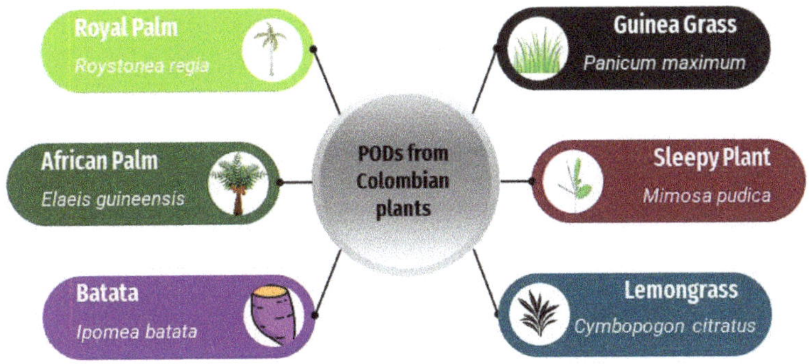

Figure 2. Main Colombian plant sources of PODs with high potential for sustainable enzyme production.

These plants produce significant agricultural by-products that can be exploited for enzyme extraction, turning waste into valuable biotechnological resources. The extraction and purification of PODs from these plants not only contribute to waste valorization but also provide a renewable source of enzymes for industrial applications [26].

Finally, the valorization of Colombian plant by-products for POD production represents a powerful example of how waste can be transformed into valuable resources within the framework of the circular bioeconomy. By harnessing the biochemical properties of peroxidases, researchers can develop innovative solutions to pressing environmental and industrial challenges. From biosensing technologies to environmental remediation, the applications of these enzymes are vast and diverse.

The purpose of this review is to provide a comprehensive overview of the current state of the research on peroxidase extraction from Colombian plant by-products, showcasing their potential as a renewable and sustainable source of enzymes for various biotechnological applications. This review highlights the potential of Colombian plant by-products as a renewable source of PODs, encouraging further research and development in this promising field. Despite the promising potential of Colombian plant-derived PODs, significant research gaps remain. First, there is a lack of comprehensive kinetic modeling to better understand the catalytic mechanisms of these enzymes, which is crucial for optimizing their performance in industrial and biosensing applications. Second, structural characterization studies, such as X-ray crystallography and molecular dynamics simulations, are limited, hindering insights into the relationship between enzyme structure and function. Finally, there is an evident scarcity of large-scale application studies aimed at transitioning these findings from laboratory settings to real-world industrial or environmental processes. Addressing these gaps is essential to fully unlocking the biotechnological potential of Colombian PODs and to fostering innovations aligned with the circular bioeconomy framework.

2. Agricultural By-Products as a Source of Peroxidases

Colombia's rich and diverse agricultural landscape is a key pillar of the country's economy, contributing significantly to both domestic markets and international trade. With its favorable climate and vast ecosystems, Colombia produces a variety of crops, generating large quantities of agricultural by-products [13,27–30]. These by-products, traditionally considered waste, are now recognized as valuable resources that can be valued for biotechnological and industrial applications. Waste valorization of these by-products not only contributes to sustainability but also adds value to agricultural production, supporting the circular bioeconomy. Several key plants and their by-products stand out for their potential in areas like energy, food, and biotechnology. Sakharov y cols., conducted a preliminary study to analyses the enzymatic activity of various Colombian plant species, including their leaves, fruits, and roots (Table 1) [31]. This research marked one of the earliest explorations into the potential of Colombian flora for biotechnological applications. The study focused on the extraction of enzymes such as PODs. The findings highlighted the rich enzymatic diversity present in Colombian plants and opened the door to further investigations into their potential for waste valorization and sustainable production. Building on this foundational research, the focus on agricultural by-products as a source of valuable enzymes has continued to grow, driving advancements in both scientific understanding and practical applications. The study identified several plant species that exhibited particularly promising enzymatic activity, making them strong candidates for further exploration in biotechnological applications. Among these, Guinea grass, royal palm, African palm, lemongrass, sleepy plant, and sweet potato stood out for their significant potential in enzyme production and waste valorization.

Table 1. Comparison of peroxidase activity across plant parts (adapted from [31]).

Plant Part	Source of POD	POD Activity (U/g)
Fruits	Almond (*Terminalia catappa*)	<1.0
	Cocoa (*Theobroma cacao*)	11.6
	Coffee (*Coffea arabica*)	22.9
	Cocoa palm (*Cocos nucifera*)	1.2
	Tree tomato (*Cyphomandra betacca*)	16.2
	Totumo (*Crescentia cujete*)	5.8
Roots	Celery (*Apium graveolens*)	58.0
	Arracacha (*Arracacia xanthorrhiza*)	<1.0
	Sweet potato (*Ipomea batatas*)	1800.0
	Coriander (*Coriandrum sativum*)	35.0
	Bore (*Colocasa esculenta*)	370.0
	Ginger (*Zingeber officinale*)	11.6
	Red radish (*Rapharus sativas*)	121.3
	Horseradish (*Armoracia rusticana*)	2600.0
	Cassava (*Manihot esculenta*)	1.7
Leaves	Oleander (*Nerium oleander*)	98.3
	Pear cactus (*Monstera delisiosa*)	179.0
	Banana (*Musa sapientum*)	49.7
	Bamboo (*Bambusa guadua*)	<1.0
	Spanish moss (*Tillandsia recurvata*)	5.2
	Boojum tree (*Cereus hexagonus*)	19.0
	Marigold (*Calendula oficionales*)	231.2
	Bottlebrush (*Callistemon lanceolatu*)	<1.0
	Sugar cane (*Sacharum officinarum*)	104.0
	Sleepy plant (*Mimosa pudica*)	460.0
	Fique (*Agave fourcroides*)	19.6
	Fern (*Adiamtum obliguum*)	<1.0
	Castor bean plant (*Ricinum communis* L.)	440.0
	Lemongrass (*Cymbopogon citratus*)	390.0
	Fan palm (*copernica pectori*)	220.0
	African oil palm (*eleais guineensis*)	566.0
	Date palm (*Phoenix dactilera*)	580.0
	Royal palm (*Roystonea regia*)	694.0
	Coconut palm (*Cocos nucifera*)	48.6
	Corozo palm (*Acrocomia aculeata*)	570.0
	Wine palm (*Scheelea butyracea*)	173.4
	Thatch palm (*Astrocarium* sp.)	220.0
	Macaw palm (*Bactris* sp.)	196.0
	Palma mararai (*Aiphanes cariotifolia*)	1145.0
	Guinea Grass (*Panicum maximum*)	980.0
	Parsley (*Petroselinum sativum*)	35.0

2.1. *Guinea Grass (Panicum maximum)*

It is widely cultivated in Colombia, particularly in the livestock sector. It serves as high-quality fodder for cattle, but the leftover biomass, such as stems and leaves, often remains underutilized [17]. Valorization of these by-products can include the production of bioenergy through anaerobic digestion, turning waste into biogas, and extraction of fibers for biodegradable packaging materials. Additionally, Guinea grass has been explored for its potential in phytoremediation, where it is used to clean contaminated soils, contributing to environmental sustainability.

2.2. *Royal Palm (Roystonea regia)*

This is another species that produces significant agricultural by-products, primarily from its fronds and seeds. Traditionally, these materials have been discarded or used as mulch, but recent advances have explored their use in biochar production, which can serve as a soil enhancer and carbon sequestration tool. Royal palm by-products can also be transformed into activated carbon, which is highly effective in water purification processes, adding environmental and economic value to this previously wasted material [18,32,33].

2.3. *African Palm (Elaeis guineensis)*

This plays a crucial role in Colombia's economy as a major source of palm oil. However, the industry generates large amounts of by-products, including empty fruit bunches, palm kernel shells, and fibers. These residues can be valorized in various ways, such as converting them into biofuels or using them in the production of biocomposites [18]. Palm oil mill effluent, a liquid by-product, is rich in nutrients and can be treated to produce biogas or used in the production of organic fertilizers, promoting a closed-loop system in agriculture.

2.4. *Lemongrass (Cymbopogon citratus)*

This is known for its essential oils, which are widely used in the fragrance and food industries. The remaining biomass, such as leaves and stalks, can be repurposed through extraction of bioactive compounds, including antioxidants and antimicrobial agents. Lemongrass waste has also shown promise in bioenergy production, where it can be converted into bioethanol or used as a raw material to produce natural fibers [33–36].

2.5. *Sleepy Plant (Mimosa pudica)*

This species, with unique movement in response to touch, is often used for medicinal purposes in Colombia. Its leaves, stems, and roots contain compounds with antibacterial, antifungal, and anti-inflammatory properties, making it a potential source for pharmaceutical and cosmetic applications. Waste valorization efforts can focus on extracting these bioactive compounds for commercial use, reducing environmental waste while creating high-value products [37–39].

2.6. *Sweet Potato (Ipomea batata)*

This is a staple crop in Colombia, and its peels and other by-products can be repurposed in various ways. Sweet potato peels are rich in starch and antioxidants, making them valuable for food additives or as a substrate for microbial fermentation in bioethanol production. The valorization of sweet potato by-products aligns with the circular bioeconomy by reducing food waste and creating new value chains in food, energy, and material science industries [20,40–43].

3. Peroxidases: Definition, Purification and Biochemical Properties

3.1. Peroxidases

PODs are a diverse group of enzymes that catalyze the oxidation of various substrates by H_2O_2 as an electron acceptor. These heme-containing enzymes play critical roles in both plants and animals, though their functions in plants are particularly significant. In plants, peroxidases are primarily involved in defense mechanisms, growth regulation, and the metabolism of reactive oxygen species (ROS) [14,44]. The biological role of peroxidases is closely linked to their ability to detoxify H_2O_2, a by-product of various metabolic processes that can cause oxidative damage to cells. By breaking down H_2O_2 into water and oxygen, PODs help mitigate oxidative stress, protecting cellular components such as lipids, proteins, and DNA from damage. In addition to their role in oxidative stress management, peroxidases are also essential for lignin biosynthesis, a process critical for cell wall formation and the structural integrity of plants. Lignin strengthens plant tissues and contributes to water transport by making cell walls less permeable to water [45]. Furthermore, PODs participate in wound healing, pathogen defense, and the modulation of hormone levels, which impacts plant growth and development. In response to biotic and abiotic stresses, peroxidases facilitate the cross-linking of cell wall components, enhancing the plant's defensive barrier against pathogens [22,46]. The enzymatic activity of PODs is defined by their ability to transfer electrons from a wide variety of donor molecules, such as phenolic compounds, to hydrogen peroxide. This reaction not only helps in the degradation of H_2O_2 but also contributes to the oxidative polymerization of organic molecules, including lignin precursors. The broad substrate specificity of peroxidases allows them to participate in diverse physiological processes, making them versatile enzymes with substantial importance in plant biology.

3.2. Extraction and Purification Techniques

The extraction and purification of PODs are crucial steps in studying their structure, function, and potential biotechnological applications. Due to the widespread occurrence of PODs in various plant tissues, isolating these enzymes involves selecting appropriate sources and employing techniques that maximize yield and purity while preserving enzymatic activity. The extraction process typically begins with the disruption of plant tissues to release intracellular enzymes, followed by a series of purification steps designed to separate PODs from other proteins and impurities. Common purification methods include precipitation, dialysis, chromatography, and ultrafiltration, each tailored to exploit the unique biochemical properties of PODs such as molecular weight, charge, and hydrophobicity. A well-designed extraction and purification protocol is essential for obtaining peroxidases in sufficient quantities and purity for further biochemical characterization and practical applications.

The purification of PODs from Colombian tropical plants has yielded promising results, with several species demonstrating high enzymatic activity. Among these, the leaves of the royal palm have proven to be a particularly rich source of POD, leading to the isolation of a novel enzyme with high purity. The purification process for this POD involved several key steps. Initially, the palm leaves were homogenized, and ammonium sulfate ($(NH_4)_2SO_4$) precipitation was used to concentrate the enzyme while removing unwanted proteins [47]. Following this, colored compounds were extracted to reduce interference during the purification process. The enzyme was then subjected to successive chromatographic steps, including hydrophobic interaction chromatography on Phenyl-Sepharose, size-exclusion chromatography using Sephacryl S100 (Cytiva, Marlborough, MA, USA), and ion-exchange chromatography on DEAE-Toyopearl. This multi-step process resulted in a highly purified peroxidase with a specific activity of 6170 U/mg. Similarly, PODs from the leaves of guinea grass have been isolated and partially purified using a biphasic polymer system consisting of polyethylene glycol (PEG) and ammonium sulfate [26]. This method allowed for an efficient separation of peroxidase from other proteins, followed by size-exclusion chromatography and ultracentrifugation to obtain a highly active and homogeneous enzyme preparation. In another approach, sweet potato peels were utilized as a POD source [20]. The purification protocol involved homogenization, removal of pigments, and subsequent chromatographic steps using Phenyl-Sepharose and DEAE-Toyopearl columns. This method produced sweet potato peroxidase (SPP) of high purity. Figure 3 shows a schematic representation of the basic stages in the purification of PODs extracted from Colombian plants. These methods underscore the versatility of purification strategies for plant PODs, highlighting the success of using both traditional and innovative techniques to achieve highly purified enzyme preparations from diverse plant sources.

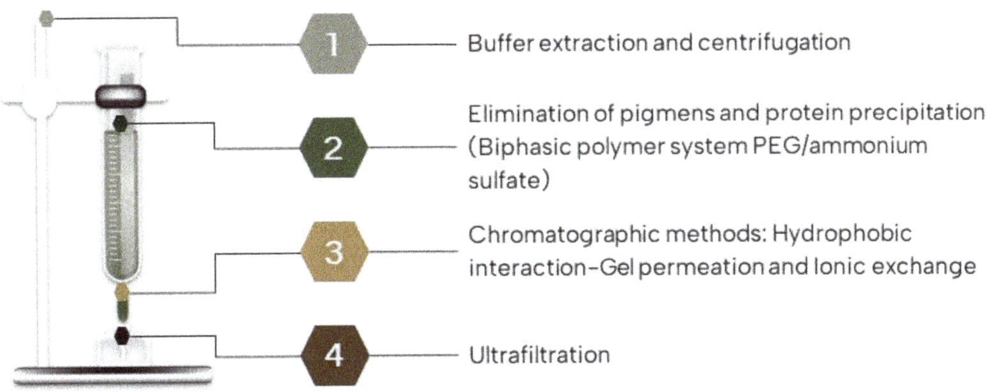

Figure 3. Stepwise protocol for POD extraction and purification from Colombian plants, illustrating innovative approaches that improve stability and scalability for biotechnological applications.

While the protocols described above have been successful in isolating highly active peroxidases from Colombian plant sources, each approach presents distinct advantages and limitations that must be considered when selecting a purification strategy. For instance, traditional precipitation methods, such as ammonium sulfate fractionation, are low-cost and simple to implement, making them suitable for small-scale laboratory extractions. However, they often result in moderate enzyme yield and can cause partial loss of enzymatic activity due to protein denaturation during salt removal steps. Chromatographic techniques, including hydrophobic interaction, ion-exchange, and size-exclusion chromatography, offer high specificity and purity, as demonstrated for royal palm and sweet potato PODs. Nevertheless, they are time-consuming, require specialized equipment, and may have limited scalability for industrial applications. Biphasic polymer systems, such as PEG/ammonium sulfate partitioning, have shown promise for Guinea grass peroxidase, providing a higher yield and preserving enzyme stability by minimizing exposure to harsh conditions. Despite these benefits, polymer-based systems can be costly and generate waste streams that require proper management. Furthermore, the choice of method directly impacts the long-term stability of the enzyme, which is critical for biosensor fabrication and industrial catalysis. Future efforts should focus on developing integrated purification workflows that balance yield, purity, cost, and environmental sustainability, potentially incorporating green extraction techniques and continuous processing to facilitate large-scale production. Table 2 illustrates the main extraction and purification techniques of Colombian plant PODs.

Table 2. Summary of extraction and purification techniques of Colombian plant peroxidases, including yield, advantages, limitations, and main biotechnological applications.

Plant Source	Extraction Technique	Yield/Specific Activity	Advantages	Drawbacks	Applications
Royal palm (*Roystonea regia*)	Homogenization → Ammonium sulfate precipitation → Hydrophobic interaction + ion-exchange chromatography	6170 U/mg [32]	High purity, excellent thermal stability	Time-consuming, high cost, not easily scalable	Electrochemical biosensors, high temperature industrial catalysis
Guinea grass (*Panicum maximum*)	Biphasic polymer system (PEG/ammonium sulfate) → Size-exclusion chromatography	2000–3000 U/mg [26]	Good stability preservation, moderate cost	Polymer disposal issues, requires optimization	Biosensors for H_2O_2, environmental monitoring
Sweet potato (*Ipomea batatas*)	Homogenization → Pigment removal → Hydrophobic interaction + ion-exchange chromatography	1800 U/mg [20]	High substrate specificity, compatible with food industry	Moderate yield, pigment interference can complicate extraction	Food biosensors, wastewater treatment
African oil palm (*Elaeis guineensis*)	Homogenization → Ammonium sulfate precipitation → Chromatographic purification	2500 U/mg [33]	Good thermal stability, wide pH tolerance	Limited studies on scalability	Environmental remediation, CLEA synthesis
Lemongrass (*Cymbopogon citratus*)	Aqueous extraction → Ammonium sulfate precipitation → Chromatography	1200 U/mg [34]	Easy implementation, accessible raw material	Enzyme unstable at pH > 7	Biosensors for H_2O_2 and phenolic compounds
Sleepy plant (*Mimosa pudica*)	Aqueous extraction → Ammonium sulfate precipitation → DEAE-Toyopearl chromatography	460 U/mg [38]	Very low detection limit with gold electrodes	Narrow pH stability range	Biosensors for sensitive biomedical detection

3.3. Biochemical Properties

PODs are versatile enzymes with biochemical properties influenced by pH, temperature, and substrate specificity, which are critical for their functionality in various applications [48]. Typically, PODs exhibit optimal activity in slightly acidic to neutral pH ranges, generally between pH 4 and 7, though some can function in broader pH conditions depending on their source. Temperature stability is another key factor, as most PODs maintain stability and high activity at moderate temperatures (25–45 °C), but their activity may diminish, or enzymes can denature at higher temperatures. Additionally, substrate specificity is a defining characteristic of PODs, as they catalyze reactions involving hydrogen peroxide with various electron donor substrates such as phenols, aromatic amines, and certain organic compounds, though preference varies across enzyme types [49]. Understanding these general properties provides a foundation for examining the unique biochemical traits of PODs derived specifically from Colombian plants, which may offer novel or enhanced attributes.

Table 3 highlights the pH and temperature optimum, inactivation constants, and substrate specificity for PODs derived from six plant sources: royal palm, African oil palm, Guinea grass, lemongrass, sweet potato, sleepy plant, and horseradish. Each enzyme's unique characteristics underscore the diversity in PODs' biochemical profiles and offer practical information for selecting specific PODs based on environmental stability and target substrate compatibility. A key observation in the table is the significant variability in the pH optima of these PODs. While many of the PODs demonstrate optimal activity in a broad range of pH values (for instance, African oil palm POD operates effectively from pH 4.0 to 9.0), others, such as sleepy plant POD, show a narrower optimal pH of 4.0. This range of pH adaptability indicates that these enzymes are well-suited for environments with fluctuating or extreme pH conditions, broadening the potential for POD applications across different industrial process. Horseradish peroxidase (HRP), commonly used as a benchmark enzyme, has a pH optimum between 6.0 and 6.5, restricting its usage in acidic conditions. By contrast, the broader pH stability of PODs like those from royal palm and African oil palm could offer enhanced versatility, particularly in biochemical processes where pH stability is a critical factor. Temperature stability, represented by the temperature optimum and inactivation constants, also varies across the POD sources. Notably, royal palm POD exhibits an impressive temperature optimum of 90 °C, significantly higher than that of HRP (25–30 °C). This high thermal tolerance makes it a promising candidate for applications in high-temperature environments, such as industrial catalysis or bioremediation in warmer climates. African oil palm and Guinea grass PODs, with optima at 72 °C and 66 °C, respectively, also show good thermal resilience, although slightly less than royal palm POD. Inactivation constants provide additional insight into thermal stability, with African oil palm and HRP showing relatively low inactivation rates (2.0×10^{-3} and 1.0×10^{-3} min^{-1}, respectively), indicating a slower rate of enzyme denaturation under prolonged exposure to heat. However, the higher inactivation constant of royal palm POD (1.5×10^{-2} min^{-1}) suggests that while it withstands high temperatures, its activity may decrease more quickly over time at these temperatures compared to HRP. Substrate specificity is another critical factor for enzyme selection, as it determines the types of reactions each POD can facilitate. All the PODs in the table show activity toward multiple substrates, with common electron donors like ABTS, ferulic acid, guaiacol, and o-dianisidine. Royal palm, African oil palm, and sweet potato PODs exhibit specificity for ferulic acid, which is valuable in phenolic compound oxidation processes often needed in environmental applications such as pollutant degradation. Lemongrass, Guinea grass, and HRP show specificity for guaiacol and o-dianisidine, indicating their suitability for different types of redox reactions commonly used in biosensing and diagnostic applications. HRP, well-known for its versatility, reacts efficiently with both ABTS and o-dianisidine, but its more limited stability under high temperatures makes it less suitable for high-temperature applications despite its broad substrate compatibility.

Beyond pH, temperature, and substrate specificity, understanding the kinetic behavior of peroxidases is essential for predicting their catalytic performance in different applications. Key kinetic parameters such as Km (Michaelis constant) and Vmax (maximum reaction velocity) provide insights into the affinity between the enzyme and its substrates. For instance, SPP has been reported with Km values ranging from 0.12 to 0.20 mM for substrates such as ABTS and o-phenylenediamine, indicating a high substrate affinity [20]. In comparison, GGP shows slightly higher Km values (0.30–0.45 mM), which correlates with its broader specificity but lower catalytic efficiency [26]. These parameters are critical for the design of biosensors where rapid and specific substrate turnover is desired. The structural stability of Colombian plant PODs has also been a topic of interest due to their ability to withstand extreme conditions. For example, royal palm peroxidase maintains over 80% of its activity at 90 °C, exhibiting a half-life of 50 min under these conditions [32]. Similarly, African oil palm peroxidase demonstrates stability across a wide pH range (4.0–9.0), which is advantageous for industrial processes involving variable reaction environments [19,33]. Such stability profiles are crucial for enzyme immobilization in biosensors and for repeated use in continuous industrial processes. Another important property is the redox potential ($E^{\circ\prime}$) of the heme active site, which determines the enzyme's ability to catalyze oxidative reactions. Colombian PODs, such as royal palm and GGP, display redox potentials between +0.85 and +0.92 V vs. Ag/AgCl, values comparable to HRP [44,48]. A higher redox potential allows these enzymes to oxidize a broader range of phenolic and aromatic amine substrates, expanding their application in pollutant degradation and biosensing technologies. The integration of kinetic data, structural stability, and redox properties provides a holistic understanding of these enzymes, allowing for the rational selection of peroxidases for specific biotechnological applications and guiding future protein engineering efforts.

Table 3. Comparative biochemical properties of peroxidases from Colombian plants.

PODs Source	pH Optimum	Temperature Optimum (°C)	Inactivation Constant (min^{-1})	Substrate Specificity	Reference
Royal palm	7.0–9.0	90	1.5×10^{-2}	Ferulic acid ABTS	[32]
African oil palm	4.0–9.0	72	2.0×10^{-3}	Ferulic acid ABTS	[19]
Guinea grass	7.0–9.0	66	8.0×10^{-3}	Guaiacol ABTS *o*-dianisidine	[26]
Lemongrass	4.0–6.0	66	1.0×10^{-2}	Guaiacol *o*-dianisidine	[34]
Sweet potato	8.0	60	7.0×10^{-3}	Ferulic acid ABTS *o*-Phenylene diamine	[20]
Sleepy plant	4.0	55	7.0×10^{-3}	-	[38]
Horseradish	6.0–6.5	25–30	1.0×10^{-3}	*o*-dianisidine ABTS	[50]

4. Biotechnological Applications of Peroxidases

4.1. Electrochemical Biosensing

Electrochemical biosensing is a powerful approach for detecting H_2O_2 and other analytes of biomedical and environmental significance [51–53]. A central element in this method is the use of PODs sourced from plants, which can catalyze reactions involving H_2O_2, producing signals measurable Via electrochemical techniques. Plant-derived PODs are ideal for biosensors due to their efficiency in redox reactions, stability under various environmental conditions, and natural availability. They catalyze the oxidation of hydrogen peroxide, producing measurable electrochemical signals that correlate with H_2O_2 concentration. This ability is especially valuable, as H_2O_2 plays crucial roles in cellular signaling and oxidative stress in biomedical fields, and it also acts as a key pollutant indicator in environmental monitoring [49].

Electrochemical biosensors work by transducing a biochemical interaction into a readable electronic signal, typically using a working electrode modified with a biorecognition element, such as plant POD, that interacts specifically with the analyte of interest. In the case of H_2O_2, the enzyme's active site catalyzes its decomposition, triggering electron transfer between the analyte and electrode surface. This interaction yields a current or voltage change, providing a quantifiable measure of H_2O_2 levels. Notably, the specificity and sensitivity of plant PODs make them versatile for designing biosensors tailored for both clinical and environmental applications. This process is beneficial because it enables low-cost, efficient, and eco-friendly monitoring of H_2O_2, providing valuable insights into various medical conditions like inflammation, cancer, and cardiovascular diseases, which are often linked to oxidative stress and cellular damage associated with abnormal H_2O_2 levels [54]. Beyond H_2O_2 detection, plant-derived peroxidases have shown significant potential for detecting other biologically and environmentally relevant analytes. For instance, they can be engineered to sense glucose, cholesterol, and uric acid, analytes critical for metabolic health monitoring. In glucose sensing, peroxidase enzymes facilitate the oxidation of glucose in the presence of H_2O_2, producing signals that allow for highly sensitive glucose measurement, an essential function in managing diabetes [55]. Likewise, cholesterol detection is possible through reactions catalyzed by PODs, enabling precise monitoring of lipid levels in blood and contributing to cardiovascular disease prevention. For environmental monitoring, POD-based sensors can detect phenolic compounds, nitrates, and heavy metals in water and soil samples [56]. Phenolic compounds, for instance, are industrial pollutants harmful to aquatic and soil ecosystems, and their detection is crucial for safeguarding environmental health.

Table 4 summarizes the performance of plant-derived POD enzymes immobilized on various electrode materials for electrochemical sensing of H_2O_2. Each plant POD demonstrates unique sensing characteristics based on its enzyme properties and electrode interface, impacting the detection limits and linear range suitable for H_2O_2 monitoring in biomedical and environmental applications. Among the PODs, the sleepy plant shows the lowest detection limit of 0.4 μM, achieved using gold nanoparticle-modified electrodes. This superior sensitivity is likely due to the excellent conductivity and high surface area of gold nanoparticles, which facilitate efficient electron transfer between the enzyme and the electrode surface. Gold nanoparticles also provide a stable platform for enzyme immobilization, reducing signal loss and improving sensor sensitivity. Consequently, MPP, combined with gold nanoparticles, may be highly advantageous for detecting low H_2O_2 concentrations in sensitive biomedical applications, such as monitoring oxidative stress markers in biological samples. Other plant sources, such as lemongrass and horseradish, also demonstrate relatively low detection limits (50 μM), though they utilize graphene and carbon paste electrodes, respectively. Graphene's high electron conductivity and large surface area contribute to this performance, enhancing electron transfer and enzyme stability on the electrode surface [57,58]. HRP, immobilized on a carbon paste electrode, displays a broader linear range of 0.05–10 mM, making it suitable for applications requiring a wider dynamic range, such as environmental pollutant detection or food safety monitoring. In contrast, royal palm and guinea grass PODs show higher detection limits of 87 μM and 150 μM, respectively, when immobilized on graphene or graphene-chitosan composite electrodes [59]. While graphene enhances electron transfer, the chitosan component may introduce some steric hindrance or diffusional limitations, affecting sensitivity. Despite this, chitosan's biocompatibility and film-forming properties make it an effective matrix for enzyme immobilization, potentially improving enzyme stability and reusability. The linear range of 0.1–5 mM for royal palm and 0.1–3.5 mM for GGP sensors suggests that they are best suited for environmental applications where H_2O_2 concentrations are generally higher [26]. SPP on graphene oxide has the highest detection limit (460 μM) among the sensors, which might be attributed to the material's functional groups. These groups enable strong enzyme binding, but their hydrophilicity can sometimes reduce electron transfer efficiency compared to more conductive materials like pure graphene or gold. This setup has a linear range of 0.25–5 mM, indicating that while sweet potato peroxidase sensors may be less suitable for ultra-trace H_2O_2 detection, they still hold promise for environmental or industrial monitoring, where a higher detection threshold is acceptable.

Table 4. Comparison of Plant-Derived Peroxidase-Based Electrochemical Sensors for Hydrogen Peroxide Detection.

Plant Source	Electrode Material	Detection Limit (μM)	Linear Range (mM)	Reference
Royal palm	Graphene/chitosan	87	0.1–5	[59]
Guinea grass	Graphene	150	0.1–3.5	[26]
Lemongrass	Graphene	50	0.5–4	[49]
Sweet potato	Graphene oxide	460	0.25–5	[20]
Sleepy plant	Gold nanoparticles	0.4	0.5–5	[37]
Horseradish	Carbon paste	50	0.05–10	[48]

PODs, often harnessed for H_2O_2 detection, exhibit a broad range of catalytic capabilities, positioning them as promising tools for detecting additional analytes, such as triclosan (TCS) [60] and pathogenic bacteria like *Staphylococcus aureus* [61], a prevalent antimicrobial agent. Thus, PODs can facilitate its degradation, making them valuable for monitoring TCS residues in water sources. A recent study demonstrated the amperometric detection of TCS using screen-printed carbon nanotube electrode modified with GGP. The system exhibited a redox potential of 370 mV and a linear response range from 20 μM to 80 μM and a limit of detection (LOD) of 3 μM, highlighting its potential utility in environmental analysis and food quality control applications. Furthermore, plant PODs hold potential for bacterial detection, especially targeting *Staphylococcus aureus*, a major cause of hospital-acquired infections. A novel approach employed GGP to detect *Staphylococcus aureus* in milk samples [61]. This approach involved modifying a screen-printed gold electrode with cysteine and GGP, enabling sensitive electrochemical detection through H_2O_2 reduction. The modified electrode successfully detected *S. aureus* in milk within a concentration range of 3×10^2 to 3×10^8 CFU/mL, achieving a detection limit as low as 10^2 CFU/mL and a rapid response time of around 20 min.

Compared to the commercial standard HRP, Colombian plant-derived PODs offer several unique advantages for biosensor development. For example, RPP exhibits exceptional thermal stability, maintaining activity at temperatures up to 90 °C, which is considerably higher than HRP's optimal range of 25–30 °C [32,50]. This property is particularly advantageous for sensors operating in harsh environmental or industrial conditions. Similarly, MPP demonstrates ultra-low detection limits when combined with gold nanoparticles (LOD = 0.4 μM), outperforming HRP-based systems in sensitive biomedical applications such as monitoring oxidative stress biomarkers. Additionally, the broad pH tolerance observed in AOP (pH 4.0–9.0) provides flexibility for sensors used in variable sample matrices, such as environmental monitoring or food safety testing. These characteristics highlight the potential of Colombian PODs as cost-effective, locally sourced alternatives that can surpass HRP in performance under specific application conditions.

4.2. Synthesis of Polyaniline

PANI is among the most thoroughly studied conducting polymers, renowned for its remarkable environmental stability and favorable electronic characteristics. Its versatility opens up numerous possibilities for applications, including organic lightweight batteries, light-emitting diodes, optical displays, anticorrosive coatings, and bioanalytical systems [15].

Emeraldine polyaniline exists in two forms: the non-conductive base and the conductive salt form. The salt is produced through the protonation of the imine sites in the emeraldine base using strong acids like organic sulfonic and phosphoric acids, a process known as "doping." Although doped PANI exhibits conductivity, it suffers from poor solubility in common solvents, limiting its processability [62]. However, PANI can form polyelectrolyte complexes by interacting with soluble polymers that carry negatively charged groups, resulting in stable dispersions of nanoparticles in aqueous media, which enhances processability. In these complexes, PANI typically adopts a doped and chiral state due to interactions between its imine groups and the polymeric anions. These polyelectrolyte complexes can be synthesized through chemical or enzymatic methods. Chemical polymerization of aniline monomers occurs under strongly acidic conditions, usually with 1 M HCl or H_2SO_4, using ammonium persulfate as the oxidant. The synthesis of PANI complexes can be achieved under environmentally friendly, kinetically controlled conditions using horseradish peroxidase (HRP) as a catalyst. However, HRP exhibits low stability at pH levels below 4.5, which coincides with the pH range suitable for forming polyelectrolyte complexes with negatively charged polymers [45]. To address this issue, alternative PODs that can efficiently polymerize aniline in acidic conditions have been explored, as demonstrated in a study that use RPP for the synthesis of conducting polyelectrolyte complexes of PANI [62,63]. The polymerization of aniline was conducted at pH 2.0 and UV-vis-NIR absorption and EPR techniques confirmed the formation of an electroactive complex similar to traditionally doped PANI. Thus, the thermostable RPP is an efficient catalyst for the polymerization of aniline to obtain PANI complexes under green conditions [64].

4.3. Chemiluminescence Assays

Chemiluminescence (CL) assays are analytical techniques that harness light emission from chemical reactions to detect and quantify various molecules with exceptional sensitivity [65,66]. In these assays, a chemiluminescent substrate, such as luminol, undergoes an oxidation reaction catalyzed by an enzyme like POD in the presence of an oxidizing agent (often hydrogen peroxide), resulting in the release of light. This emitted light is captured by sensitive detectors, with the intensity directly proportional to the concentration of the target analyte. Due to their high sensitivity and low background noise, chemiluminescence assays are commonly used in clinical diagnostics, environmental monitoring, and food safety testing, where they facilitate the detection of low-abundance molecules, pathogens, or specific biomarkers. Compared to fluorescence or colorimetric assays, chemiluminescence assays offer advantages such as reduced interference from background signals and enhanced detection limits. However, these assays require careful optimization of reaction conditions (e.g., pH, temperature, and reagent concentrations) to maximize light yield and maintain enzyme stability, factors that can impact assay reproducibility and performance [65].

HRP-catalyzed CL is a widely used method for detecting low concentrations of analytes due to its high sensitivity and low background signal [67]. HRP is commonly used to catalyze the oxidation of luminol or other substrates in the presence of hydrogen peroxide, which produces light detectable by photomultiplier tubes or other light-sensitive devices. This light output is proportional to the concentration of the target analyte, making HRP-based CL assays particularly useful in immunoassays, DNA detection, and various biochemical analyses [68]. However, despite its popularity, HRP has several limitations. One significant disadvantage is its sensitivity to environmental conditions, such as pH and temperature; HRP can quickly lose activity outside of its optimal pH range (around pH 7) or under high temperatures, which limits its utility in harsh or variable assay conditions.

POD from African oil palm, for example, has demonstrated potential for enhanced stability and reactivity in specific pH and temperature ranges, which can be advantageous for assays requiring durability under varying conditions [69]. Studies indicate that this enzyme can withstand higher temperatures compared to HRP, making it a valuable alternative for applications where thermal stability is essential. Meanwhile, POD from the royal palm offers distinct advantages in terms of substrate affinity, particularly with substrates like 3,3′,5,5′-tetramethylbenzidine (TMB) and luminol [70]. The efficiency of these enzymes is affected by factors such as ionic strength, pH, and the presence of cofactors, which influence their conformational state and active site accessibility, thereby impacting their chemiluminescent output. Optimizing these conditions can yield stronger luminescent signals, enhancing assay sensitivity.

While HRP remains the most widely used enzyme in chemiluminescence (CL) assays, its activity declines sharply under extreme pH or elevated temperatures, limiting its robustness. In contrast, Colombian PODs such as RPP retain over 80% activity at pH 3 and 90 °C, providing a more stable catalytic platform for CL systems exposed to variable reaction environments [32,69]. This increased stability reduces assay variability and enhances reproducibility, making these enzymes suitable for low-cost diagnostic kits in regions where controlled laboratory conditions may not be feasible.

4.4. Cross-Linked Enzymatic Aggregates

CLEAs are innovative biocatalytic materials formed by aggregating enzymes through precipitation, followed by cross-linking to create stable, insoluble enzyme clusters [16]. This approach enhances enzyme stability and reusability, making CLEAs valuable for applications in industrial biocatalysis, environmental remediation, and biosensing. Unlike conventional enzyme immobilization, CLEAs do not require a solid support, which simplifies the process and reduces production costs. CLEAs are applied in fields where enzymes must withstand harsh conditions, including organic synthesis, wastewater treatment, and biotransformation of complex substrates [71].

When CLEAs are synthesized with PODs, they offer further benefits for oxidative reactions. Peroxidase-CLEAs can be used in chemiluminescence assays, biosensors for detecting hydrogen peroxide, and pollutant degradation, where they catalyze oxidation reactions with improved stability under extreme pH, temperature, or organic solvents. This stability is crucial for long-term, repeated use in bioelectrochemical sensors and diagnostic kits, enhancing their efficiency and cost-effectiveness.

HRP has been extensively used to form CLEAs due to its high catalytic activity and compatibility with a variety of substrates. However, HRP-CLEAs have limitations, including sensitivity to denaturation under extreme conditions like high temperatures or fluctuating pH levels, which can reduce enzyme activity over time [72]. These factors have driven interest in exploring alternative peroxidase sources that could provide greater resilience and cost efficiency. To address these limitations, researchers are investigating plant-derived peroxidases from species like the RPP and GGP. For example, RPP was subject to a study focus in its immobilization through CLEAs to enhance its stability and activity. The resulting RPTP-CLEAs showed remarkable activity, maintaining 40% of maximum activity even at pH 3, where free RPTP is inactive. In thermal stability tests, the RPTP-CLEAs retained high stability similar to the free enzyme, with a half-life of 50 min at 90 °C and pH 7. Unlike the free enzyme, which undergoes subunit dissociation at pH 3, RPTP-CLEAs avoided this instability, showing significant thermostabilization [73]. Additionally, RPTP-CLEAs also exhibited good stability with low hydrogen peroxide concentrations (10 mM), though stability declined at higher concentrations (300 mM), where immobilization provided limited improvement. In practical applications, the RPTP-CLEAs were effective in decolorizing methyl orange using 5 mM hydrogen peroxide for four cycles (4 h each) without noticeable activity loss, achieving around 50% substrate degradation. With 225 mM hydrogen peroxide, activity gradually decreased across cycles but allowed complete colorant degradation [72]. These findings suggest that RPTP-CLEAs can function under challenging conditions, such as pH 3 and high hydrogen peroxide levels, where the free enzyme would typically be inactive, supporting their potential use in various industrial and environmental applications.

But not only was RPTP studied; GGP was also investigated for immobilization through CLEAs for the decolorization of indigo carmin (IC) [74]. The biocatalyst was prepared using 50% v/v ethanol and 0.88% w/v glutaraldehyde, with stirring for 1 h, achieving an immobilization yield of 93.74% and a specific activity of 36.75 U mg^{-1}. This immobilized form demonstrated 61% higher activity than the free enzyme at its optimal pH (pH 6 for both), with activity levels nearly 10 times higher at a pH of 9. GGP-CLEAs also showed significantly greater thermal stability, with improvements of 2–4 times compared to the free enzyme, and were 2–3 times more resistant to hydrogen peroxide. The GGP-CLEAs effectively removed over 80% of 0.05 mM indigo carmine at pH 5 in the presence of 0.55 mM H_2O_2 after 60 min, outperforming the free enzyme. However, operational stability tests indicated a reduction in enzyme activity of over 60% after 4 cycles, likely due to suicide inhibition [74].

These PODs offer potentially more sustainable, cost-effective, and environmentally resilient alternatives for CLEA applications. Studies suggest that PODs from these plants exhibit stability across a broader range of environmental conditions, which can be advantageous for applications requiring robust catalytic activity in varied settings. By creating CLEAs with RPP and GGP, it may be possible to develop biocatalysts that maintain high efficiency and stability in applications like biosensors, pollutant degradation, and chemiluminescent assays while reducing dependency on traditional HRP sources.

Colombian PODs also demonstrate superior performance when incorporated into CLEAs compared to traditional HRP. For instance, RPP-CLEAs maintained high activity across four decolorization cycles at pH 3, a condition under which free HRP and HRP-CLEAs would typically lose activity [73]. Similarly, GGP-CLEAs displayed 2–3 times greater resistance to hydrogen peroxide inactivation than free enzymes or HRP-CLEAs, making them more suitable for industrial wastewater treatment and other challenging oxidative processes [74]. These findings emphasize the potential of Colombian PODs to serve as resilient, sustainable alternatives for industrial biocatalysis while reducing dependency on imported HRP.

While CLEAs significantly improve enzyme stability and reusability compared to free enzymes, several limitations remain. One key challenge is operational stability, as repeated reaction cycles often result in gradual activity loss due to partial enzyme inactivation or structural degradation of the aggregates. For example, GGP-CLEAs exhibited a >60% reduction in activity after four cycles of indigo carmine degradation, likely caused by suicide inactivation in the presence of excess hydrogen peroxide [74]. Similarly, RPP-CLEAs, while stable at low H_2O_2 concentrations, showed diminished stability under high oxidative stress, limiting their long-term utility in industrial processes [73]. Another important issue is recyclability, which directly impacts process economics and environmental sustainability. Although CLEAs are theoretically reusable, repeated recovery steps may cause physical losses or partial fragmentation of the aggregates, reducing their effectiveness over time. This highlights the need for strategies to enhance mechanical robustness and improve immobilization methods. To address these limitations, advanced engineering approaches should be considered. Protein engineering through site-directed mutagenesis or directed evolution could generate POD variants with higher intrinsic resistance to oxidative stress and extreme pH or temperature conditions. Additionally, integrating PODs with nanozymes—nanomaterials with enzyme-mimicking activity—offers a promising hybrid strategy. For instance, coupling PODs with graphene oxide or metal nanoparticles could enhance electron transfer, improve stability, and provide self-regenerative catalytic activity, thus extending the functional lifespan of the biocatalyst [24,57]. These hybrid

CLEA-nanozyme systems could also enable multifunctionality, combining biocatalytic specificity with the robustness of inorganic materials. Future research should focus on scalable, green synthesis approaches for these hybrid systems to ensure environmental compatibility and economic feasibility.

5. Sustainability and the Circular Bioeconomy in the Context of Colombian Plants Peroxidases

Sustainability and the circular bioeconomy provide the conceptual framework for POD valorization in Colombia. Agricultural by-products such as palm fronds, guinea grass leaves, or sweet potato peels are abundant and frequently discarded. Their repurposing into enzyme sources reduces waste while generating added value. This approach aligns with the Sustainable Development Goals (SDGs), particularly responsible production, climate action, and innovation in green technologies [10,74–76].

The valorization of Colombian agricultural by-products for POD extraction not only contributes conceptually to the circular bioeconomy but also yields quantifiable environmental benefits. For instance, Colombia generates an estimated 3.5–4.0 million tons of agricultural residues annually, with a significant proportion coming from crops such as sugarcane, palm oil, and tubers like sweet potato [13,30]. Repurposing even 10% of these residues for biotechnological processes could prevent approximately 350,000 tons of organic waste from being landfilled or burned each year, reducing methane emissions associated with anaerobic decomposition. From a climate perspective, substituting traditional chemical processes or imported commercial enzymes with locally produced PODs offers meaningful CO_2 savings. The carbon footprint of industrial enzyme production, primarily HRP derived from horseradish, has been estimated at 8–10 kg CO_2 per kilogram of purified enzyme when factoring in cultivation, transportation, and processing [10]. By sourcing PODs from local agricultural waste streams, transportation-related emissions could be reduced by up to 40–50%, while valorizing waste biomass also sequesters carbon that would otherwise be released during open burning. Moreover, POD-based processes, such as wastewater treatment using CLEAs, have demonstrated a 30–45% reduction in chemical oxidant usage compared to conventional treatment methods [11,74]. This translates to lower secondary pollution and reduced energy requirements for chemical production. For example, implementing POD-CLEA systems at a medium-sized textile facility could reduce annual CO_2 emissions by 120–150 metric tons, primarily by decreasing the demand for synthetic oxidants like hydrogen peroxide and chlorine compounds. Quantifying these benefits provides a clearer perspective on how Colombian POD-based biotechnologies can move beyond laboratory-scale innovation to become measurable contributors to sustainability goals, including the United Nations Sustainable Development Goals (SDGs 12 and 13).

6. Conclusions

The valorization of Colombian agricultural by-products for POD extraction offers a powerful pathway to sustainable biotechnological innovation. This review highlights how plant-derived PODs can be harnessed for diverse applications, including biosensing, advanced material synthesis, environmental remediation, and health monitoring while reducing waste and supporting local economies.

Looking ahead, three main research priorities emerge:

(i) Scaling up POD production: Future studies should focus on optimizing extraction and purification methods for large-scale, cost-effective production. This includes developing continuous processing technologies, green extraction approaches, and robust immobilization strategies to meet industrial demands.

(ii) Structural characterization: Detailed studies using X-ray crystallography, cryo-EM, and computational modeling are needed to understand the structural basis of the exceptional thermal stability and substrate specificity of Colombian PODs. These insights will enable rational protein engineering and design of tailored biocatalysts.
(iii) Integration into circular bioeconomy policies: Collaboration with policymakers, industries, and local communities is essential to incorporate POD-based technologies into Colombia's circular bioeconomy framework, promoting sustainable waste valorization and contributing to national and global climate action goals.

By advancing these research areas, Colombian plant PODs can transition from laboratory-scale innovations to impactful technologies, fostering environmental sustainability, economic growth, and global leadership in green biotechnology.

Funding: This research was funded by [Vicerrectoría de Investigaciones, Universidad Industrial de Santander] grant number [3923].

Acknowledgments: We would like to acknowledge the Universidad Industrial de Santander for financial support.

Conflicts of Interest: The author declares no conflicts of interest.

References

1. Cui, Z.; Li, Y.; Zhang, H.; Qin, P.; Hu, X.; Wang, J.; Wei, G.; Chen, C. Lighting Up Agricultural Sustainability in the New Era through Nanozymology: An Overview of Classifications and Their Agricultural Applications. *J. Agric. Food Chem.* **2022**, *70*, 13445–13463. [CrossRef]
2. Nesterov, D.; Barrera-Martínez, I.; Martínez-Sánchez, C.; Sandoval-González, A.; Bustos, E. Approaching the circular economy: Biological, physicochemical, and electrochemical methods to valorize agro-industrial residues, wastewater, and industrial wastes. *J. Environ. Chem. Eng.* **2024**, *12*, 113335. [CrossRef]
3. Capanoglu, E.; Nemli, E.; Tomas-Barberan, F. Novel Approaches in the Valorization of Agricultural Wastes and Their Applications. *J. Agric. Food Chem.* **2022**, *70*, 6787–6804. [CrossRef] [PubMed]
4. Costa, J.R.; Tonon, R.V.; Cabral, L.; Gottschalk, L.; Pastrana, L.; Pintado, M.E. Valorization of Agricultural Lignocellulosic Plant Byproducts through Enzymatic and Enzyme-Assisted Extraction of High-Value-Added Compounds: A Review. *Am. Chem. Soc.* **2020**, *8*, 13112–13125. [CrossRef]
5. Sánchez, A. A Perspective of Solid-State Fermentation As Emergent Technology for Organic Waste Management in the Framework of Circular Bioeconomy. *ACS Sustain. Resour. Manag.* **2024**, *1*, 1630–1638. [CrossRef]
6. Chen, Z.; Lu, W.; Paneru, R.; Yang, Q.; Gong, W.; Tjeng, S.T.; Goroncy, A.; Dai, Q.; Zhang, J.; Kammen, D.M.; et al. Transformative and sustainable approach to waste plastic mixture valorization. *Chem. Eng. J.* **2024**, *499*, 156558. [CrossRef]
7. Zhang, J.; Kang, Z.; Jiang, W.; Zhang, Q.; Sun, P. Life-Cycle Greenhouse Gas Emissions and Primary Energy Demand of Agricultural Greenhouse Plastics: Proposed Optimization toward Agricultural Plastic Sustainability. *ACS Sustain. Chem. Eng.* **2024**, *12*, 8415–8424. [CrossRef]
8. Mubayi, V.; Ahern, C.B.; Calusinska, M.; O'Malley, M.A. Toward a Circular Bioeconomy: Designing Microbes and Polymers for Biodegradation. *Am. Chem. Soc.* **2024**, *13*, 1978–1993. [CrossRef]
9. Jin, C.; Hu, J.; Wu, J.; Liang, H.; Li, J. Innovative and Economically Beneficial Use of Corn and Corn Products in Electrochemical Energy Storage Applications. *Am. Chem. Soc.* **2021**, *9*, 10678–10703. [CrossRef]
10. Sheldon, R.A.; Basso, A.; Brady, D. New frontiers in enzyme immobilisation: Robust biocatalysts for a circular bio-based economy. *Chem. Soc. Rev.* **2021**, *50*, 5850–5862. [CrossRef]
11. Svetozarević, M.; Šekuljica, N.; Knežević-Jugović, Z.; Mijin, D. Agricultural waste as a source of peroxidase for wastewater treatment: Insight in kinetics and process parameters optimization for anthraquinone dye removal. *Environ. Technol. Innov.* **2021**, *21*, 101289. [CrossRef]
12. Lui, M.Y.; Wong, C.Y.Y.; Choi, A.W.T.; Mui, Y.F.; Qi, L.; Horváth, I.T. Valorization of Carbohydrates of Agricultural Residues and Food Wastes: A Key Strategy for Carbon Conservation. *ACS Sustain. Chem. Eng.* **2019**, *7*, 17799–17807. [CrossRef]
13. Gonzalez, L.V.P.; Gómez, S.P.M.; Giraldo Abad, P.A. Exploitation of Agroindustrial Waste in Colombia. *Rev. Investig. Agrar. Ambient.* **2017**, *8*, 141–150. [CrossRef]
14. Mathé, C.; Barre, A.; Jourda, C.; Dunand, C. Evolution and expression of class III peroxidases. *Arch. Biochem. Biophys.* **2010**, *500*, 58–65. [CrossRef]

15. El-naggar, A.M.; Alhaqbani, N.; Mohamed, M.B.; Kamal, A.M.; Albassam, A.A.; Lakshminarayana, G. Structural optical, dielectr and electrical characteristics of flexible blended polymers based on PMMA/PVAc/TBAI and milled PANI for energy storag applications and optoelectronic devices. *J. Mol. Liq.* **2024**, *414*, 126131. [CrossRef]
16. Sheldon, R.A. Cleas combi-cleas and 'smart' magnetic cleas: Biocatalysis in a bio-based economy. *Catalysts* **2019**, *9*, 261. [CrossRe
17. Asrafi, R.; Kumar, Y.; Bist, Y.; Saxena, D.C.; Sharanagat, V.S. Esterified porous starch from guinea grass seed for enhanced faci microencapsulation of bioactive materials. *Carbohydr. Polym. Technol. Appl.* **2024**, *7*, 100490. [CrossRef]
18. Yuan, M.; Zhao, H.; Huang, Q.; Liu, X.; Zhou, Y.; Diao, X.; Li, Q.X. Comparison of three palm tree peroxidases expressed b Escherichia coli: Uniqueness of African oil palm peroxidase. *Protein Expr. Purif.* **2021**, *179*, 105806. [CrossRef]
19. Skaharov, I.; Vesga-Blanco, K.; Sakharova, I. Substrate Specificity of African Oil Palm Tree Peroxidase. *Biochemistry* **2002**, *6* 1043–1047. [CrossRef]
20. Leon, J.C.; Alpeeva, I.S.; Chubar, T.A.; Galaev, I.Y.; Csoregi, E.; Sakharov, I.Y. Purification and substrate specificity of peroxidas from sweet potato tubers. *Plant Sci.* **2002**, *163*, 1011–1019. [CrossRef]
21. Sheldon, R.A.; Woodley, J.M. Role of Biocatalysis in Sustainable Chemistry. *Chem. Rev.* **2018**, *118*, 801–838. [CrossRef] [PubMec
22. de Oliveira, F.K.; Santos, L.O.; Buffon, J.G. *Mechanism of Action, Sources, and Application of Peroxidases*; Elsevier Ltd.: Amsterdan The Netherlands, 2021. [CrossRef]
23. Pandey, V.P.; Awasthi, M.; Singh, S.; Tiwari, S.; Dwivedi, U.N. A Comprehensive Review on Function and Application of Plan Peroxidases. *Biochem. Anal. Biochem.* **2017**, *6*, 308. [CrossRef]
24. Li, Y.; Schluesener, H.J.; Xu, S. Gold nanoparticle-based biosensors. *Gold Bull.* **2010**, *43*, 29–41. [CrossRef]
25. Ferreira, L.M.C.; Lima, D.; Marcolino-Junior, L.H.; Bergamini, M.F.; Kuss, S.; Campanhã Vicentini, F. *Cutting-Edge Biorecog nition Strategies to Boost the Detection Performance of COVID-19 Electrochemical Biosensors: A Review*; Elsevier B.V.: Amsterdam The Netherlands, 2024. [CrossRef]
26. Centeno, D.A.; Solano, X.H.; Castillo, J.J. A new peroxidase from leaves of guinea grass (*Panicum maximum*): A potentia biocatalyst to build amperometric biosensors. *Bioelectrochemistry* **2017**, *116*, 33–38. [CrossRef]
27. Kor, L.; Diazgranados, M. Identifying important plant areas for useful plant species in Colombia. *Biol. Conserv.* **2023**, *284*, 11018 [CrossRef]
28. Sánchez, M.; Castañeda, R.; Castañeda, S.M. Usos y potencialidad de la Higuerilla (*Ricinus communis*) en sistemas agroforestale en Colombia. *Pubvet* **2016**, *10*, 507–512. [CrossRef]
29. Jaramillo, M.A.; Reyes-Palencia, J.; Jiménez, P. Floral biology and flower visitors of cocoa (*Theobroma cacao* L.) in the uppe Magdalena Valley, Colombia. *Flora* **2024**, *313*, 152480. [CrossRef]
30. Garcia-Vallejo, M.C.; Alzate, C.A.C. Life cycle assessment of the cassava simplified value chain in Colombia and the use o cassava residues as energy carriers. *Ind. Crop. Prod.* **2024**, *210*, 118135. [CrossRef]
31. Sakharov, I.Y.; Ardila, G.B.; Sakharova, I.V. Peroxidasa de plantas tropicales. *Rev. Colomb. Quim.* **1999**, *28*, 97–106.
32. Sakharov, I.Y.; Vesga, M.K.; Galaev, I.Y.; Sakharova, I.V.; Pletjushkina, O.Y. Peroxidase from Leaves of Royal Palm Tree Roystone Regia: Purification and Some Properties. 2001. Available online: www.elsevier.com/locate/plantsci (accessed on 6 October 2025)
33. Rodríguez, A.; Pina, D.G.; Yélamos, B.; León, J.J.C.; Zhadan, G.G.; Villar, E.; Gavilanes, F.; Roig, M.G.; Sakharov, I.Y.; Shnyrov, V.L Thermal stability of peroxidase from the African oil palm tree Elaeis guineensis. *Eur. J. Biochem.* **2002**, *269*, 2584–2590. [CrossRef
34. Pandey, S.; Sharma, K.; Gundabala, V. Development of a Lemongrass/Silver Nanocomposite for Controlling a Foodborn Pathogen—Escherichia coli. *ACS Food Sci. Technol.* **2022**, *2*, 1850–1861. [CrossRef]
35. Don, S.M.; Rambli, M.; Nore, B.F. Antioxidant content following fermentation of lemongrass for herbal beverage development *Food Sci. Technol.* **2024**, *61*, 1–14. [CrossRef]
36. Tazi, A.; Zinedine, A.; Rocha, J.M.; Errachidi, F. Review on the pharmacological properties of lemongrass (*Cymbopogon citratus*) as a promising source of bioactive compounds. *Pharmacol. Res.—Nat. Prod.* **2024**, *3*, 100046. [CrossRef]
37. Dhanush, C.; Aravindh, S.; Jesreena, J.S.; Nagadharshini, R.; Jano, N.; Almeer, R.; Velu, S.K.P. Biomimetic Synthesis of Carbor Dots from Mimosa pudica Leaves for Enhanced Bioimaging. *Waste Biomass Valorization* **2024**, *16*, 713–721. [CrossRef]
38. Hagihara, T.; Mano, H.; Miura, T.; Hasebe, M.; Toyota, M. Calcium-mediated rapid movements defend against herbivorous insects in Mimosa pudica. *Nat. Commun.* **2022**, *13*, 1–9. [CrossRef] [PubMed]
39. Adurosakin, O.E.; Iweala, E.J.; Otike, J.O.; Dike, E.D.; Uche, M.E.; Owanta, J.I.; Ugbogu, O.C.; Chinedu, S.N.; Ugbogu, E.A *Ethnomedicinal Uses, Phytochemistry, Pharmacological Activities and Toxicological Effects of Mimosa Pudica—A Review*; Elsevier B.V. Amsterdam, The Netherlands, 2023. [CrossRef]
40. Collado, L.S.; Mabesa, R.C.; Corke, H. Genetic variation in the physical properties of sweet potato starch. *J. Agric. Food Chem* **1999**, *47*, 4195–4201. [CrossRef] [PubMed]
41. Wang, J.; Chen, P.; Zhao, T.; Huang, X.; Zong, J.; Luo, Q.; Peng, C.; Wu, X.; Qiu, F.; Zhao, D.; et al. Biosynthesis of Scopoletin in Sweet Potato Confers Resistance against Fusarium oxysporum. *J. Agric. Food Chem.* **2024**, *72*, 7749–7764. [CrossRef] [PubMed]

Arrazola-Paternina, G.; Alvis-Bermúdez, A.; García-Mogollon, C. Efecto del tratamiento de escaldado sobre la actividad enzimática de la polifenoloxidasa en dos variedades de batata (*Ipomoea batatas* Lam.). *Rev. Colomb. Cienc. Hortícolas* **2016**, *10*, 80–88. [CrossRef]

Jiménez-Villalba, K.; Arrieta-Banquet, L.; Salcedo-Mendoza, J.; Contreras-Lozano, K. Characterization of batatas flours and starches (*Ipomoea batatas* Lam.) from the colombian caribbean coast. *Rev. U.D.C.A Actual. Divulg. Cient.* **2019**, *22*, e1185. [CrossRef]

Ayala, M.; Roman, R.; Vazquez-Duhalt, R. A catalytic approach to estimate the redox potential of heme-peroxidases. *Biochem. Biophys. Res. Commun.* **2007**, *357*, 804–808. [CrossRef]

Škulj, S.; Kožić, M.; Barišić, A.; Vega, A.; Biarnés, X.; Piantanida, I.; Barisic, I.; Bertoša, B. Comparison of two peroxidases with high potential for biotechnology applications—HRP vs. APEX2. *Comput. Struct. Biotechnol. J.* **2024**, *23*, 742–751. [CrossRef]

Minibayeva, F.; Beckett, R.P.; Kranner, I. *Roles of Apoplastic Peroxidases in Plant Response to Wounding*; Elsevier Ltd.: Amsterdam, The Netherlands, 2015. [CrossRef]

Watanabe, L.; Nascimento, A.S.; Zamorano, L.S.; Shnyrov, V.L.; Polikarpov, I. Purification, crystallization and preliminary X-ray diffraction analysis of royal palm tree (Roystonea regia) peroxidase. *Acta Crystallogr. Sect. F Struct. Biol. Cryst. Commun.* **2007**, *63*, 780–783. [CrossRef] [PubMed]

Dequaire, M.; Limoges, B.; Moiroux, J.; Savéant, J.M. Mediated electrochemistry of horseradish peroxidase. Catalysis and inhibition. *J. Am. Chem. Soc.* **2002**, *124*, 240–253. [CrossRef]

Guarin-Guio, P.A.; Cano-Calle, H.D.; Castillo-León, J.J. Detección electroquímica de peróxido de hidrógeno usando peroxidasa de pasto Guinea (*Panicum maximum*) inmovilizada sobre electrodos serigrafiados de puntos cuánticos. *Rev. Ion* **2019**, *32*, 67–76. [CrossRef]

Solanki, P.R.; Kaushik, A.; Ansari, A.A.; Sumana, G.; Malhotra, B.D. Horse radish peroxidase immobilized polyaniline for hydrogen peroxide sensor. *Polym. Adv. Technol.* **2011**, *22*, 903–908. [CrossRef]

Stepanov, E.V.; Shcherbakov, I.A. Physicochemical Methods of Studying Hydrogen Peroxide for Biomedical Applications. *Phys. Wave Phenom.* **2023**, *31*, 92–97. [CrossRef]

Barbosa, L.M.M.; Carneiro, T.d.S.; Favoreto, M.W.; Borges, C.P.F.; Reis, A.; Meireles, S.S.; Loguercio, A.D. Whitening toothpastes with hydrogen peroxide concentrations vs. at-home bleaching. *Clin. Oral. Investig.* **2024**, *28*, 436. [CrossRef]

Malevich, D.; Mypati, S.; Ray, S.G.; Dinh, C.T.; Barz, D.P.J. Surfactant-tolerant cathodes for electrochemical generation of hydrogen peroxide for wastewater treatment. *J. Appl. Electrochem.* **2024**, *55*, 231–241. [CrossRef]

Alpeeva, I.S.; Niculescu-Nistor, M.; Leon, J.C.; Csöregi, E.; Sakharov, I.Y. Palm tree peroxidase-based biosensor with unique characteristics for hydrogen peroxide monitoring. *Biosens. Bioelectron.* **2005**, *21*, 742–748. [CrossRef]

Castillo, J.; Gáspár, S.; Sakharov, I.; Csöregi, E. Bienzyme biosensors for glucose, ethanol and putrescine built on oxidase and sweet potato peroxidase. *Biosens. Bioelectron.* **2003**, *18*, 705–714. [CrossRef] [PubMed]

Forzato, C.; Vida, V.; Berti, F. Biosensors and Sensing Systems for Rapid Analysis of Phenolic Compounds from Plants: A Comprehensive Review. *Biosensors* **2020**, *10*, 105. [CrossRef] [PubMed]

Castillo, J.J.; Orduz, A.E.; Rozo, C.E. Characterization of the non-covalent conjugate graphene-folic acid using Raman spectroscopy and computational methods. *Rev. Acad. Colomb. Cienc. Exactas Fis. Nat.* **2018**, *42*, 96–103. [CrossRef]

Vallés, C.; Zhang, X.; Cao, J.; Lin, F.; Young, R.J.; Lombardo, A.; Ferrari, A.C.; Burk, L.; Mülhaupt, R.; Kinloch, I.A. Graphene/Polyelectrolyte Layer-by-Layer Coatings for Electromagnetic Interference Shielding. *ACS Appl. Nano Mater.* **2019**, *2*, 5272–5281. [CrossRef]

Villamizar, E.N.; Ríos, C.A.; Castillo, J.J. A hydrogen peroxide biosensor based on the immobilization of the highly stable royal palm tree peroxidase (*Roystonea regia*) with chitosan and glutaraldehyde on screen-printed graphene electrodes. *J. Mex. Chem. Soc.* **2016**, *60*, 135–140. [CrossRef]

Orduz, A.E.; Gutiérrez, J.A.; Blanco, S.I.; Castillo, J.J. Amperometric detection of triclosan with screen-printed carbon nanotube electrodes modified with Guinea Grass (*Panicum maximum*) peroxidase. *Univ. Sci.* **2019**, *24*, 363–379. [CrossRef]

Guarín, P.; Cristancho, J. Rapid electrochemical detection of Staphylococcus aureus based on screen-printed gold electrodes modified with cysteine and Guinea grass (*Panicum maximum*) peroxidase. *Rev. Acad. Colomb. Cienc. Exactas Físicas Nat.* **2020**, *44*, 835–844. [CrossRef]

Sakharov, I.Y.; Vorobiev, A.C.; Leon, J.J.C. Synthesis of polyelectrolyte complexes of polyaniline and sulfonated polystyrene by palm tree peroxidase. *Enzym. Microb. Technol.* **2003**, *33*, 661–667. [CrossRef]

Mazhugo, Y.M.; Caramyshev, A.V.; Shleev, S.V.; Sakharov, I.Y.; Yaropolov, A.I. Enzymatic synthesis of a conducting complex of polyaniline and poly(2-acrylamido-2-methyl-1-propanesulfonic acid) using palm tree peroxidase and its properties. *Appl. Biochem. Microbiol.* **2005**, *41*, 247–250. [CrossRef]

Caramyshev, A.V.; Evtushenko, E.G.; Ivanov, V.F.; Barceló, A.R.; Roig, M.G.; Shnyrov, V.L.; van Huystee, R.B.; Kurochkin, I.N.; Vorobiev, A.K.; Sakharov, I.Y. Synthesis of conducting polyelectrolyte complexes of polyaniline and poly(2-acrylamido-3-methyl-1-propanesulfonic acid) catalyzed by pH-stable palm tree peroxidase. *Biomacromolecules* **2005**, *6*, 1360–1366. [CrossRef]

65. Blau, R.; Shelef, O.; Shabat, D.; Satchi-Fainaro, R. Chemiluminescent probes in cancer biology. *Nat. Rev. Bioeng.* **2023**, *1*, 648–6 [CrossRef]
66. Zvereva, M.V.; Zhmurova, A.V. *The Use of a Chemiluminescence in the Assessment of the Nanomaterials Antioxidant Activity*; Sprin Science and Business Media Deutschland GmbH: Berlin/Heidelberg, Germany, 2023. [CrossRef]
67. Yan, X.L.; Xue, X.-X.; Deng, X.-M.; Jian, Y.-T.; Luo, J.; Jiang, M.-M.; Zheng, X.-J. Chemiluminescence strategy induced HRP-sandwich structure based on strand displacement for sensitive detection of DNA methyltransferase. *Microchem. J.* **20** *158*, 105183. [CrossRef]
68. Chen, L.; Zhang, Z.; Zhang, P.; Zhang, X.; Fu, A. An ultra-sensitive chemiluminescence immunosensor of carcinoembryo antigen using HRP-functionalized mesoporous silica nanoparticles as labels. *Sens. Actuators B Chem.* **2011**, *155*, 557–5 [CrossRef]
69. Sakharov, I. Long-term chemiluminescent signal is produced in the course of luminol peroxidation catalyzed by peroxida isolated from leaves of african oil palm tree. *Biochemistry* **2001**, *66*, 515–519. [CrossRef] [PubMed]
70. Alpeeva, I.S.; Sakharov, I.Y. Luminol oxidation catalyzed by royal palm leaf peroxidase. *Appl. Biochem. Microbiol.* **2007**, *43*, 25– [CrossRef]
71. Parveen, S.; Asgher, M.; Bilal, M. Lignin peroxidase-based cross-linked enzyme aggregates (LiP-CLEAs) as robust biocataly materials for mitigation of textile dyes-contaminated aqueous solution. *Environ. Technol. Innov.* **2021**, *21*, 101226. [CrossRef]
72. Morales, A.; Barbosa, O.; Rueda, N.; Fonseca, Z.; Torres, R.; Rodrigues, R.C.; Ortiz, C.; Fernandez-Lafuente, R. Optimization a characterization of CLEAs of the very thermostable dimeric peroxidase from Roystonea regia. *RSC Adv.* **2015**, *5*, 53047–530 [CrossRef]
73. Terres, J.; Battisti, R.; Andreaus, J.; De Jesus, P.C. Decolorization and degradation of Indigo Carmine dye from aqueous soluti catalyzed by horseradish peroxidase. *Biocatal. Biotransform.* **2014**, *32*, 64–73. [CrossRef]
74. Perez, A.V.; Gaitan-Oyola, J.A.; Vargas-Delgadillo, D.P.; Castillo, J.J.; Barbosa, O.; Fernandez-Lafuente, R. Synthesis a Characterization of Cross-Linked Aggregates of Peroxidase from Megathyrsus maximus (Guinea Grass) and Their Applicati for Indigo Carmine Decolorization. *Molecules* **2024**, *29*, 2696. [CrossRef]
75. Andhalkar, V.V.; Ahorsu, R.; De María, P.D.; Winterburn, J.; Medina, F.; Constantí, M. Valorization of Lignocellulose by Produci Polyhydroxyalkanoates under Circular Bioeconomy Premises: Facts and Challenges. *Am. Chem. Soc.* **2022**, *10*, 16459–164 [CrossRef]
76. Türker, Y.Ö. The impact of the right of access to information on sustainable development goals under the Aarhus Conventi *J. Environ. Manag.* **2024**, *370*, 122918. [CrossRef]

processes

MDPI

Article

Cost-Effective Optimization of the Transfructosylation Activity of an Invertase Produced from *Aspergillus carbonarius* PC-4 Using Pineapple Crown and Determination of Its Biochemical Properties

Ryhára Dias Batista [1], Gustavo Carvalho do Nascimento [1], Nayara Bezerra Carvalho [1], Paula Candido Leite [2], Rodrigo Correa Basso [2], Sergio Andres Villalba Morales [1,2], Michelle da Cunha Abreu Xavier [1], Rafael Firmani Perna [2,*] and Alex Fernando de Almeida [1,*]

[1] Graduate Program in Food Science and Technology, Federal University of Tocantins (UFT), Palmas 77001-090, Brazil; ryharabatista@hotmail.com (R.D.B.); gustavocarvalho081294@hotmail.com (G.C.d.N.); nayara.bezerra@mail.uft.edu.br (N.B.C.); sergio.morales@mail.uft.edu.br (S.A.V.M.); michellecax@mail.uft.edu.br (M.d.C.A.X.)

[2] Graduate Program in Chemical Engineering, Institute of Science and Technology, Federal University of Alfenas (UNIFAL-MG), Poços de Caldas 37715-400, Brazil; paula.leite@sou.unifal-mg.edu.br (P.C.L.); rodrigo.basso@unifal-mg.edu.br (R.C.B.)

* Correspondence: rafael.perna@unifal-mg.edu.br (R.F.P.); alexfernando@mail.uft.edu.br (A.F.d.A.)

Abstract: Fructooligosaccharides are prebiotic sugars that are widely used in the production of functional foods, which can be produced enzymatically by the transfructosylation reaction of sucrose. This work aimed to optimize the production of an invertase with high transfructosylation activity from *Aspergillus carbonarius* PC-4 using pineapple crown as the inducer substrate and evaluate its biochemical properties. The culture medium was optimized using a Plackett–Burman experimental design and a central composite rotatable design, resulting in a maximum transfructosylation activity of 65.33 U/mL at 72 h of cultivation. The cultivation parameters were $Y_{p/s}$ = 1070.75 U/g and P_P = 2771.48 U/h, which showed an increase of 5.2-fold in the enzyme produced. The optimum temperature (50 °C) and pH (5.0) for the enzymatic activity were obtained by a CCR design. The enzyme showed a half-life of 60 min at 40 °C. In conclusion, the invertase produced from *A. carbonarius* PC-4 using agro-industrial waste (pineapple crown) and an inorganic nitrogen source (ammonium nitrate) exhibits high transfructosylation activity that can be used as a potential source for the production of fructooligosaccharides.

Keywords: transfructosylation activity; *Aspergillus*; invertase; agro-industrial waste; enzyme activity; submerged cultivation

1. Introduction

Invertases (β-fructofuranosidase, E.C. 3.2.1.26) are enzymes that belong to the carbohydrase class (family GH32) and catalyze the hydrolysis of the α-1,4-glycosidic bond from sucrose into glucose and fructose in equimolar proportions of inverted sugar at a concentration of approximately 10% substrate. These enzymes can be obtained from a wide variety of microorganisms, including animals, plants, bacteria, yeasts, and fungi. However, fungi stand out because they have attracted the attention of different sectors of the industry due to their biotechnological potential and because they are considered saccharolytic, that is, they ferment various carbohydrates [1,2]. The fungi that stand out in the production of invertases belong to the genera *Penicillium, Aerobasidium, Fusarium*, and, mainly, *Aspergillus* [3–5]. In addition, invertases can perform a transfructosylation reaction when exposed to a range of sucrose concentrations from 20 to 85%, thus also being classified as fructosyltransferases (E.C. 2.4.1.9), a subclass of transferases [1,6]. Fructosyltransferases (FTases) act on the β-(1-2) bonds of sucrose and transfer the fructosyl radical to another sucrose molecule, forming fructooligosaccharides (FOSs), or transfer the fructosyl radical to an FOS by lengthening the chain by a fructose unit, releasing glucose in both situations [3,7].

Transfructosylation carried out by invertases has wide applications in several industries. In the food industry, it is used to produce fructooligosaccharides (FOSs), which act as prebiotics and improve the texture and stability of food products [8]. In the pharmaceutical industry, the resulting oligosaccharides are incorporated into prebiotic supplements and other formulations due to their benefits for intestinal health [9,10]. In biotechnology, this enzymatic reaction is exploited to synthesize new functional sugars and modify biomolecules [11]. The cosmetics industry uses products derived from transfructosylation as humectants in moisturizing formulations. Furthermore, in the agricultural industry, FOSs can be added to animal feed to promote digestive health. These applications highlight the versatility of transfructosylation in improving processes and products in several areas [9,12].

FOSs are commonly designated as 1-kestose (GF2), 1-nystose (GF3), and 1F-β-fructofuranosylnystose (GF4) [3]. They are classified as prebiotics, defined as non-digestible food ingredients that are resistant to hydrolysis by human digestion, because of the β conformation in the anomeric carbon of fructose monomers [13,14]. These biomolecules have beneficial effects on human and animal health, since they promote good absorption of minerals in the body, regulate blood glucose and cholesterol levels, promote the proliferation of beneficial bacteria in the large intestine (particularly Bifidobacteria, which regulate the intestinal microbiota), prevent the onset of colon cancer, relieve constipation, and increase immunity [15,16]. FOSs are widely used in the food industry and can be safely consumed by diabetics, since they have about one-third of the sweetening power of sucrose and are low in calories [3,7,16]. They are commonly used in dairy products, cookies, breads, confectionery products, and functional products (to promote a symbiotic effect with probiotic microorganisms), among others. Additionally, they can be used in animal feed for the same purpose as prebiotics and can also minimize the formation of tooth decay, since they are not consumed by *Streptococcus mutans* [1,17].

Enzymes can be produced by submerged cultivation or solid-state cultivation; nevertheless, most industrial enzymes are produced by submerged cultivation, since it is an efficient method for enzyme production and due to the greater ease in the control of the physicochemical parameters [18,19]. The use of agro-industrial waste for the production of microbial enzymes has been widely adopted as a substitute for pure carbon sources, since it represents a valuable and rich source of energy and other nutrients (lignocellulose, proteins, carbohydrates, lipids, etc.), and it is also a low-cost biomass, which would otherwise be discarded into the environment and cause major problems of solid waste pollution [15,20]. One of the residues that causes major environmental issues is the waste from pineapple cultivation. Brazil is the second largest producer of pineapple (*Ananas comosus*) in the world, producing around 1.56 billion pineapples per year [21]. The by-products generated from pineapple correspond to residual pulp, peels, crowns, stems, and leaves [22].

Using a statistical approach to optimize enzyme production is of the utmost importance, since it involves the analysis of different variables, such as carbon, nitrogen, salts, and physicochemical factors, in the search for optimal conditions in the production process. In this sense, Plackett and Burman designs allow for the screening of the most important parameters and the response surface for the achievement of optimal conditions [16,18,23]. Previous studies have shown that a strain of *Aspergillus* sp. isolated from canned peach syrup was able to produce high amounts of fructosyltransferase when grown in a submerged medium, using pineapple crown and raffinose as the carbon source and soy protein and ammonium nitrate as the nitrogen source. Thus, the present work aimed to optimize the production of an invertase with high transfructosylation activity produced from *A. carbonarius* PC-4 under submerged conditions using Plackett and Burman and DCCR experimental designs and to characterize the biochemical properties of the enzyme produced in the crude extract.

2. Materials and Methods

2.1. Materials

The pineapple crown was purchased from local commerce (Gurupi, Brazil). Potato dextrose agar (PDA) was purchased from Merck (Rahway, NJ, USA). The glucose oxidase–peroxidase kit was purchased from Sigma-Aldrich (St. Louis, MO, USA). Citric acid*H_2O, $ZnSO_4$*$7H_2O$, $Fe(NH_4)_2(SO_4)_2$*$6H_2O$, $CuSO_4$*$5H_2O$, $MnSO_4$*H_2O, H_3BO_3, Na_2MoO_4*$2H_2O$, sodium citrate*$5H_2O$, KH_2PO_4, NH_4NO_3, $MgSO_4$*$7H_2O$, $CaCl_2$*$2H_2O$, 0,1 mg/mL biotin solution, glucose, sucrose, and sodium acetate were purchased from Labynth® (Diadema, Brazil). All chemicals used were analytical grade.

2.2. Methods

2.2.1. Microorganism and Maintenance

A black *Aspergillus carbonarius* strain PC-4 was isolated from peach syrup and maintained in the Laboratory of Biotechnology, Food Analysis and Products (LABAP), Habite—Biotechnology Companies Incubator, Federal University of Tocantins—UFT, Gurupi, Tocantins, Brazil [17]. *A. carbonarius* PC-4 was cultivated on PDA for 3 days at 28 °C and then stored at 4 °C in a PDA slant. *A. carbonarius* PC-4 was also preserved in sterile distilled water [24]. The dishes (approximately 5 mm) containing a small portion of the culture medium and sporulated mycelium were aseptically transferred into sterile 6 mL flasks filled with 4 mL of sterile distilled water and sealed with a rubber stopper. The flasks were stored at 4 °C, and the viability of the strains was verified every six months.

2.2.2. Submerged Culture Conditions

A liquid medium was prepared using Vogel's medium (Merck, Rahway, NJ, USA) [25]. The trace element solution (solution A) was prepared containing (g/L) the following ingredients: citric acid*H_2O, 50; $ZnSO_4$*$7H_2O$, 50; $Fe(NH_4)_2(SO_4)_2$*$6H_2O$, 10; $CuSO_4$*$5H_2O$, 2.5; $MnSO_4$*H_2O, 0.05; H_3BO_3, 0.05; and Na_2MoO_4*$2H_2O$, 0.05. The salt solution (solution B) was prepared containing (g/L) the following ingredients: sodium citrate*$5H_2O$, 150; KH_2PO_4, 250; NH_4NO_3, 100; $MgSO_4$*$7H_2O$, 10; $CaCl_2$*$2H_2O$, 5 and biotin solution (0.1 mg/mL), 5 mL; and solution A, 5 mL. The solutions were maintained at 4 °C. The medium preparation consisted of a 50-fold dilution of solution B, replacing glucose with other carbon sources, and adjusting the final pH to 6.0.

The cultures were performed in Erlenmeyer flasks (100 mL) containing 20 mL of culture medium. All media were autoclaved at 121 °C for 20 min. The inocula were prepared using 3-day-old cultures. The media were inoculated with 1 mL of a conidia suspension (1×10^7 spores or cells per mL) and incubated at 28 °C, 180 rpm, for 3 and 5 days. The biomass was separated from the fermentation broth by filtration in muslin. The cell-free broth was used for fructosyltransferase activity assays. The results were assayed for fructosyltransferase activity (TFA), fructosyltransferase yield on the substrate (Yp/s), and fructosyltransferase productivity (Pp). The parameters Yp/s (U/g) and Pp (U/h) were calculated using Equations (1) and (2), respectively.

$$Y_{p/s} = P_f - \left(\frac{P_0}{S_0}\right) \quad (1)$$

$$Pp = TFA/t \quad (2)$$

where P_f is the final product, P_0 is the initial product, S_0 is the initial substrate (pineapple crown waste), and t is the time of cultivation.

2.2.3. The Transfructosylation Activity of the Invertase from *A. carbonarius* PC-4

The transfructosylation activity was determined according to Rawat et al. [26]. A total of 100 microliters of culture filtrate with 400 μL of sucrose (20% *w*/*v* in 0.1 M sodium acetate buffer pH 5.0) was heated at 50 °C for 1 h in a water bath. The reaction was stopped by boiling the mixture in a water bath at 100 °C for 10 min. The transfructosylation activity was estimated by taking 20 μL of the appropriately diluted reaction mixture and mixing it with 2 mL of the test reagent (Glucose oxidase–peroxidase kit, Sigma-Aldrich, St. Louis, MO, USA). The glucose released was measured at 505 nm. One unit of transfructosylation activity was defined as the amount of enzyme required to produce 1 mol of glucose per minute under the assay conditions.

2.2.4. Optimization of the Production of Transfructosylation Activity

Plackett–Burman Design

The Plackett–Burman experimental design [27] was used to evaluate the relative importance of carbon and nitrogen in the production of an invertase with high transfructosylation activity from *A. carbonarius* PC-4 after 72 h and 120 h of cultivation. Raffinose and pineapple crown were used as carbon sources, while ammonium nitrate and soybean protein were used as nitrogen sources (Table 1). Each variable represented three levels—high concentration (1), low concentration (−1), and intermediate concentration (0)—in eight trials (Table 1). The response variable analyzed was enzyme activity.

Table 1. Experimental variables and levels used for the production of an invertase with high transfructosylation activity from *A. carbonarius* PC-4 using the Plackett–Burman design.

Factors	Code	−1	0	1
Pineapple crown	X_1	0	5	10
Raffinose	X_2	0	5	10
Soy protein	X_3	0	1	2
Ammonium nitrate	X_4	0	1	2

Note: the values are expressed in g/L.

Central Composite Rotatable Design

After the identification of the carbon and nitrogen sources affecting enzyme production in the Plackett–Burman design, a response surface methodology of a central composite rotatable design (CCRD) was used to discover the optimal combination of the independent variables for invertase production. The two main independent variables chosen for this experiment were pineapple crown (X_1) and ammonium nitrate (X_2) with 4 trials under the axial conditions and 3 repetitions at the central point, totaling 11 trials (Table 2). The response variable analyzed was enzyme activity.

Table 2. Experimental variables and levels using a CCRD for the production of an invertase with high transfructosylation activity from *A. carbonarius* PC-4.

Factors	Code	−1.41	−1	0	1	1.41
Pineapple crown	X_1	6	10	20	30	34
Ammonium nitrate	X_2	0.5	3	9	15	17.5

Note: the values are expressed in g/L.

All experiments were conducted as previously described, and invertase production was considered to be the independent variable or response (Y). The second-order polynomial coefficients were obtained and evaluated statistically by analysis of variance (ANOVA). The model's accuracy in predicting the maximum transfructosylation activity was confirmed by a triplicate experiment in the optimized conditions. The predicted and experimental values of transfructosylation activity were confirmed using the optimal values for the significant variables generated by CCRD.

2.2.5. The Biochemical Properties of the Invertase

Effect of pH and Temperature on Invertase Activity

The optimal conditions for transfructosylation activity in different ranges of pH and temperature were determined in a test tube immersed in a water bath, containing 20% (*w*/*v*) sucrose, in McIlvaine buffer, with a reaction time of up to 60 min. This experiment was carried out using the response surface methodology of CCRD, in which pH was defined as X_1 and temperature as X_2 (Table 3). Each independent variable was studied at five coded levels (Table 3). The response variable analyzed was enzyme activity.

Table 3. Experimental variables and levels using the CCRD for the influence of pH and temperature on the activity of the invertase with high transfructosylation activity from *A. carbonarius* PC-4.

Factors	Code	−1.41	−1	0	1	1.41
pH	X_1	2.17	3	5	7	7.83
Temperature (°C)	X_2	14.64	25	50	75	85.36

All experiments were conducted as previously described, and invertase production was considered to be the independent variable or response (Y). The second-order polynomial coefficients were obtained and evaluated statistically by analysis of variance (ANOVA). The model's accuracy in predicting the maximum transfructosylation activity was confirmed by a triplicate experiment in the optimized conditions. The predicted and experimental values of transfructosylation activity were confirmed using the optimal values for the significant variables generated by CCRD.

The Effects of pH and Temperature on the Stability of the Transfructosylation Activity

The effect of pH on the enzyme stability was tested using the McIlvaine buffer with pH values ranging from 3.0 to 8.0. The enzyme preparation was diluted in each buffer (1:2, *v*/*v*) and incubated for 7 h and 24 h at 15 °C, without substrate.

Thermal stability assays were conducted by incubating the crude extract, without substrate, at the temperatures of 40 °C, 50 °C, and 60 °C for up to 150 min, at the previously determined pH value.

Aliquots were withdrawn at specific time intervals and maintained in an ice bath for 5 min. The residual activity was determined as previously described, using the McIlvaine buffer with 20% of sucrose (*w*/*v*) for 60 min and at 50 °C. Results were expressed as relative activity, considering the initial activity (t = 0) to be 100%.

2.2.6. Statistical Analysis

The experimental design was evaluated using the software "Protimiza Experimental Design" (https://experimental-design.protimiza.com.br, accessed on 9 August 2024) [28]. The polynomial models with 90% and 95% confidence levels were evaluated by analysis of variance (ANOVA), and Student's t-test and Fischer's test (F) were used to determine the statistical significance of the regression coefficients and to obtain the second-order model equation, respectively. In turn, the quality of the fit polynomial model was assessed by the coefficient of determination (R^2).

3. Results and Discussion

3.1. Screening of Carbon and Nitrogen Sources by the Plackett–Burman Design

A. carbonarius PC-4 has been previously identified as the producer of an invertase with high transfructosylation activity under submerged conditions using pure and complex carbon and nitrogen sources [17]. Under these conditions, the maximum enzyme production was obtained using Vogel's salt medium supplemented with raffinose and pineapple crown as carbon sources and ammonium nitrate and soybean protein as nitrogen sources (44.40 U/mL) after 168 h of cultivation. Sequential optimization approaches were applied in this study, initially by screening the nutritional factors that affected the production of the invertase with transfructosylation activity using the Plackett–Burman design after three and five days of cultivation (Table 4). The results of enzyme production were given in units per mL (U/mL), production yield ($Y_{P/S}$), and productivity (P_P). In this sense, a large variation was observed, from 0.02 to 46.26 U/mL after 72 h of cultivation, and from 0 to 52.20 U/mL after 120 h of cultivation. The mean effects of the factors examined for enzymatic activity are presented in the Pareto plot (Figure 1).

Table 4. CCRD for the transfructosylation activity of the invertase produced from *A. carbonarius* PC-4.

Run	Pineapple Crown (X_1, g/L)	Ammonium Nitrate (X_2, g/L)	TFA (U/mL)	*Yp/s* (U/g)	*Pp* (U/h)
1	10	3	35.18 ± 1.50	2526.17	7.02
2	30	3	16.73 ± 0.35	409.49	3.41
3	10	15	29.88 ± 5.42	1711.80	4.75
4	30	15	40.83 ± 7.61	941.26	7.84
5	6	9	24.92 ± 3.23	2891.45	4.82
6	34	9	16.73 ± 3.58	309.41	2.92
7	20	0.5	32.76 ± 0.69	1443.03	8.02
8	20	17.5	65.86 ± 0.12	2958.73	16.44
9	20	9	68.98 ± 3.92	2916.05	16.20
10	20	9	69.44 ± 3.00	2657.67	14.76
11	20	9	52.48 ± 3.35	2233.18	12.41

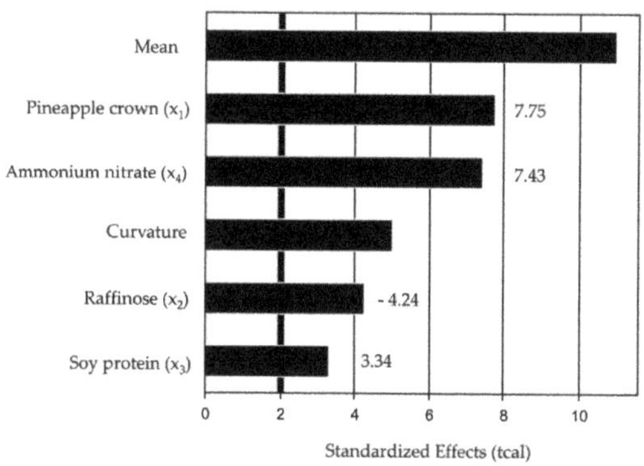

(A)

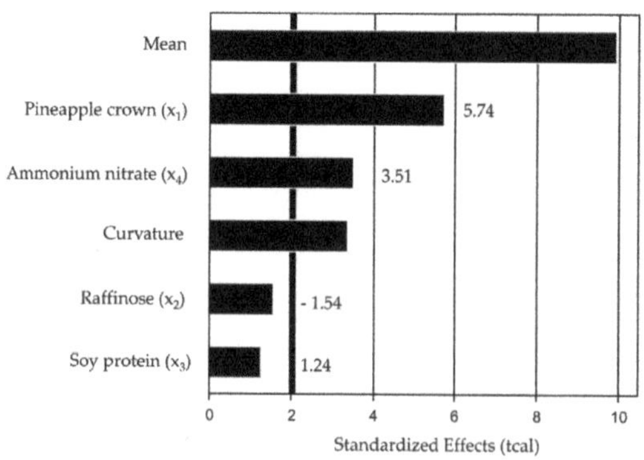

(B)

Figure 1. Pareto chart of the effects of independent variables on the response variable of the transfructosylation activity of invertase, (**A**) 72 h and (**B**) 120 h.

The analysis of the cultivation parameters of the transfructosylation activity of the invertase produced using *A. carbonarius* PC-4 with the Plackett–Burman design showed that the enzyme production (46.26 U/mL) was not reduced after three days of cultivation. As a comparison, the initial cultivations carried out using the parametric technique of culture optimization with carbon and nitrogen sources showed maximal production after 168 h of cultivation [17]. According to the results obtained using the Plackett–Burman design, the variables pineapple crown, ammonium nitrate, and soy protein had a significant positive effect ($p < 0.10$), while raffinose had a significant negative effect, at the 72 h time point. At the 120 h time point, only the variables pineapple crown and ammonium nitrate had a significant positive effect ($p < 0.10$) (Figure 1). These results suggest that higher concentrations of these components lead to increased enzymatic activity for the variables with a positive effect. Conversely, for the variable with a negative effect, lower concentrations result in higher enzymatic activity. Furthermore, a medium of the following composition is expected to lead to similar results: 20 g/L pineapple crown, 4 g/L ammonium nitrate, and 4 g/L soy protein. Under these conditions, $Y_{P/S}$ was 3700.44 U/g of the substrate and P_P was 10.28 U/h. The results showed a 1.59-fold increase in enzyme productivity while maintaining the production yield. In this study, a decrease in the duration of the cultivation to 72 h was achieved, which represents an important reduction in energy costs to produce the invertase from *A. carbonarius* PC-4 under submerged conditions using agro-industrial waste and a mineral nitrogen source.

Organic and inorganic nitrogen sources are essential for enzyme synthesis. Inorganic nitrogen can be utilized quickly, while organic sources provide various cell growth factors and amino acids that are essential for cell metabolism and enzyme production [29]. Ademakinwa et al. [18] observed that ammonium ions can influence fructosyltransferase production from *Aureobasidium pullulans* using the Plackett–Burman design. Ammonium nitrate has been used as a nitrogen source for the production of xylanase from *Aspergillus candidus* [30], amylase from *Aspergillus niger* [31], and lipase from *Candida viswanathii* [32].

Agro-industrial waste is economically feasible for enzyme production, with a reduction in operational costs, and it is environmentally friendly. Pineapple waste contains a considerable amount of soluble sugars, such as sucrose, which makes it suitable for use as a substrate in microbial fermentation [33,34]. Therefore, agro-industrial waste, such as pineapple crown, are potentially suitable substrates for the production of value-added biomolecules when used in the composition of microbial culture media [17,28]. This substrate has been used to produce β-glucosidase and xylanase from *Trichoderma viride* [22,35], cellulases from *Trichoderma ressei* [36], and invertase from *A. niger* [34].

3.2. Medium Composition Optimization by Central Composite Rotational Design (CCRD)

For the optimization experiment using CCRD and RSM methodologies, and according to previous results from the Plackett–Burman design, at the 72 h time point, despite the soy protein having a significant positive effect on the enzymatic activity, only ammonium nitrate was selected as the nitrogen source due to its more pronounced positive effect. Pineapple crown was chosen as the sole carbon source, because raffinose had a negative effect on the enzymatic activity. The response data based on the independent variables were obtained from the experiments and are depicted in Table 4.

The factors analyzed showed that the concentration of ammonium nitrate had a positive linear effect and a negative quadratic effect, indicating a tendency for maximum FTase production near the central point, while the concentration of the pineapple crown had a negative quadratic effect, indicating that an increase or decrease in the value of this variable would lead to a reduction in FTase production [37] (Table 5).

Table 5. Estimates of the coefficient of independent variables on invertase with transfructosylation activity production using the CCRD to determine the transfructosylation activity of invertase.

Factors	Coefficient	Error	t	*p*-Value
Média	63.63	4.66	13.65	0.000
X1	−2.38	2.85	−0.84	0.441
$X1^2$	−22.51	3.40	−6.63	0.001
X2	8.20	2.85	2.87	0.035
$X2^2$	−8.26	3.40	−2.43	0.059
X1.X2	7.35	4.04	1.82	0.128

A second-order equation was fitted to the data by multiple regression analysis, which generated the reparametrized model that describes the measured responses for the significant independent variables (pineapple crown and ammonium nitrate). The mathematical model was expressed with the following equation:

$$\text{TFA } (U/mL) = 63.63 - 22.51\, X_1^2 + 8.20\, X_2 - 8.26\, X_2^2 \quad (3)$$

The experimental model was validated by the analysis of variance (ANOVA) with a coefficient of determination $R^2 = 0.8533$, an F value calculated from the regression to be 13.6 (greater than the tabulated F value of 5.27), and an *F* lack of adjustment value of 0.9 (not significant), making the model valid in the 90% confidence interval (Table 6).

Table 6. Analysis of variance (ANOVA) for transfructosylation activity of the invertase.

Variation Source	Sum of Squares	Degree of Freedom	Mean Square	F_{cal}	*p*-Value
Regression	3415.5	3	1138.5	13.6	0.00265
Residue	587.4	7	83.9		
Lack of fit	400.7	5	80.1	0.9	0.61566
Pure error	186.7	2	93.4		

$F_{tab\ regression/residue}$ (3; 7; 0.10): 3.07; $F_{tab\ lack\ of\ fit/pure\ error}$ (5; 2; 0.10): 9.29. R^2: 85.33%.

A response surface plot (Figure 2) was generated from the reparametrized model equation, indicating that the maximum transfructosylation activity of the invertase was achieved at the midpoint of the experimental design (pineapple crown, 2.0%, *w*/*v*, and ammonium nitrate, 1.0%, *w*/*v*) after 72 h of cultivation. The increase in pineapple crown causes a decrease in the enzymatic activity. This fact was explained by Amim et al. [38], according to whom the gradual increase in substrate concentration will cause the enzyme production to increase at a directly proportional rate until the medium becomes saturated with the substrate. After reaching the saturation point, the addition of extra substrate will no longer make a difference.

Park et al. [39] stated that increasing the amount of nitrate has no significant effect on the enzymatic activity of fructosyltransferase. This fact can be observed, using other nitrogen sources, as it was in the study conducted by Ademakinwa et al. [23], who performed a response surface experiment to evaluate the variables sucrose, NH_4Cl, and yeast extract in the production of FTase from *Aureobasidium pullulans*. By increasing the sucrose concentration and maintaining the NH_4Cl concentration, there was an increase in the enzymatic activity of fructosyltransferase; on the other hand, the increase in yeast extract had a negative effect on the activity of fructosyltransferase. The same behavior was observed when the concentration of yeast extract was kept constant and the concentration of NH_4Cl varied, resulting in a decline in the enzymatic activity.

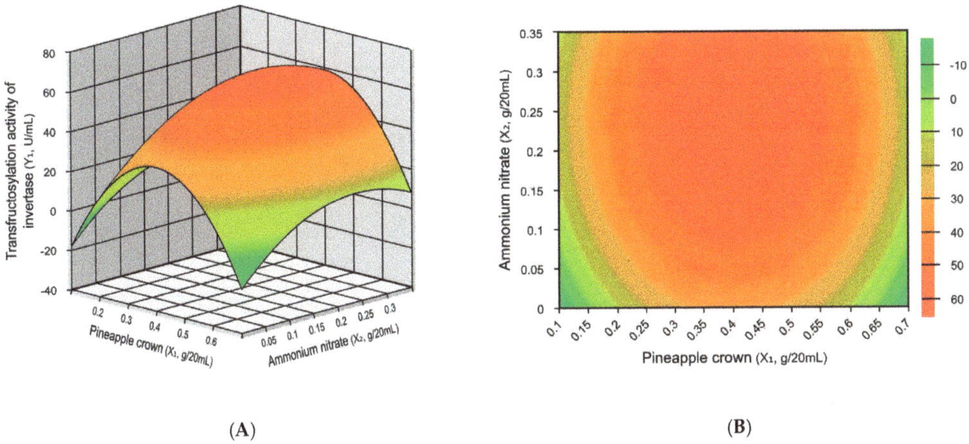

Figure 2. Invertase production with transfructosylation activity influenced by the interaction between pineapple crown (X1) and ammonium nitrate (X2). (**A**) Response surface and (**B**) contour curve.

In this study, a 5-fold increase in enzyme production was observed compared to the initial production of 13.38 U/mL during 72 h of cultivation [17], and there was also an increase in yield from 1070.75 U/g to 2771.48 U/g and a 5.19-fold increase in productivity. Although many researchers have investigated various effects on fructosyltransferase production [17,23,37], as far as we know, no optimization study has used the combination of ammonium nitrate and pineapple crown, which successfully increased enzyme production.

3.3. Validation

The results predicted by the model suggested that the maximum transfructosylation activity of the invertase produced from *A. carbonarius* PC-4 would be 65.33 ± 4.62 U/mL with the supplementation of 0.40 g of pineapple crown and 0.21 g of ammonium nitrate. The obtained results yielded an average FTase production of 66.46 ± 2.67 U/mL (Table 7). According to the predicted and experimental results, the model was validated based on the existence of the optimum point. There was a 1.77-fold increase compared to the best result for enzymatic activity (3 days of cultivation) of the Plackett and Burman design and 3.82-fold compared to the result obtained by Nascimento et al. [5] (17.36 U/mL).

Table 7. Validation of the culture conditions for the production of the invertase with transfructosylation activity from *A. carbonarius* PC-4.

Variable	Experimental Conditions	Predicted Value	Experimental Value
Pineapple crown Ammonium nitrate	20 g/L 10.5 g/L	65.33 ± 4.62 U/mL	66.46 ± 2.67 U/mL

3.4. The Physical and Chemical Properties of the Transfructosylation Activity

3.4.1. Influence of Temperature and pH on Enzyme Activity

The effect of pH and temperature on the enzymatic activity was analyzed using a central composite rotational design (Table 8). The relative activity values were presented in relation to the maximum activity value, considered to be 100%. Thus, it was observed that pH and temperature values at different levels strongly influenced the transfructosylation activity of the enzyme produced from *A. carbonarius* PC-4. According to Ghazi et al. [40], there was no significant fructosyltransferase activity at pH values below 3.5 or above 9.5, and temperatures higher than 65 °C inactivated the fructosyltransferase.

Table 8. Relative activity at different pH values and temperatures of transfructosylation activity in the invertase using CCRD.

Run	pH X_1	Temperature (°C) X_2	TFA (U/mL)	Relative Activity (%)
1	3	25	0.00	0.00
2	7	25	2.01	3.49
3	3	75	0.00	0.00
4	7	75	0.86	1.47
5	2.17	50	0.01	0.01
6	7.83	50	1.36	2.35
7	5	14.64	2.09	3.62
8	5	85.36	0.09	0.15
9	5	50	54.55	89.48
10	5	50	57.65	94.62
11	5	50	51.59	100

The factors analyzed showed that the pH and temperature are significant variables in quadratic terms, and both have negative effects, indicating that an increase in the value of these variables above the studied limits would lead to a decrease in invertase production (Table 9). A second-order equation was fitted to the data by multiple regression analysis, generating a reparametrized model that describes the measured responses for the significant independent variables (pH and temperature). The mathematical model was expressed with the following equation:

$$TFA\ (U/mL) = 54.60 - 27\ X_1^2 - 26.80\ X_2^2 \quad (4)$$

Table 9. Estimates of the coefficients of independent variables on invertase production with transfructosylation activity using the CCRD for transfructosylation activity.

Factors	Coefficient	Error	t	*p*-Value
Mean	54.60	1.12	48.64	0.000
X_1	0.60	0.69	0.87	0.4243
X_1^2	**−27.00**	**0.82**	**−33.00**	**0.0000**
X_2	−0.50	0.69	−0.73	0.4997
X_2^2	**−26.80**	**0.82**	**−32.75**	**0.0000**
$X_1.X_2$	−0.29	0.97	−0.30	0.7778

Factors are in bold when $p < 0.05$.

The experimental model was validated by analysis of variance (ANOVA) with a coefficient of determination $R^2 = 99.62\%$, an F value calculated from the regression as 1048.5 (greater than the tabulated F value of 4.46), and an F value for lack of adjustment (0) that was not significant, making the model valid in the 95% confidence interval (Table 10).

Table 10. Analysis of variance (ANOVA) for transfructosylation activity of the invertase.

Variation Source	Sum of Squares	DF	Mean Square	Fcal	*p*-Value
Regression	6314.5	2	3157.3	1048.5	0.00000
Residue	24.1	8	3.0		
Lack of fit	5.7	6	1.0	0.0	0.99683
Pure error	18.4	2	9.2		
Total	6338.6	10			

$F_{tab\ regression/residue}$ (2; 8; 0.05): 4.46; $F_{tab\ lack\ of\ fit/pure\ error}$ (6; 2; 0.05): 19.33. R^2: 99.62%.

The maximum transfructosylation activity was reached at the central point of the experimental design (pH of 5 and temperature of 50 °C) (Figure 3), where the ionization state and the established temperature stabilize the conformation of the enzyme, as well as the adequate binding of the substrate to the active site. Similar results were observed by Nemukula et al. [41], who characterized the fructosyltransferase from *Aspergillus aculeatus* and found that it has optimal activity at a pH of 6 and temperature of 60 °C. Regarding temperature, Aguiar-Oliveira and Maugeri [42] conducted a study on fructosyltransferase and stated that the highest transfructosylation rates occur at temperatures between 45 °C and 65 °C. Kashyap et al. [43] found that the relative activity of the fructosyltransferase from *A. aculeatus* increased as the pH increased to 4.5 at the temperature of 55 °C and subsequently declined and became constant.

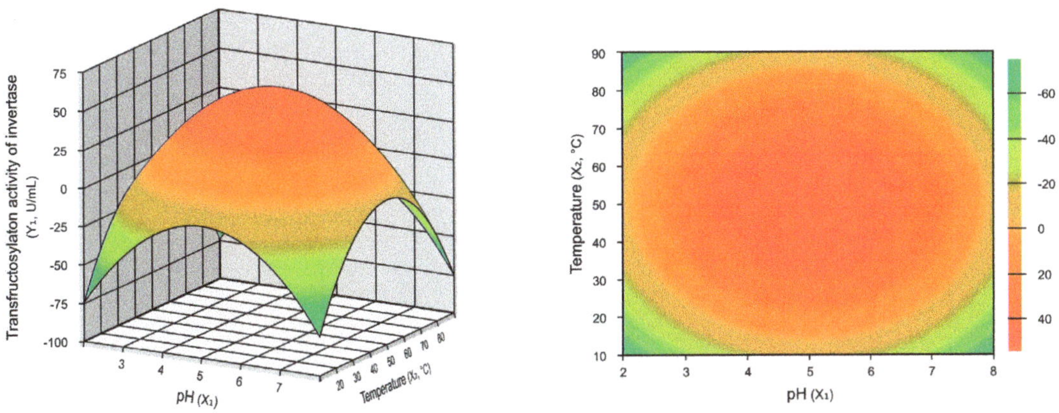

(A) (B)

Figure 3. Transfructosylation activity in interaction between pH (X_1) and temperature (X_2). (**A**) Response surface (**B**) contour curves.

For the purified enzyme, L'Hocine et al. [44] demonstrated that the best pH and temperature of fructosyltransferase from *A. niger* are 5.8 and 50 °C, respectively. Zeng et al. [45] reported that different microbial species can produce different molecular structures and active sites of the enzyme, leading to different optimal initial reaction pH values.

3.4.2. Validation

To confirm the model's accuracy in predicting the maximum transfructosylation activity, an additional experiment was performed in triplicate under the optimized conditions. The model suggested that the maximum activity is 54.60 ± 1.12 U/mL, which can be achieved when the process conditions include a pH = 5.0 and a temperature of = 50 °C. The results obtained yielded a maximum transfructosylation activity of 53.85 U/mL. According to the predicted and experimental results, the model was validated based on the existence of the optimum point.

3.5. Thermal Stability and pH Stability

The FTase produced from *A. carbonarius* PC-4 was stable at 40 °C, where 50% of its activity was verified after 60 min of incubation and remained at around 30% after 155 min. On the other hand, at the temperatures of 50 °C and 60 °C, the half-life of the enzyme was reached after 15 min of incubation. The enzyme was not stable at 60 °C, and only 17% of its activity was verified after 60 min of incubation, while at 50 °C, the FTase retained 35% of its activity. After 155 min, both temperatures led to activity below 10% (Figure 4A).

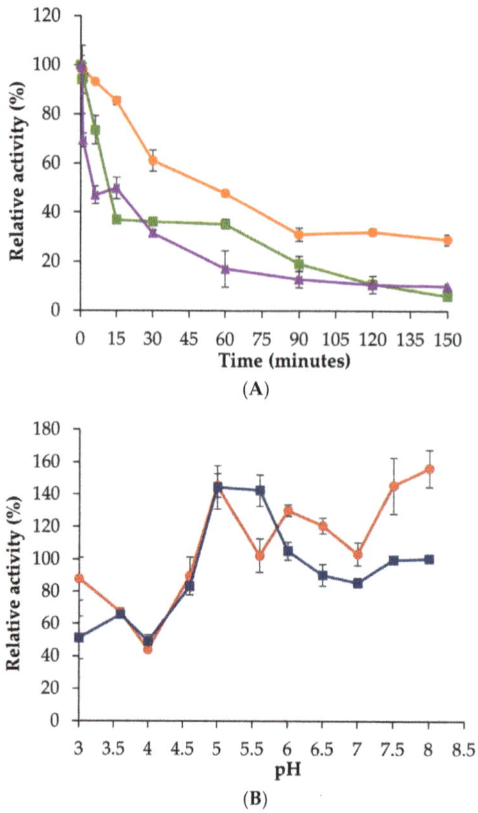

Figure 4. Thermal stability of the invertase at (**A**) 40 °C (•) orange line, 50 °C (■) green line, and 60 °C (▲) purple line for different periods and pH stabilities after (**B**) 7 h (•) red line and 24 h (■) blue line at 15 °C.

Similar results were achieved by Yang et al. [46], who found that fructosyltransferase purified from *A. niger* was more stable at 40 °C for 60 min; at 50 °C, it retained 60% of its activity, and at 60 °C, the enzyme was not stable, with a rapid decline in its activity. The fructosyltransferase from *A. aculeatus* was stable at the temperatures of 25 to 50 °C; nevertheless, it decreased sharply when incubated at 60 °C and was completely inactivated when subjected to the temperature range from 65 °C to 70 °C for 60 min [40]. The invertase with transfructosylation activity was more stable in the temperature range from 25 to 30 °C for 60 min [37].

In this work, the transfructosylation activity of the invertase from *A. carbonarius* PC-4 was more stable at pH 5, reaching a maximum of 144.40% of its activity at 24 h of incubation and 156.134% of its activity when incubated at pH 8 for 7 h. This increase may be related to the ionization state of the enzyme, which, when incubated at pH 5 for 24 h and at pH 8 for 7 h, was better at stabilizing the protein conformation [47]. On the other hand, this fact may be related to the enzyme being present in the crude extract and being influenced by factors such as metal ions, the presence of other enzymes, cofactors, and others.

For the pH range of 3–5, only at pH 4 was the relative activity below 50%. This fact may be related to the pH influencing the kinetic parameters of the enzymatic reaction and being able to change the stability of the enzyme–substrate complex [48]. For the pH ranges 5–5.5 and 6.5–8, the activity was maintained above 90% (Figure 4B). According to Yang et al. [46], a fructosyltransferase from *A. aculeatus* reached the ideal stability at pH 6.0 and retained more than 90% of its activity in the pH range of 4.0–9.0 after 24 h of incubation. Furthermore, it also retained approximately 80% of activity in pH values below 2.0 or above 11.0, indicating that FTase is stable in a wide pH range, favoring its production, storage, and industrial applications.

4. Conclusions

This study demonstrates the cost-effective optimization of an invertase from *A. carbonarius* PC-4 with high transfructosylation activity using pineapple crown as a carbon inducer source and ammonium nitrate as an inorganic nitrogen source. The experimental design of this study allowed a 1.77-fold increase in the transfructosylation activity after 72 h of cultivation. However, this combination is not found in the literature and may serve as a model for further studies. A partial characterization of the enzyme in the crude extract showed that the reaction conditions of the enzyme for the maximum transfructosylation activity occurred at pH 5.0 and a temperature of 50 °C. The enzyme showed thermal stability at 40 °C after 1 h of incubation and was stable over the wide pH range of 3.0–8.0. These parameters are important for the development of a successful bioprocess, which may favor its production, storage, and industrial applications. Low-cost agro-industrial waste, in conjunction with ammonium nitrate, has the potential to be used in the production of invertases with the aim of optimizing their transfructosylation activity for application in the production of fructooligosaccharides.

Author Contributions: Conceptualization, R.D.B. and A.F.d.A.; methodology, R.D.B., A.F.d.A., R.C.B., and R.F.P.; software, R.D.B., N.B.C., and M.d.C.A.X.; formal analysis, S.A.V.M.; investigation, R.D.B. and G.C.d.N.; resources, A.F.d.A. and R.F.P.; data curation, R.D.B. and P.C.L.; writing—original draft preparation, R.D.B. and A.F.d.A.; writing—review and editing, S.A.V.M., M.d.C.A.X., R.C.B., R.F.P., and A.F.d.A.; supervision, A.F.d.A.; project administration, A.F.d.A. All authors have read and agreed to the published version of the manuscript.

Funding: This research received no external funding.

Data Availability Statement: Data are available on request.

Acknowledgments: This study was financed in part by the Coordenação de Aperfeiçoamento de Pessoal de Nível Superior—Brasil (CAPES)—Finance Code 001. R.D.B. thanks CAPES for his student fellowship. A.F.A. thanks Fundação de Amparo à Pesquisa do Tocantins—FAPT/Governo do Tocantins, Brazil. The authors gratefully acknowledge the financial support from Fundação de Amparo à Pesquisa do Estado de Minas Gerais—FAPEMIG/Governo de Minas Gerais/Brazil (Process Number: APQ-05218-23) by publication of this work in an open access journal.

Conflicts of Interest: The authors declare no conflicts of interest.

References

1. Manoochehri, H.; Hosseini, N.F.; Saidijam, M.; Taheri, M.; Rezaee, H.; Nouri, F. A review on invertase: Its potentials and applications. *Biocatal. Agric. Biotechnol.* **2020**, *25*, 101599–101610. [CrossRef]
2. Panetta, J.C.; Barbuto, O.J.M.; Riccetti, R.V.; Moreno, A.G. Ocorrência de microrganismos responsáveis pela deterioração de um produto cárneo de baixa acidez. *Rev. Fac. Med. Vet. Zootec. Univ. São Paulo* **1976**, *13*, 241–247. [CrossRef]
3. Karkeszová, K.; Polakovic, M. Production of Fructooligosaccharides Using a Commercial Heterologously Expressed *Aspergillus* sp. Fructosyltransferase. *Catalysts* **2023**, *13*, 843. [CrossRef]
4. Han, S.; Ye, T.; Leng, S.; Pan, L.; Zeng, W.; Chen, G.; Liang, Z. Purification and biochemical characteristics of a novel fructosyltransferase with a high FOS transfructosylation activity from *Aspergillus oryzae* S719. *Protein Expr. Purif.* **2020**, *167*, 105549–105558. [CrossRef]
5. Nascimento, G.C.; Batista, R.D.; Santos, C.C.A.D.A.; Silva, E.M.; Paula, F.C.; Mendes, D.B.; Oliveira, D.P.; Almeida, A.F. β-Fructofuranosidase and β-D-Fructosyltransferase from New Aspergillus carbonarius PC-4 Strain Isolated from Canned Peach Syrup: Effect of Carbon and Nitrogen Sources on Enzyme Production. *Sci. World J.* **2019**, *1*, 6956202. [CrossRef]
6. Osiebe, O.; Adewale, I.O.; Omafuvbe, B.O. Production and characterization of intracellular invertase from *Saccharomyces cerevisiae* (OL629078.1), using cassava-soybean as a cost-effective substrate. *Sci. Rep.* **2023**, *13*, 16295–16304. [CrossRef]
7. Michel, M.R.; Flores-Gallegos, A.C.; Villarreal-Morales, S.L.; Aguilar-Zárate, P.; Aguilar, C.N.; Riutort, M.; Rodríguez-Herrera, R. Fructosyltransferase production by *Aspergillus oryzae* BM-DIA using solid-state fermentation and the properties of its nucleotide and protein sequences. *Folia Microbiol.* **2021**, *66*, 469–481. [CrossRef]

8. Belmonte-Izquierdo, Y.; Salomé-Abarca, L.F.; González-Hernández, J.C.; Francisco, L.; López, M.G. Fructooligosaccharides (FO production by microorganisms with fructosyltransferase activity. *Fermentation* **2023**, *9*, 968. [CrossRef]
9. Correa, A.C.; Lopes, M.S.; Perna, R.F.; Silva, E.K. Fructan-type prebiotic dietary fibers: Clinical studies reporting health impac and recent advances in their technological application in bakery, dairy, meat products and beverages. *Carbohydr. Polym.* **202** *323*, 121396. [CrossRef]
10. Ho, J.; Nicolucci, A.C.; Virtanen, H.; Schik, A.; Meddings, J.; Reimer, R.A.R.; Huang, C. Effect of prebiotic on microbiota, intestin permeability, and glycemic control in children with type 1 diabetes. *J. Clin. Endocrinol. Metab.* **2019**, *104*, 4427–4440. [CrossRef]
11. Sheu, D.-C.; Chang, J.-Y.; Chen, Y.-J.; Lee, C.-W. Production of high-purity neofructooligosaccharides by culture of *Xanthophy lomyces dendrorhous*. *Bioresour. Technol.* **2013**, *132*, 432–435. [CrossRef] [PubMed]
12. Dominguez, A.L.; Rodrigues, L.R.; Lima, N.M.; Teixeira, J.A. An Overview of the recent developments on fructooligosacchari production and applications. *Food Bioprocess Technol.* **2014**, *7*, 324–337. [CrossRef]
13. Choukade, R.; Kango, N. Production, properties, and applications of fructosyltransferase: A current appraisal. *Crit. Rev. Biotechnc* **2021**, *41*, 1178–1193. [CrossRef] [PubMed]
14. Van der Meulen, R.; Avonts, L.; De Vuyst, L. Short fractions of oligofructose are preferentially metabolized by *Bifidobacteriu animalis* DN-173 010. *Appl. Environ. Microbiol.* **2004**, *70*, 1923–1930. [CrossRef] [PubMed]
15. De La Rosa, O.; Flores-Gallegos, A.C.; Muñiz-Márquez, D.B.; Ochoa-Zarzosa, A.; Rodríguez-Herrera, R.; Aguilar, C.N. Fru tooligosaccharides production from agro-wastes as alternative low-cost source. *Trends Food Sci. Technol.* **2019**, *91*, 139–14 [CrossRef]
16. Ganaie, M.A.; Soni, H.; Naikoo, G.A.; Oliveira, L.T.S.; Rawat, H.K.; Mehta, P.K.; Narain, N. Screening of low-cost agricultura wastes to maximize the fructosyltransferase production and its applicability in generation of fructooligosaccharides by solid stat fermentation. *Int. Biodeterior. Biodegrad.* **2017**, *118*, 19–26. [CrossRef]
17. Ojwach, J.; Kumar, A.; Mutanda, T.; Mukaratirwa, S. Fructosyltransferase and inulinase production by indigenous coprophilou fungi for the biocatalytic conversion of sucrose and inulin into oligosaccharides. *Biocatal. Agric. Biotechnol.* **2020**, *30*, 101867–10187 [CrossRef]
18. Uday, U.S.P.; Choudhury, P.; Bandyopadhyay, T.K.; Bhunia, B. Classification, mode of action and production strategy of xylanas and its application for biofuel production from water hyacinth. *Int. J. Biol. Macromol.* **2016**, *82*, 1041–1054. [CrossRef]
19. Maiorano, A.E.; Piccoli, R.M.; Silva, E.S.; Rodrigues, M.F.A. Microbial production of fructosyltransferases for synthesis o pre-biotics. *Biotechnol. Lett.* **2008**, *30*, 1867–1877. [CrossRef] [PubMed]
20. Kavuthodi, B.; Sebastian, D. Biotechnological valorization of pineapple stem for pectinase production by *Bacillus subtilis* BKDS Media formulation and statistical optimization for submerged fermentation. *Biocatal. Agric. Biotechnol.* **2018**, *16*, 715–72 [CrossRef]
21. IBGE—Instituto Brasileiro de Geografia e Estatística. Produção Agrícola. Lavoura Temporária. 2023. Available online: https //cidades.ibge.gov.br/brasil/pesquisa/14/0 (accessed on 28 August 2024).
22. Almeida, J.M.; Lima, V.A.; Lima, P.C.G.; KNOB, A. Effective and low-cost saccharification of pineapple peel by *Trichoderma virid* crude extract with enhanced beta-glucosidase activity. *BioEnergy Res.* **2016**, *9*, 701–710. [CrossRef]
23. Ademakinwa, A.N.; Ayinla, Z.A.; Agboola, F.K. Strain improvement and statistical optimization as a combined strategy fo improving fructosyltransferase production by *Aureobasidium pullulans* NAC8. *J. Genet. Eng. Biotechnol.* **2017**, *15*, 345–35 [CrossRef] [PubMed]
24. Castellani, A. Maintenance and cultivation of the common pathogenic fungi of man in sterile distilled water. *J. Trop. Med. Hyg* **1967**, *70*, 181–184.
25. Vogel, H.J. A convenient growth medium for Neurospora crassa (medium N). *Microbiol. Genet. Bull.* **1956**, *13*, 42–43.
26. Rawat, H.K.; Ganaie, M.A.; Kango, N. Production of inulinase, fructosyltransferase and sucrase from fungi on low-valu inulin-rich substrates and their use in generation of fructose and fructo-oligosaccharides. *Antonie Van Leeuwenhoek* **2015**, *107* 799–811. [CrossRef]
27. Plackett, R.L.; Burman, J.P. The design of optimum multifactorial experiments. *Biometrika* **1946**, *33*, 305–325. [CrossRef]
28. Rodrigues, M.I.; Iemma, A.F. *Experimental Design and Process Optimization*, 1st ed.; CRC Press: Boca Raton, FL, USA, 2014 pp. 1–336. [CrossRef]
29. Tan, T.; Zhang, M.; Xu, J.; Zhang, J. Optimization of culture conditions and properties of lipase from *Penicillium camembertii* Thom PG-3. *Process Biochem.* **2004**, *39*, 1495–1502. [CrossRef]
30. Garai, D.; Kumar, V. A Box-Behnken design approach for the production of xylanase by *Aspergillus candidus* under solid state fermentation and its application in saccharification of agro residues and *Parthenium hysterophorus* L. *Ind. Crops Prod.* **2013**, *44* 352–363. [CrossRef]
31. Suganthi, R.; Benazir, J.F.; Santhi, R.; Ramesh Kumar, V.; Hari, A.; Meenakshi, N.; Nidhyia, K.A.; Kavitha, G.; Lakshmi, R. Amylase production by *Aspergillus niger* under solid state fermentation using agroindustrial wastes. *Int. J. Eng. Sci. Technol.* **2011**, *3* 1756–1760.
32. Almeida, A.F.; Tauk-Tornisielo, S.M.; Carmona, E.C. Influence of carbon and nitrogen sources on lipase production by a newly *Candida viswanathii* strain. *Ann. Microbiol.* **2013**, *63*, 1225–1234. [CrossRef]
33. Siti Roha, A.M.; Zainal, S.; Noriham, A.; Nadzirah, K.Z. Determination of sugar content in pineapple waste variety N36. *Int. Food Res. J.* **2013**, *20*, 1941–1943.

Oyedeji, O.; Bakare, M.K.; Adewale, I.O.; Olutiola, P.O.; Omoboye, O.O. Optimized production and characterization of thermostable invertase from *Aspergillus niger* IBK1, using pineapple peel as alternate substrate. *Biocatal. Agric. Biotechnol.* **2017**, *9*, 218–223. [CrossRef]

Knob, A.; Fortkamp, D.; Prolo, T.; Izidoro, S.C.; Almeida, J.M. Agro-residues as alternative for xylanase production by filamentous fungi. *Bioresour. Technol.* **2014**, *9*, 5738–5773.

Saravanan, P.; Muthuvelayudham, R.; Viruthagiri, T. Enhanced production of cellulase from pineapple waste by response surface methodology. *J. Eng.* **2012**, *2012*, 1–8. [CrossRef]

Nascimento, A.K.C.; Nobre, C.; Cavalcanti, M.T.H.; Teixeira, J.A.; Porto, A.L.F. Screening of fungi from the genus *Penicillium* for production of β-fructofuranosidase and enzymatic synthesis of fructooligosaccharides. *J. Mol. Catal. B Enzym.* **2016**, *134*, 70–78. [CrossRef]

Amin, F.; Bhatti, H.N.; Rehman, S. Optimization of growth parameters for lipase production by *Ganoderma lucidum* using response surface methodology. *Afr. J. Biotechnol.* **2011**, *10*, 5514–5523.

Park, J.P.; Bae, J.T.; Yun, J.W. Critical effect of ammonium ions on the enzymatic reaction of a novel transfructosylating enzyme for fructooligosaccharide production from sucrose. *Biotechnol. Lett.* **1999**, *21*, 987–990. [CrossRef]

Ghazi, I.; Fernandez-Arrojo, L.; Garcia-Arellano, H.; Ferrer, M.; Ballesteros, A.; Plou, F.J. Purification and kinetic characterization of a fructosyltransferase from *Aspergillus aculeatus*. *J. Biotechnol.* **2007**, *128*, 204–211. [CrossRef]

Nemukula, A.; Mutanda, T.; Wilhelmi, B.S.; Whiteley, C.G. Response surface methodology: Synthesis of short chain fructooligosaccharides with a fructosyltransferase from *Aspergillus aculeatus*. *Bioresour. Technol.* **2009**, *100*, 2040–2045. [CrossRef]

Aguiar-Oliveira, E.; Maugeri, F. Characterization of the Immobilized Fructosyltransferase from *Rhodotorula* sp. *Int. J. Food Eng.* **2010**, *6*, 1–21. [CrossRef]

Kashyap, R.; Palai, T.; Bhattacharya, P.K. Kinetics and model development for enzymatic synthesis of fructo-oligosaccharides using fructosyltransferase. *Bioprocess Biosyst. Eng.* **2015**, *38*, 2417–2426. [CrossRef] [PubMed]

L'Hocine, L.; Wang, Z.; Jiang, B.; Xu, S. Purification and partial characterization of fructosyltransferase and invertase from *Aspergillus niger* AS0023. *J. Biotechnol.* **2000**, *81*, 73–84. [CrossRef] [PubMed]

Zeng, X.-A.; Zhou, K.; Liu, D.-L.; Brennan, C.S.; Brennan, M.; Zhou, J.-S.; Yu, S.-J. Preparation of fructooligosaccharides using *Aspergillus niger* 6640 whole-cell as catalyst for bio-transformation. *Food Sci. Technol.* **2016**, *65*, 1072–1079. [CrossRef]

Yang, H.; Wang, Y.; Zhang, L.; Shen, W. Heterologous expression and enzymatic characterization of fructosyltransferase from *Aspergillus niger* in *Pichia pastoris*. *New Biotechnol.* **2016**, *33*, 164–169. [CrossRef] [PubMed]

Nelson, D.L.; Cox, M.M. *Princípios de Bioquímica de Lehninger*, 5th ed.; Artmed: Porto Alegre, Brasil, 2011; pp. 189–193.

Keramat, A.; Kargari, A.; Sohrabi, M.; Mirshekar, H.; Sanaeepur, H. Kinetic model for invertase-induced sucrose hydrolysis: Initial time lag. *Chem. Eng. Technol.* **2017**, *40*, 529–536. [CrossRef]

processes

Article

Optimization of Cellulase Production from Agri-Industrial Residues by *Aspergillus terreus* NIH2624

Elen Ayumi Kadoguchi [1], Josman Velasco [2], Silvio Silvério da Silva [1], Avinash P. Ingle [3], Fernando Segato [1] and Anuj Kumar Chandel [1,*]

[1] Department of Biotechnology, Engineering School of Lorena, University of São Paulo (EEL-USP), Lorena 12602-810, SP, Brazil
[2] Departamento de Ciencias Biologicas, Universidad de los Andes, Bogotá 111711, Colombia; j.velascomendoza@uniandes.edu.co
[3] Biotechnology Centre, Department of Agricultural Botany, Dr. Panjabrao Deshmukh Agricultural University, Akola 444 104, India
* Correspondence: anuj10@usp.br or anuj.kumar.chandel@gmail.com

Abstract: The objective of this study was to assess the cellulase production of four fungi: *Aspergillus terreus* NIH2624, *Aspergillus clavatus* NRRL1, *Aspergillus versicolor* CBS583.65 and *Aspergillus phoenicis* ATCC3157, under submerged cultivation conditions. When these fungi were cultured in shake flasks using Mandels and Weber's minimal medium with 1% sugarcane bagasse as a carbon source and 1.8 g/L of rice bran extract as a nitrogen source, *A. terreus* showed maximum cellulase production (filter paper activity (FPase) 3.35 U/mL; carboxymethyl cellulase activity (CMCase) 1.69 U/mL). Consequently, *A. terreus* was selected for the optimization study for cellulase production. Among the different tested carbon sources, *A. terreus* showed higher CMCase activity when it was cultivated on delignified sugarcane bagasse (1.64 U/mL) and higher FPase activity on sugarcane straw (7.95 U/mL). Regarding the nitrogen sources, the maximum FPase activity was observed when using rice bran (FPase, 8.90 U/mL) and soybean meal (FPase, 9.63 U/mL). The optimized fermentation medium (minimal medium with delignified sugarcane bagasse and rice bran as carbon and nitrogen sources, respectively) resulted in an enzymatic cocktail mainly composed of xylanases, with a maximum activity of 1701.85 U/mL for beechwood xylan, 77.12 U/mL for endoglucanase and 21.02 U/mL for cellobiohydrolase. Additionally, the enzymatic cocktail showed efficient activities for β-glucosidase, β-xylanase, arabinofuranosidase and lytic polysaccharide monoxygenases (LPMOs). This cellulase enzyme solution has the potential to efficiently hydrolyze lignocellulosic biomass, producing second-generation sugars in biorefineries.

Keywords: *Aspergillus* sp.; agro-industrial by-products; cellulases; LPMOs; fermentation

1. Introduction

The limited availability of gasoline and its consequent impacts on the environment are important concerns that highlight the urgent demand for sustainable gasoline alternatives. One of the main challenges in the renewable industry is the conversion of lignocellulosic biomass into fermentable sugars at a low cost [1]. Among the strategies proposed to reduce the cost of cellulase production, the use of agro-industrial residues from feedstock shows great promise due to their wide availability and low cost [2]. Agricultural residues such as sugarcane bagasse, sugarcane straw, corn cob, rice straw, etc. have been recognized as viable substrates to produce fungal enzymes [3]. These substrates are abundantly available throughout the year in many agricultural countries, including Brazil, the USA, China and India. Therefore, such lignocellulosic biomasses can be utilized to develop sustainable cellulase production processes in fermentation industries, holding significant economic importance [4].

Lignocellulosic biomass usually primarily consists of cellulose, hemicellulose and lignin. However, the interaction between these three components in the plant cell wall renders the biomass rigid, complex and recalcitrant. Consequently, an effective biomass pre-treatment becomes extremely necessary to enable the enzyme access to biomass during saccharification. The sugars derived from enzymatic hydrolysis are referred to as second-generation (2G) and serve as building blocks in lignocellulose biorefineries to produce renewable fuel, biomaterials and other high value-added chemicals [5].

An ideal cellulolytic enzyme cocktail should contain a good amount of exoglucanases, endoglucanases, β-glucosidase and other auxiliary enzymes for efficient enzyme hydrolysis of the lignocellulosic biomass [4]. Cellulase enzymes are not only of great interest in biorefineries but also in the textile, beverage, cleaning product and pulp and paper manufacturing industries. Moreover, cellulases are being used in the degradation and smoothing of fabric fibers, aging of jeans, production of fruit juice, production of detergent and in winemaking, the animal feed industry and in the pulp and paper industries [6].

It is evident that cellulases are enzymes that exhibit different specificities for cellulose degradation, converting into soluble sugars that are then assimilated by microorganisms for fuels and specialty chemical products. The complete enzymatic degradation of cellulose requires the coordinated action of hydrolytic and oxidative enzymes. Hydrolytic enzymes include endoglucanases (responsible for the hydrolysis of the internal regions of the cellulose), exoglucanases (acting at the ends of the microcrystalline cellulose molecule, releasing cellobiose units) and β-glucosidases (which hydrolyze cellobiose and some glucose-soluble oligosaccharides). Oxidative enzymes, such as lytic polysaccharide monoxygenases (LPMOs), act in synergy with cellulases to potentiate cellulose degradation, being activated by enzymes that act as electron donors, such as cellobiose dehydrogenase (CDH) [7,8].

According to Florencio et al. [9], among the microorganisms capable of producing cellulolytic enzymes that efficiently degrade plant biomass, filamentous fungi stand out, especially *Trichoderma reesei* and *Aspergillus niger* strains. In this study, we chose to an *Aspergillus* species, as these fungi are well-known to produce a complete cellulase cocktail, including cellobiohydrolases, endoglucanases, β-glucosidases, β-xylosidases, endoxylanases, xyloglucanases and α-arabinofuranosidases. *Aspergillus* spp. are robust fungi that thrive on a variety of low-cost carbon and nitrogen sources, yielding high titers of plant biomass-degrading enzymes. It is evident from the literature that *A. niger* produces more effective hemicellulases and β-glucosidases than *Trichoderma* spp., with strong resistance to phenolic compounds from lignin and deactivators. Florecio et al. [9] studied the proteomic analysis of the *A. niger* strain and *T. reesei* and found that the former showed a secretome with a greater number of identified proteins and greater titers of cellulase enzymes.

The production of cellulase enzymes by *Aspergillus* sp. and *Trichoderma* sp. has been well-documented; however, there are only a few reports available on the production of cellulase by *A. terreus*. To the best of our knowledge, this study is first to report a comparison of enzyme production potentials in four different species viz. *Aspergillus clavatus, A. versicolor, A. terreus* and *A. phoenicis* growing on agro-industrial residues as carbon and nitrogen sources in a submerged fermentation process.

2. Materials and Methods

2.1. Microorganisms

Four different filamentous fungi viz. *A. clavatus* NRRL1, *A. terreus* NIH2624, *A. versicolor* CBS583.65 and *A. phoenicis* ATCC3157 were kindly provided by the Synthetic and Molecular Biology Laboratory at the Department of Biotechnology-EEL/USP, Lorena, São Paulo, Brazil for the production of cellulase.

2.2. Inoculum Preparation

Spores from all four *Aspergillus* strains were transferred to a pre-inoculum with 50 mL of growth medium (2% D-glucose, 2% malt extract, 1% peptone, pH: 5.5) in an orbital shaker (30 °C and 200 rpm) for 48 h. Subsequently, 1 mL of pre-inoculum was transferred to an Erlenmeyer flask containing 100 mL of the minimal medium (2 g/L of KH_2PO_4, 1.4 g/L of $(NH_4)_2SO_4$, 0.3 g/L of $MgSO_4.7H_2O$, 0.3 g/L of $CaCl_2$, 0.3 g/L of urea, 2 ml/L of trace elements (5 mg/L of $FeSO_4.7H_2O$, 1.56 mg/L of $MnSO_4.H_2O$, 1.4 mg/L of $ZnSO_4.7H_2O$, 2 mg/L of $CoCl_2$)) with 1% sodium carboxymethylcellulose (CMC) and a pH of 5.5, as described by Mandels and Weber [10], and kept at 30 °C for 96 h under agitation at 200 rpm. Samples were withdrawn after every 24 h with 5 min of rest for decanting, and 2 mL of the supernatant was removed for the cellulase assay.

2.3. Carbon and Nitrogen Sources in the Production Medium

For cellulase production, two different parameters were used: the carbon source and the nitrogen source (defined and non-defined). The carbon sources consisted of sugarcane bagasse, sugarcane straw, corn cob and pequi mesocarp, as these are agro-industrial residues and have different concentrations of cellulose, lignin and hemicellulose. The defined nitrogen sources were based on the medium described by Mandels and Weber [10], where each compound (urea, peptone and ammonium sulfate) was tested separately. The non-defined nitrogen sources consisted of rice straw, soybean bran and rice bran.

2.4. Alkaline Pre-Treatment of Carbon Sources

The native biomass samples were alkaline pre-treated using a 4% NaOH solution (w/v) in an autoclave at 121 °C for 40 min. Briefly, 10% lignocellulosic biomass (sugarcane bagasse, sugarcane straw, corn cob and pequi mesocarp) was added to the 4% NaOH solution. After the end of the pre-treatment, the biomass was filtered under a vacuum pump until most of the liquid was removed. Subsequently, the pre-treated material was washed with distilled water until the yellow color disappeared to ensure the removal of the remaining lignin present and to reach a neutral pH. After this procedure, the biomass was subjected to drying at room temperature and grinding in a knife mill to obtain a size smaller than a 20 mesh (0.841 mm). All samples were stored in a cold room at 4 °C.

2.5. Fermentation Assay under Optimized Conditions

Fermentation conditions, such as the pH (5.5), temperature (30 °C), agitation frequency (200 rpm) and culture medium (except for the carbon and nitrogen sources), were the same in all analyzed fermentations. To prepare the medium to select the best carbon source, the carboxymethyl cellulose (CMC) was replaced with 1% of a single carbon source (sugarcane bagasse or sugarcane straw or corn cob or pequi mesocarp) and the rest of the components followed the minimal medium protocol described above.

To select the best nitrogen source, synthetic nitrogen source substrates were added to the medium with a defined equimolar fraction as well as to the minimal medium already described, obtaining a total weight of 2.25 g/L for urea and ammonium sulfate and 2.7 g/L for peptone. The non-synthetic nitrogen sources were used at a concentration of 1.8 g/L of the total weight. Sugarcane bagasse was used as a major carbon source in this test due to its better performance, as shown in previous assays. For both carbon and nitrogen selection, fermentation was carried out using the same procedure used in the study of potential cellulolytic enzyme-producing fungi but, this time, varying only the carbon and nitrogen sources.

The *A. terreus* fungus was transferred to a pre-inoculum in 50 mL of medium in an orbital shaker (30 °C, 200 rpm) for 48 h. Subsequently, 2 mL were transferred to an Erlenmeyer flask containing 200 mL of minimal medium with 1% sugarcane bagasse and 1.8 g/L of rice bran, then kept at 30 °C for 96 h while agitated at 200 rpm. After fermentation, the contents of the Erlenmeyer flask were centrifuged, and the liquid fraction was used later for protein quantification and to determine enzyme concentration and activity.

2.6. Carboxymethyl Cellulase (CMCase) Activity

The CMC test indicates the presence of endoglucanases in the enzyme solution. In this step, 2 mL of the sample, obtained after the cultivation of fungi from the best carbon and nitrogen sources, was centrifuged at 10,000 rpm and 4 °C. Then, 1 mL of the supernatant was taken for analysis. The CMCase activity was determined by adding 0.5 mL of the crude enzyme extract into 0.5 mL of the 1% sodium carboxymethylcellulose solution in an acetate buffer (0.05 M, pH 5.0) followed by incubation in a water bath at 50 °C for 60 min. Periodically, the substrate-enzyme system was shaken to keep the cellulose in suspension. Then, 1 mL of a dinitrosalicylic acid (DNS) reagent was added, and the mixture was subjected to a water bath for 10 min at 100 °C. It was then cooled in an ice bath for 5 min, and 3.5 mL of distilled water was added. Finally, the absorbance was read in a spectrophotometer at 540 nm after calibrating the device with a blank composed of DNS reacted with the substrate without crude enzyme, which was replaced by distilled water. The enzyme activity tests of the enzyme solutions obtained from all four fungal strains were performed in triplicate.

Subsequently, CMCase activity tests were also performed on Greiner microplates to obtain enzymatic cocktail production profiles. In this case, 50 µL of the 0.5% CMC solution, 40 µL of a citrate buffer solution (pH 6) and 10 µL of the enzymatic extract were added in microtubes. The same was done for the blank, however, without the addition of the enzyme extract. Then the samples were placed in a dry bath at 50 °C for 30 min. After that, 100 µL of the DNS reagent was added to the samples and 10 µL of the enzymatic extract was added to the blank. The samples were submitted to a dry bath for 5 min at 100 °C and later added to Greiner microplates and analyzed in a plate reader at 540 nm.

The CMCase activity was determined in terms of glucose released (µmoles of reducing sugar produced per minute, using per ml of enzyme extract (U/mL) from the carboxymethylcellulose (substrate; CMC) at a pH of 6.0 and temperature of 50 °C) following the statistical analysis proposed by Triola et al. [11].

2.7. FPase Activity

FPase activity, i.e., filter paper activity, is determined based on the degradation of a strip of Whatman No. 1 filter paper (1.0 × 6.0 cm) by a mixture of exoglucanases and endoglucanases. In the tube containing the reaction assay, 1 mL of sodium citrate buffer solution (pH 4.8 to 50 mM), 0.5 mL of enzymatic extract and a strip of filter paper were added. In another tube, the reaction control was carried out by adding 1 mL of the same buffer solution and 0.5 mL of enzymatic extract; 1.5 mL of buffer solution and a strip of filter paper were added to the third tube, which was compared to the control. The samples were incubated in a water bath at 50 °C for 60 min, and the reaction was stopped with the addition of 3 mL of DNS reagent. The tubes were placed in boiling water for 5 min, and then 20 mL of distilled water was added for subsequent measurement of the absorbance in a spectrophotometer at 540 nm. The FPase activity was determined in terms of glucose released (µmoles of reducing sugar produced per minute, using per ml of enzyme extract (U/mL) from the Whatman filter paper (substrate) at a pH of 4.8 and temperature of 50 °C).

2.8. Biomass Characterization

Native and pre-treated sugarcane bagasse were characterized in terms of structural polymeric fractions (cellulose, hemicellulose, lignin), ash and extractives based on the analytical procedures established by the National Renewable Energy Laboratory (NREL), CO, USA [12].

2.9. Protein Quantification

Protein quantification was performed before and after concentrating the enzymatic extract using the Bio-Rad DC II kit, a colorimetric assay for protein concentration after detergent solubilization [13]. To prepare the blank, in duplicate, 20 µL of the minimal medium were added to microplates with rice bran. Then, 10 µL of reagent A (2% solution of Na_2CO_3 in 0.1 M of NaOH) and 80 µL of reagent B (0.5% solution of $CuSO_4.5H_2O$ and 1% sodium citrate) were added. The plates were left to rest for 15 min, and then the absorbance was measured in the plate reader at 750 nm. As for the samples, in triplicate, the same procedure mentioned above was performed, replacing the minimal medium with 20 μL of the enzymatic extract.

2.10. Concentration of the Crude Enzyme Extract

The enzymatic extract, obtained from the optimized fermentation, was filtered through filter paper and concentrated up to 3 or 10 times by ultrafiltration in an Amicon stirred cell apparatus (Merck-Millipore, São Paulo, Brazil) with a 10 KDa cut-off membrane.

2.11. Xylanase Assay Using Beechwood and Birchwood Xylan

The xylanase activity of the enzymatic solution was performed using beechwood and birchwood as substrates. The substrates beechwood and birchwood were each added to microtubes followed by 50 μL of xylan 1%, 40 μL of citrate buffer (pH 4.8) and 10 μL of the enzyme extract. The same was done for the blank, replacing the enzymatic extract with the buffer. After that, the samples were incubated in a dry bath at 50 °C for 30 min. Then 100 μL of DNS reagent was added to the samples while 100 μL of DNS and 10 μL of enzyme extract were added to the blank. The samples were placed in a dry bath at 100 °C for 5 min and then diluted to a ratio of 1:4 (*v*/*v*) using distilled water before being transferred to Greiner microplates and analyzed in a plate reader at 540 nm. The activity value was calculated by considering 1 international unit (IU) equivalent to 1 μmol of xylose released per minute, per ml of enzyme (U/mL) using beechwood and birchwood as substrates at a pH of 4.8 and temperature of 50 °C.

2.12. Assay with Phosphoric Acid Swollen Cellulose (PASC)

For the PASC's preparation, 1 g of Avicel was added first to 25 mL of phosphoric acid (85% w/v) in an ice bath and stirred for 1 h. Then 400 mL of distilled water was added and stirred for another 1 h. After that, the solution was filtered with filter paper and washed extensively with 2 L of distilled water. The solution was then neutralized with 700 mL of a 1% $NaHCO_3$ solution and washed again with 1.5 L of distilled water. The PASC was removed with the aid of a spatula and resuspended in a buffer until use.

Samples were made in triplicate by adding 250 μL of PASC (0.5%) to 200 μL of citrate buffer (0.5 M, pH 4.8) with 50 μL of enzyme extract. For the blanks, a sample without substrate and another without the enzymes were made as controls. The citrate buffer was used to replace the substrate and enzymes, respectively, in these two cases. The assay was performed in a shaker bath at 50 °C for 60 min at 1000 rpm. Afterwards, the samples (reaction mixtures) were heated to 100 °C for 5 min to stop the reaction. Thereafter, the samples were cooled and centrifuged at 12,500 rpm for 5 min. After centrifugation, 100 μL of the supernatant was mixed with 100 μL of DNS reagent and incubated in a water bath at 100 °C for 5 min. The absorbance was then read by a spectrophotometer using a plate reader at 540 nm.

For the analysis of lytic polysaccharide monoxygenases (LPMOs), the same procedure as described above was used, with the addition of 1 mM of ascorbic acid in the final concentration. Therefore, 250 μL of PASC, 150 μL of citrate buffer, 50 μL of enzyme extract and 50 μL of ascorbic acid were used for the samples. For these reactions, a reaction containing all the reagents except the enzyme extract was used as a blank.

2.13. Assays with Para-Nitrophenyl (pNP)-Labeled Substrates

The enzymatic extract was used for a multi-enzyme assay. For this, pNP-glucose, pNP-cellobiose, pNP-xylose and pNP-arabinofuranose were taken as substrates to test for the presence of β-glucosidase, cellobiohydrolase, β-xylosidase and arabinofuranosidase, respectively.

For this, 40 μL of the substrate (1 mM), 10 μL of the enzyme extract and 50 μL of the citrate buffer (0.5 M, pH 4.8) were added to the samples. As for the blank, which was made in duplicate, 40 μL of the substrate and 60 μL of the citrate buffer were used. The reaction was incubated at 50 °C for 30 min, then 100 μL of 1 M sodium carbonate was added and the solution was transferred to microplates for absorbance readings at 405 nm by a UV-visible spectrophotometer. After the 30 min incubation, there was a clear linearity in enzyme activity. The same method was used for each substrate and activity calculations were performed considering 1 international unit (IU) as equivalent to 1 nmol of pNP released per minute per ml of enzyme (U/mL) using the specific substrates at a pH of 4.8 and temperature of 50 °C.

3. Results and Discussion

Pre-treated sugarcane bagasse was used in this study as a primary carbon source for the four *Aspergillus* strains (i.e., *A. clavatus* NRRL1, *A. phoenicis* 275 ATCC3157, *A. versicolor* CBS583.65 and *A. terreus* NIH2624). The characterization of native sugarcane bagasse and alkaline pre-treated sugarcane bagasse is demonstrated in Table 1, showing the amount of total lignin (soluble and insoluble), glucose, xylan, arabinose and ash.

Table 1. Chemical composition (% dry wt.) of native and alkaline pre-treated (4% NaOH, 10% bagasse concentration, 120 °C, 30 min) sugarcane bagasse (SCB).

SCB (native)						
Sample	**Total lignin**	**Glucan**	**Xylan**	**Arabinosyl**	**Ashes**	**Total**
A	30.88	39.92	22.33	9.73	3.46	106.31
B	33.42	40.62	20.64	10.79	3.66	109.15
C	31.62	41.02	24.52	9.12	3.52	109.81
Media	31.62	40.62	22.33	9.73	3.52	109.15
Pre-Treated SCB						
Sample	**Total lignin**	**Glucan**	**Xylan**	**Arabinosyl**	**Ashes**	**Total**
A	6.78	66.65	27.8	6.24	1.53	109
B	7.35	62.25	26.72	6.88	0.79	103.99
C	8.38	54.88	23.77	6.08	0.69	93.8
Media	7.58	60.77	25.78	6.16	0.74	101.03

The characterization data of biomass, i.e., native sugarcane bagasse and bagasse pre-treated with sodium hydroxide (NaOH), showed that the concentration of total lignin and arabinose was found to be less in pre-treated sugarcane bagasse compared to native sugarcane bagasse. The cellulosic fraction rationally increased in the substrate as lignin was removed from the pre-treated biomass. The higher concentration of glucose in the pre-treated bagasse is due to lignin removal. Similarly, the concentration of xylan was also found to be higher in pre-treated biomass but cannot be considered significant (variance less than 10%). Table 1 also confirms the presence of a higher composition of glucose in the pre-treated sugarcane bagasse because of the removal of lignin and a fraction of hemicellulose.

The results recorded in the present study showed a resemblance with observations recorded in previous studies [14–16] where an alkaline treatment with NaOH was found to be the most efficient method to delignify agricultural residues, increasing the internal surface area and decreasing the degree of polymerization and crystallinity, in addition to separating the structural bonds between lignin and carbohydrates by breaking the lignin structure. The disadvantage of this technique is that it also degrades a fraction of the hemicellulose [15]. Other types of pre-treatments, on the other hand, have little effect on reducing lignin content and do not show a profound impact on cell wall compactness, eventually reducing the accessibility of microorganisms to cellulose entities during cultivation.

The enzymatic activity (CMCase and FPase) of all four test *Aspergillus* strains (i.e., *A. clavatus*, *A. versicolor*, *A. terreus* and *A. phoenicis*) was evaluated and is shown in Figure 1.

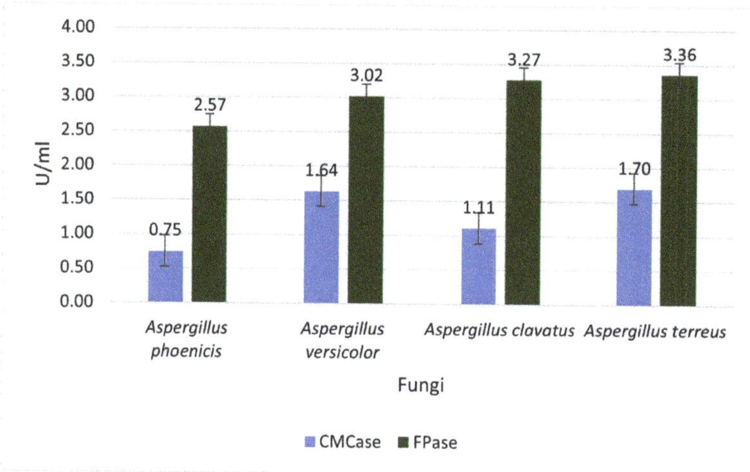

Figure 1. Cellulase production potential of filamentous fungi: *A. clavatus* NRRL1, *A. phoenicis* ATCC3157, *A. versicolor* CBS583.65 and *A. terreus* NIH2624.

The analysis demonstrated that *A. terreus* NIH2624 showed the maximum enzymatic activity (CMCase activity of 1.70 U/mL and FPase activity of 3.36 U/mL) compared to other strains (Figure 1). Therefore, *A. terreus* NIH2624 was selected for the further optimization of various carbon and nitrogen sources for cellulase production. The FPase activity (3.35 U/mL) reported in the present study was found to be significantly higher compared to previous studies, whereas CMCase activity (1.69 U/mL) was found to be lower. For example, Hui et al. [17] obtained an FPase value of 1.40 U/mL. Shahriarinour et al. [18] obtained an FPase of 0.69 U/mL and a CMCase of 7.41 U/mL for *A. terreus*, using peptone as a source of nitrogen in the minimum medium and using cellulose as carbon source. Sohail et al. [19] found lower values of FPase (0.15 U/mL) and CMCase (0.295 U/mL) for *A. terreus* activity with a mineral salt medium while employing solid-state fermentation. The CMCase value (1.32 U/mL) of this study is like the value found by Silva et al. [20] that used the mutant strain of *T. reesei* RP698.

After the selection of *A. terreus* NIH2624 as the fungus of study, four different carbon sources, i.e., corn cob, pequi mesocarp, sugarcane straw and sugarcane bagasse, were evaluated for cellulase production. The cellulase production profile of *A. terreus* NIH2624 growing on these carbon sources is presented in Figure 2.

Figure 2 shows the maximum CMCase (1.64 U/mL) and FPase (7.95 U/mL) production from sugarcane bagasse and sugarcane straw, respectively. Because sugarcane straw showed low CMCase production (0.29 U/mL), this biomass was not used further as a main carbon feedstock for cellulase production and, as the sugarcane bagasse showed a considerably higher production of cellulase, it was further selected as a primary carbon source in fermentation reactions.

The cellulase production by *A. terreus* NIH2624 can be compared with existing reports documented in the scientific literature. For instance, Corrêa [21] evaluated other *A. terreus* strains and found that *A. terreus* BLU24 produced 0.30 U/mL of CMCase and 0.50 U/mL of FPase, whereas Sohail et al. [19] found that *A. terreus* MS105 produced 0.726 IU/L/h of CMCase activity when grown on sugarcane bagasse. After the selection of *A. terreus* NIH2624 and the carbon source (sugarcane bagasse), the nitrogen sources were tested separately.

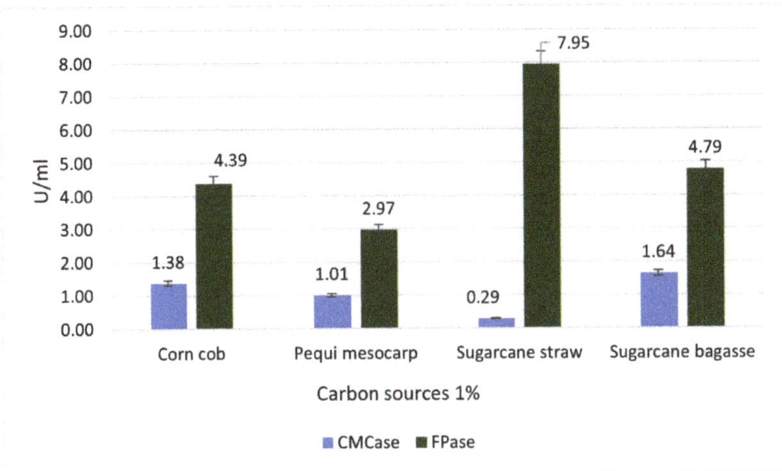

Figure 2. Cellulase production profile of *A. terreus* NIH2624 when grown on four different carbon sources (corn cob, pequi mesocarp, sugarcane straw and sugarcane bagasse).

As shown in Figure 3, higher CMCase activity was observed when using rice bran (2.35 U/mL) and higher FPase activity was observed when using soybean bran (9.63 U/mL) while using pre-treated sugarcane bagasse as a carbon source. Considering that an enzyme cocktail must contain, mainly, endoglucanase and exoglucanase, rice bran was chosen as the best source of nitrogen.

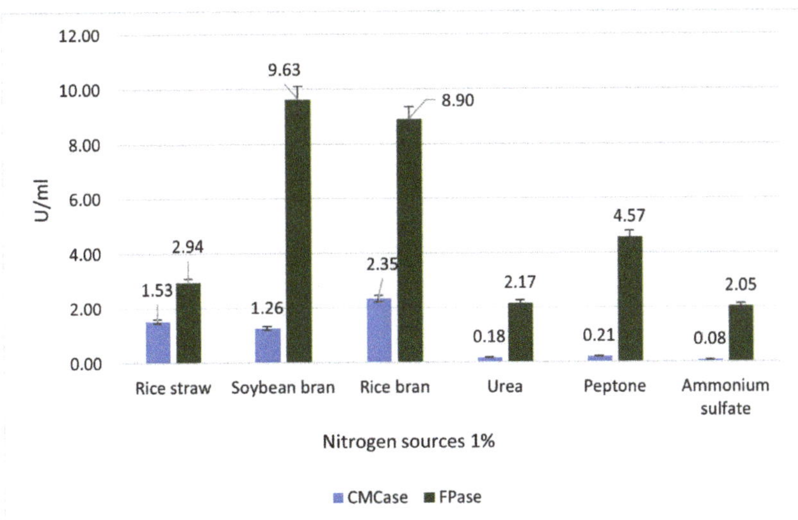

Figure 3. Effect of various nitrogen sources on cellulase production by *A. terreus* NIH2624 when grown on sugarcane bagasse as a primary carbon source.

The FPase values of this study are promising when compared to the literature. Latifian et al. [22] found FPase values of 1.163 U/mL for *T. reesei* QM9414 cellulases. In another study using rice bran and husk, a strain of *Rhizopus oryzae* showed an activity of 0.92 U/mL and 0.43 U/mL for CMCase and FPase, respectively, while the *T. reesei* strain showed an activity of 0.97 U/mL and 0.32 U/mL for CMCase and FPase, respectively [23]. *Aureoba-*

sidium pullulans LB83 showed maximum cellulase activity (FPase of 2.27 U/mL; CMCase of 7.42 U/mL) on sugarcane bagasse and, while using soybean meal as a non-defined nitrogen source also showed maximum cellulase activity (FPase of 2.45 U/mL; CMCase of 6.86 U/mL) after 60 h [24].

To have a better understanding of the enzymatic cocktail profile, fermentation was carried out employing optimized conditions (i.e., growing *A. terreus* on a production medium containing alkaline pre-treated sugarcane bagasse as a carbon source and dilute acid pre-treated rice bran as an organic nitrogen source) (Table 2). The enzymatic extract obtained was concentrated from 0.353 µg/µL of protein to 0.575 µg/µL and used to evaluate the presence of different enzyme families through a substrate panel to analyze the auxiliary and plant cell wall-degrading activities.

Table 2. Plant cell wall-degrading enzymes produced by *A. terrus* NIH2624 growing on a production medium consisting of alkaline pre-treated sugarcane bagasse (carbon source) and rice bran (nitrogen source) and employing standard conditions.

Substrate	U/mL (µmol/(min·mL))	Enzymes
CMC	77.12 ± 2.8	Endoglucanase
Xylan from beechwood	1701.85 ± 98.8	Xylanases
Xylan from birchwood	1559.27 ± 31	Xylanases
Phosphoric acid swollen cellulose	21.03 ± 1.4	Endoglucanase, Cellobiohydrolase
Substrate	**U/mL (nmol/(min·mL))**	**Enzymes**
para-nitrophenyl-glucose	23.58 ± 0.1	β-glucosidase
para-nitrophenyl-cellobiose	8.46 ± 0.2	Cellobiohydrolase
para-nitrophenyl-xylose	4.45 ± 0.4	β-xylosidase
para-nitrophenyl-arabinofuranose	10.73 ± 0.4	Arabinofuranosidase

It can be noted that the concentrated enzyme cocktail has large amounts of xylanases (1701.85 U/mL and 1559.26 U/mL for beechwood xylan and birchwood xylan, respectively). These xylanase values are much higher when compared to the literature. A secretomic analysis study of *T. ressei* RUT-C30 and *A. niger* A12, which aimed to produce cellulolytic enzymes and hydrolyze sugarcane bagasse, that was carried out by Florencio et al. [9] showed xylanase activities of 7.9 IU/mL and 7.8 IU/mL for *T. reesei* RUT-C30 and *A. niger* A12, respectively. In addition, compared to the study of Florencio et al. [9], the endoglucanase activities shown in the present work were higher than the ones Florencio et al. [9] found of 1.6 IU/mL and 0.6 IU/mL for *T. reesei* RUT-C30 and *A. niger* A12, respectively. Zhao et al. [25] found activities for endoglucanase (EG), cellobiohydrolase (CBH) and β-glucosidase of 430.45 mg/h/mL, 10.09 mg/h/mL and 0.25 µmol/min/mL, respectively. Compared to the values obtained in the present work (EG: 832.93 mg/h/mL; CBH: 227.09 mg/h/mL; β-glucosidase: 0.02µmol/min/mL), the activities of EG and CBH were 1.9 and 22.5 times higher, respectively. Thus, *A. terreus* is notable for its ability to produce cellulolytic enzymes.

The PASC test was also performed by adding ascorbic acid to analyze the presence of LPMOs, important enzymes that have revolutionized our understanding of the biological degradation of plant cell walls. The PASC test can indicate the presence of endoglucanase and cellobiohydrolase [26]. The addition of ascorbic acid to the test and the observation of increased activity strongly indicates the presence of LPMOs since LPMOs are activated in the presence of an electron donor, which is, in this case, ascorbic acid. Comparing the activity with and without ascorbic acid, we noted an increase of 17.84% in the activity (Figure 4), which suggests the presence of LPMOs in the obtained enzymatic cocktail.

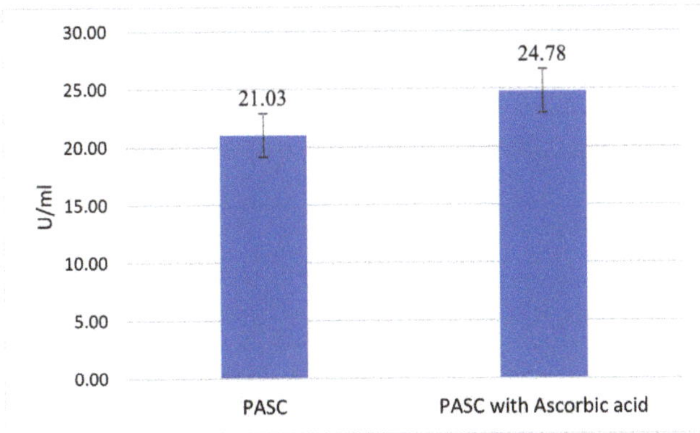

Figure 4. Increase in the saccharification power of the *A. terreus* NIH2624 cocktail on phosphoric acid swollen cellulose (PASC) by the addition of an electron donor (ascorbic acid) for lytic polysaccharide monooxygenases (LPMOs).

The boosting effect of LPMOs acting on cellulose in synergy with cellulases is well known but little explored for *A. terreus* enzymes. The *A. terreus* genome harbors 12 genes that encode LPMOs, making it an important source for this type of enzyme [27]. The diversity of proteins produced by *A. terreus* was also evidenced in SDS-PAGE gels, where it was possible to observe band patterns of different sizes and intensities. The bands with the greatest intensities correspond to approximate sizes of 100 and 25 KDa, which are frequently sizes associated with cellobiohydrolases, beta-glucosidases (~100 KDa) [28], xylanases, endoglucanases and LPMOs (~25 kDa) [29].

4. Conclusions

A. terreus NIH2624 showed a higher production of cellulase and hemicellulose enzymes compared to the other tested fungi. When this microorganism was grown in the production medium containing sugarcane bagasse (as a carbon source) and rice bran (as a nitrogen source), it showed improved production of endoglucanases, exoglucanases and xylanases. Furthermore, the enzyme cocktail from *A. terreus* NIH2624 showed mainly xylanase activity, with a potential to complement cellulolytic enzyme cocktails of other known fungi, such as *T. reesei* and other *Aspergillus* species. *A. terreus* NIH2624 showed higher endoglucanase and CBH activities compared to the enzyme activity reported with other filamentous fungi. In addition to these enzymes, activities for cellobiohydrolases, β-xylosidases, arabinofuranosidases and LPMOs were also obtained. The use of this fungus shows promising results for holistic cellulolytic enzyme cocktail production in lignocellulose biorefineries, supporting the effective hydrolysis of biomasses to produce second-generation sugars.

Author Contributions: E.A.K. collected samples, performed experiments, and wrote the first draft of the manuscript; J.V. performed the enzyme assays, analyzed the data and jointly wrote the manuscript; S.S.d.S. analyzed data and reviewed the manuscript; A.P.I. analyzed the data and edited the original draft; F.S. provided microbial strains and performed the LPMOS analysis; A.K.C. planned the experiments, supervised the research, and reviewed and edited the manuscript. All authors have read and agreed to the published version of the manuscript.

Funding: This research received no external funding.

Data Availability Statement: The original contributions presented in the study are included in the article, further inquiries can be directed to the corresponding author.

Acknowledgments: A.K.C. gratefully acknowledges The Brazilian National Council for Scientific and Technological Development (CNPq), Brazil for the scientific productivity program (Process number: 309214/2021-1) and the Universidad de los Andes FAPA project PR.3.2024.10867.

Conflicts of Interest: The authors declare no conflict of interest.

References

1. Reis, C.E.R.; Libardi, N., Jr.; Bento, H.B.S.; de Carvalho, A.K.F.; de Souza Vandenberghe, L.P.; Soccol, C.R.; Aminabhavi, T.M Chandel, A.K. Process strategies to reduce cellulase enzyme loading for renewable sugar production in biorefineries. *Chem. En J.* **2023**, *451*, 138690. [CrossRef]
2. Ellilä, S.; Fonseca, L.; Uchima, C.; Cota, J.; Goldman, G.H.; Saloheimo, M.; Sacon, V.; Siika-aho, M. Development of a low-cos cellulase production process using Trichoderma reesei for Brazilian biorefineries. *Biotechnol. Biofuels* **2017**, *10*, 30. [CrossRef]
3. Sasaki, C.; Matsuura, K.; Omasa, T. Cellulase production on easy-to-handle solid media containing agricultural waste and it application for enzymatic hydrolysis of cellulosic biomass. *Biomass Convers. Biorefinery* **2022**. [CrossRef]
4. Arora, R.; Reis, C.E.R.; Chandel, A.K. Key takeaways on the cost-effective production of cellulosic sugars at large scale. *Processe* **2024**, *12*, 1496. [CrossRef]
5. Chandel, A.K.; Garlapati, V.K.; Jeevan Kumar, S.P.; Hans, M.; Singh, A.K.; Kumar, S. The role of renewable chemicals and biofuel in building a bioeconomy. *Biofuels Bioprod. Biorefining* **2020**, *14*, 830–844. [CrossRef]
6. Bhardwaj, N.; Kumar, B.; Agrawal, K.; Verma, P. Current perspective on production and applications of microbial cellulase A review. *Bioresour. Bioprocess.* **2021**, *8*, 95. [CrossRef] [PubMed]
7. Lynd, L.R.; Weimer, P.J.; van Zyl, W.H.; Pretorius, I.S. Microbial Cellulose Utilization: Fundamentals and Biotechnology. *Microbic Mol. Biol. Rev.* **2002**, *66*, 506–577. [CrossRef] [PubMed]
8. Beeson, W.T.; Vu, V.V.; Span, E.A.; Phillips, C.M.; Marletta, M.A. Cellulose Degradation by Polysaccharide Monooxygenase *Annu. Rev. Biochem.* **2015**, *84*, 923–946. [CrossRef]
9. Florencio, C.; Cunha, F.M.; Badino, A.C.; Farinas, C.S.; Ximenes, E.; Ladisch, M.R. Secretome analysis of Trichoderma reesei an Aspergillus niger cultivated by submerged and sequential fermentation processes: Enzyme production for sugarcane bagass hydrolysis. *Enzym. Microb. Technol.* **2016**, *90*, 53–60. [CrossRef]
10. Mandels, M.; Weber, J. The Production of Cellulases. In *Cellulases and Their Applications*; American Chemical Society: Washingtor DC, USA, 1969; pp. 391–414. [CrossRef]
11. Triola, M.F. *Introdução à Estatística*; LTC: Rio de Janeiro, Brazil, 2008.
12. Sluiter, A.; Hames, B.; Ruiz, R.; Scarlata, C.; Sluiter, J.; Templeton, D.; Crocker, D. *Determination of Structural Carbohydrates an Lignin in Biomass*; NREL/TP-510-42618; National Renewable Energy Laboratory: Golden, CO, USA, 2008.
13. Lowry, O.H.; Rosebrough, N.J.; Farr, A.L.; Randall, R.J. Protein measurement with the Folin phenol reagent. *J. Biol. Chem.* **1951** *193*, 265–275. [CrossRef]
14. Kumar, S.; Paritosh, K.; Pareek, N.; Chawade, A.; Vivekanand, V. De-construction of major Indian cereal crop residues through chemical pretreatment for improved biogas production: An overview. *Renew. Sustain. Energy Rev.* **2018**, *90*, 160–170. [CrossRef
15. Sharma, S.; Nandal, P.; Arora, A. Ethanol Production from NaOH Pretreated Rice Straw: A Cost-Effective Option to Manage Ric Crop Residue. *Waste Biomass Valorization* **2019**, *10*, 3427–3434. [CrossRef]
16. Vaibhav, V.; Vijayalakshmi, U.; Roopan, S.M. Agricultural waste as a source for the production of silica nanoparticles. *Spectrochim Acta Part A Mol. Biomol. Spectrosc.* **2015**, *139*, 515–520. [CrossRef]
17. Hui, Y.S.; Amirul, A.A.; Yahya, A.R.M.; Azizan, M.N.M. Cellulase production by free and immobilized *Aspergillus terreus*. *World J Microbiol. Biotechnol.* **2010**, *26*, 79–84. [CrossRef]
18. Shahriarinour, M.; Wahab, M.N.; Mohamad, R.; Mustafa, S.; Ariff, A.B. Effect of medium composition and cultural condition or cellulase production by *Aspergillus terreus*. *Afr. J. Biotechnol.* **2011**, *10*, 7459–7467.
19. Sohail, M.; Ahmad, A.; Khan, S.A. Production of cellulase from *Aspergillus terreus* MS105 on crude and commercially purifiec substrates. *3 Biotech* **2016**, *6*, 103. [CrossRef] [PubMed]
20. Silva, J.C.R.; Salgado, J.C.S.; Vici, A.C.; Ward, R.J.; Polizeli, M.L.T.M.; Guimarães, L.H.S.; Furriel, R.P.M.; Jorge, J.A. A nove Trichoderma reesei mutant RP698 with enhanced cellulase production. *Braz. J. Microbiol.* **2020**, *51*, 537–545. [CrossRef]
21. Corrêa, C.L. Estudo do Transcritoma Global do Fungo *Aspergillus terreus* Quando Cultivado em Resíduos Agroindustriais [Study of Global Transcriptome Analysis of *Apergillus terrus* Fungus when Cultivated on Agro-Industrial Residues] [Programa de Pós-Graduação em Biologia Molecular-Post-Graduation Program of Molecular Biology at University of Brasilia, Brazil]. Ph.D Thesis, Universidade de Brasília, Brasília, Brazil, 2016.
22. Latifian, M.; Hamidiesfahani, Z.; Barzegar, M. Evaluation of culture conditions for cellulase production by two *Trichoderma reese* mutants under solid-state fermentation conditions. *Bioresour. Technol.* **2007**, *98*, 3634–3637. [CrossRef]
23. Kupski, L.; Pagnussatt, F.A.; Buffon, J.G.; Furlong, E.B. Endoglucanase and Total Cellulase from Newly Isolated *Rhizopus oryzae* and *Trichoderma reesei*: Production, Characterization, and Thermal Stability. *Appl. Biochem. Biotechnol.* **2014**, *172*, 458–468 [CrossRef]

Vieira, M.M.; Kadoguchi, E.A.; Segato, F.; da Silva, S.S.; Chandel, A.K. Production of cellulases by *Aureobasidium pullulans* LB83: Optimization, characterization, and hydrolytic potential for the production of cellulosic sugars. *Prep. Biochem. Biotechnol.* **2021**, *51*, 153–163. [CrossRef]
Zhao, C.; Deng, L.; Fang, H. Mixed culture of recombinant *Trichoderma reesei* and *Aspergillus niger* for cellulase production to increase the cellulose degrading capability. *Biomass Bioenergy* **2018**, *112*, 93–98. [CrossRef]
Gonçalves, A.L.; Cunha, P.M.; da Silva Lima, A.; dos Santos, J.C.; Segato, F. Production of recombinant lytic polysaccharide monooxygenases and evaluation effect of its addition into *Aspergillus fumigatus* var. niveus cocktail for sugarcane bagasse saccharification. *Biochim. Biophys. Acta—Proteins Proteom.* **2023**, *1871*, 140919. [CrossRef] [PubMed]
Velasco, J.; Sepulchro, A.G.V.; Higasi, P.M.R.; Pellegrini, V.O.A.; Cannella, D.; de Oliveira, L.C.; Polikarpov, I.; Segato, F. Light Boosts the Activity of Novel LPMO from *Aspergillus fumigatus* Leading to Oxidative Cleavage of Cellulose and Hemicellulose. *ACS Sustain. Chem. Eng.* **2022**, *10*, 16969–16984. [CrossRef]
Tiwari, P.; Misra, B.N.; Sangwan, N.S. β -Glucosidases from the fungus Trichoderma: An efficient cellulase machinery in biotechnological applications. *Biomed Res. Int.* **2013**, *2013*, 203735. [CrossRef]
Støpamo, F.G.; Røhr, Å.K.; Mekasha, S.; Petrović, D.M.; Várnai, A.; Eijsink, V.G.H. Characterization of a lytic polysaccharide monooxygenase from *Aspergillus fumigatus* shows functional variation among family AA11 fungal LPMOs. *J. Biol. Chem.* **2021**, *297*, 101421. [CrossRef]

processes

Article

Enzymatic Pretreatment of Slaughterhouse Wastewater: Application of Whole Lipolytic Cells of *Rhizopus oryzae* Produced from Residual Vegetable Oil

Willian S. M. Reis [1], Heitor B. S. Bento [2,*], Ana K. F. Carvalho [3,*] and Ernandes B. Pereira [4]

1 Department of Biotechnology, Engineering School of Lorena, University of Sao Paulo, Lorena 12602-810, SP, Brazil; willian.matias@usp.br
2 Department of Engineering of Bioprocesses and Biotechnology, School of Pharmaceutical Sciences, São Paulo State University (UNESP), Araraquara 14800-903, SP, Brazil
3 Department of Basic and Environmental Sciences, Engineering School of Lorena, University of Sao Paulo, Lorena 12602-810, SP, Brazil
4 Faculty of Pharmaceutical Sciences, Federal University of Alfenas, Alfenas 37130-001, MG, Brazil; ernandes.pereira@unifal-mg.edu.br
* Correspondence: heitor.bento@unesp.br (H.B.S.B.); anacarvalho@usp.br (A.K.F.C.)

Abstract: This study assessed the application of whole lipolytic cells in the pretreatment of slaughterhouse wastewater to reduce its lipid content. The fungal biomass of *Rhizopus oryzae* was evaluated in the hydrolysis of slaughterhouse wastewater containing high lipid concentrations, focusing on the biomass's concentration and the effect of using an emulsifier and surfactant. The use of the whole-cells lipase of *Rhizopus oryzae* grown in a residual vegetable oil medium proved effective in the hydrolysis of slaughterhouse wastewater, generating concentrations of free fatty acids (FFA) ranging from 40.36 to 90.14 mM. The action of lipase in the hydrolysis of slaughterhouse residues indicated its effectiveness in pretreating lipid-rich liquid residues, potentially boosting the microbiota of this anaerobic treatment. The results showed that lipase activity without surfactant exhibited a similar performance to that of Triton X-100 in the hydrolysis of liquid residues. However, the combination of lipase and surfactant could represent a promising strategy to optimize free fatty acid production from slaughterhouse residues, strengthening anaerobic treatment processes and potentially enhancing the overall efficiency of waste management systems.

Keywords: whole cell; lipase; hydrolysis

1. Introduction

The growth of the world's population, coupled with improving economies in developing countries, is rapidly driving global food demand [1]. The global supply of meat is expected to increase to meet rising demand, reaching 377 million tons by 2031, with Brazil as one of the primary leaders in the global export of poultry and beef. This growth is driven by a favorable exchange rate and an abundance of grains for feed. Brazil is predicted to maintain and expand its position as the leading exporter of poultry and beef throughout the projected period, until 2031 [2]. The growth in meat production is driving the increase in slaughterhouse waste, raising concerns about waste generation and pollution.

Slaughterhouses are places where animals are slaughtered to meet the growing demand for meat for human consumption. The waste generated in these places is mostly byproducts from animal processing [3,4]. The meat processing industry is a major consumer of fresh water (2.5 to 40 m^3 of water per metric ton of produced meat), generating large volumes of effluents. Their composition includes fats, proteins, and fibers from the slaughtering process. These residues contain contaminants, primarily blood, stomach, and intestinal mucus, along with high levels of organic products, microorganisms, and cleaning agents [5,6].

The wastewater discharged after proper treatment must comply with local regulations for the safe disposal of effluents. In the case of organically rich wastewater, and especially effluents from slaughterhouses, biological treatment is generally preferred over other treatment options like electrocoagulation, membrane separation, and advanced oxidation [7]. However, waste from dairies, slaughterhouses, and meat processing, while rich in nutrients and organic matter, also contains high levels of fats and oils, which are challenging for biological treatments. A prior separation of fats and oils is essential to optimize this treatment [8].

Anaerobic digestion is a biological treatment method employed for wastewater from slaughterhouses. It involves a community of microorganisms performing different tasks to convert organic matter into biogas. Initially, organic macromolecules (carbohydrates, lipids, proteins) undergo hydrolysis into monomers. These monomers are subsequently converted into volatile fatty acids during the acidogenesis phase. Following acidogenesis, acetogenesis occurs, where volatile fatty acids are transformed into acetic acid, carbon dioxide, and hydrogen gas (H_2). Finally, in methanogenesis, acetic acid and a portion of H_2 are converted into methane and carbon dioxide [9–11].

The primary reason for the removal of oils and fats is that an excess of these elements can accumulate on the sludge surface, reducing the transfer rates of soluble substrates to biomass and oxygen due to aerobic microorganisms. This inhibits sludge activity and the development of filamentous microorganisms, hindering sludge settlement and leading to biomass losses due to reactor overflows. Additionally, long-term challenges such as blockage occurrence and the generation of unpleasant odors caused by fats and oils in wastewater are evident [8,12,13]. Therefore, the pretreatment process is necessary to hydrolyze fats and oils, enhancing efficiency of the subsequent biological treatment of wastewater.

The inhibitory effects of lipids during the biodigestion process are also associated with interference in the electron transport chain, by compromising nutrient uptake, inhibiting specific enzymatic activities, or generating peroxidation products. Since inhibition is reversible, it is partially driven by the adsorption of lipid onto biomass. Methanogenic activity can resume once the lipids accumulated in the biomass are progressively metabolized through pretreatments [14,15].

An alternative treatment method involves utilizing a biochemical pathway, and particularly lipases, due to their clean application and low environmental impact. Lipases can be applied to a large variety of biotechnological applications, including the treatment of effluents with high fat contents. The biological anaerobic treatment of this kind of effluent has some problems, which are caused by high fat contents [16]. Thus, a pretreatment with enzymes has been proposed as an alternative or a complement to conventional biological processes. Another alternative is the use of biosurfactants that can make fats and oils more available to microbial biomasses [17].

The application of lipases in the treatment of wastewater with a high lipid content faces challenges such as high production costs, purification issues, and stability concerns under ideal conditions. Specific operational conditions and factors like a high organic load, temperature, pH, and the presence of metallic ions can limit the effectiveness of lipases in treating industrial effluents. Although enzyme immobilization may enhance their stability, its scalability for wastewater treatment is still underexplored [16]. Low-cost enzymatic products for wastewater treatment are crucial because high-cost commercial lipase products would render the process economically unfeasible. As an alternative, there is the production of whole-cell biomass from filamentous fungi with high lipolytic activity, which can be used for wastewater treatment, eliminating the need for the recovery and purification of these enzymes [18].

Given the scarcity of studies involving the application of commercial lipases and/or lipolytic cells in the pretreatment of slaughterhouse wastewater, the current study aims to produce whole cells with high hydrolytic activity and evaluate their application in the pretreatment of poultry and swine slaughterhouse wastewater (*SSW*) to hydrolyze the present oils and fats. The fungus *Rhizopus oryzae* has been highlighted as one of the most promising fungal species in the production of whole cells with mycelium-bound lipase, as well as for its efficient application in the hydrolysis reactions of substrates containing different compositions of fatty acids. This underscores the potential of this fungus to be applied as a biocatalyst in the pretreatment of slaughterhouse wastewater.

2. Materials and Methods

2.1. Microorganism

The strain used was *Rhizopus oryzae* CCT3759, obtained from the André Tosello Tropical Research and Technology Foundation (Campinas, SP, Brazil). In order to obtain and maintain culture spores, fungal cells had been previously inoculated on Sabouraud agar medium under aseptic conditions. The cultures were incubated at 30 °C for 72 h or until they reached their highest sporulation status.

2.2. Materials

Sabouraud agar (HIMEDIA®, Kennett, MI, USA); soy peptone (HIMEDIA®, Kennett, MI, USA); magnesium sulfate heptahydrate (Vetec®, Duque de Caxias, Brazil); olive oil (Carbonell®, Córdoba, Spain); gum arabic powder (Dinâmica®, Indaiatuba, Brazil); disodium phosphate dibasic (Dinâmica®, Indaiatuba, Brazil); sodium hydroxide (Vetec®, Duque de Caxias, Brazil); ethyl alcohol; Triton™ X-100 (70% v/v) (Vetec®, Duque de Caxias, Brazil); acetone (Synth®, Diadema, Brazil); phenolphthalein (Synth®, Diadema, Brazil). Slaughterhouse wastewater (SWW) was obtained from a local slaughterhouse farm focused on poultry and pork production (Alfenas, Minas Gerais, Brazil). *SWW* samples were collected before and after, from a flotation tank located at the treatment plant itself. Slaughterhouse waste samples were then frozen and maintained at −20 °C prior to utilization.

2.3. Physicochemical Characterization of *SWW*

For the characterization of the raw effluent, its pH, total solids (TSs), fixed solids (TFSs), volatile solids (TVSs), free fatty acids (FFAs), acidity index, and saponification were analyzed. All analyses were conducted following procedures outlined in the Standard Methods for the Examination of Water and Wastewater [19]. Fatty acid composition of both synthetic and real effluents was determined as fatty acid methyl ester (FAME) by gas chromatography according to the American Oil Chemists' Society (AOCS) official method [20].

2.4. Enzymatic Activity

Mycelium-bound lipase activity was assessed in terms of its dry biomass concentration (g L^{-1}) and hydrolytic activity (U g^{-1}), using the method of olive oil emulsion hydrolysis. Enzyme activity (U g^{-1}) is defined as the amount of dry biomass required to release 1 µmol of free fatty acids per minute under experimental conditions (0.1 g of biomass at a 37 °C reaction temperature, 100 mM sodium phosphate buffer, and at a pH of 7.0 for a 5 min reaction) [18].

2.5. Culture Medium and Conditions

The culture medium consisted of 30 g L^{-1} of residual frying oil after vacuum filtration, 70 g L^{-1} of soy peptone, 1 g L^{-1} of $NaNO_3$, 1 g L^{-1} of KH_2PO_4, and 0.5 g L^{-1} of $MgSO_4 \cdot 7H_2O$, all previously autoclaved (121 °C for 15 min) [18]. After autoclaving, Erlenmeyer flasks were cooled and olive oil (3% w/v) was added in a sterile manner. The cultures were established in 250 mL Erlenmeyer flasks containing 100 mL of autoclaved medium and inoculated with a suspension of 1×10^6 spores at 30 °C, with orbital agitation at 180 rpm. The spore concentration was determined by counting the cells in a Neubauer chamber using an Olympus® binocular microscope (Hicksville, NY, USA). At the end of the cultivation, the produced biomass was separated from its medium by vacuum filtration, washed with water and acetone and quantified for its hydrolytic activity [21]. Subsequently, the fungal biomass was stored at 4 °C before use.

2.6. Enzymatic Pretreatment of Slaughterhouse Wastewater in Stirred Tank Reactors

In 250 mL glass-lined reactors, 100 mL of SWW was used as substrate for a hydrolysis reaction that used 2.0 g of dry biomass. The tests were carried out at 40 °C and 600 rpm of mechanical agitation, which was carried out using a suspended agitator motor with a steel helical impeller for up to 24 h. A 50:50 (v/v) mixture of acetone and ethanol was added to the aliquots (0.5 g), which were removed periodically, and the FFA concentration was quantified by titration with 20 mM of sodium hydroxide (NaOH) solution using phenolphthalein as the indicator. The concentration of free fatty acids (FFAs) (mM) was calculated using Equation (1).

$$\text{FFA (mM)} = \frac{(V_a - V_b) * C_{NaOH} * 1000}{m} \tag{1}$$

where V_a is the volume of NaOH in the sample (mL); V_b is the volume of NaOH in the control (mL); C_{NaOH} is the molar concentration of NaOH (20 mM); and m is the sample mass (0.5 g).

Initial reaction rates were analyzed by the formation of FFAs (mM) in the initial 12 h of the reaction. Results were plotted using the software Origin Pro version 5.0 so as to obtain a linear equation for the initial hydrolysis reaction rates of the *SWW*.

2.7. Variation in Biomass Mass during the Enzymatic Pretreatment of Slaughterhouse Wastewater

Different initial masses of fungal biomass were evaluated as biocatalysts in the enzymatic pretreatment of *SWW*. The assessed masses were 0.5, 1.0, and 2.0 g of dry biomass, corresponding to an average hydrolytic activity of 100, 200, and 400 U, respectively. The produced lipase was evaluated for its ability to generate free fatty acids (FFAs) by hydrolyzing the triglycerides present in the *SWW* pretreatment.

2.8. Evaluation of pH Adjustment in the Enzymatic Pretreatment of SWW

The need for a pH adjustment was assessed to determine the influence of the natural pH of slaughterhouse wastewater on the performance of the produced lipase. The pH was adjusted using a concentrated HCl solution to reach a pH of 6.0, known as the optimal pH for the activity of the lipase bound to the mycelium of the fungus *Rhizopus oryzae* CCT3759.

2.9. Influence of Surfactants and Emulsifiers on the Enzymatic Pretreatment of SWW

The influence of a surfactant and an emulsifier was evaluated in the enzymatic pretreatment in association with lipase-catalyzed hydrolysis from *Rhizopus oryzae* biomasses. Both the surfactant and the emulsifier were assessed at a concentration of 3% (w/v), with Triton X-100 evaluated as the surfactant and arabic gum as the emulsifier. Both were applied individually and in combination.

3. Results and Discussion

3.1. Characterization of Slaughterhouse Wastewater

The meat industry utilizes significant amounts of water in its industrial processes, generating considerable volumes of effluents characterized by high organic loads and concentrations of suspended solids. The characteristics of these effluents vary depending on the type of industrial process adopted [3,5]. In this study, effluent from slaughterhouses (birds and pigs), collected from two sectors of the slaughterhouse treatment plant, was used. One sample was taken from raw slaughterhouse wastewater (*RSWW*), prior to it entering the main flotation tank, and another sample from within the flotation tank (*SWWF*). The characterization of both samples is described in Table 1.

Table 1. Physical–chemical characterization of raw slaughterhouse wastewater (*RSWW*) and slaughterhouse wastewater obtained from the flotation tank (*SWWF*).

Parameter	*RSWW*	*SWWF*
pH	6.15 ± 0.06	7.59 ± 0.35
Total solids (mg L^{-1})	18,609.17 ± 661.98	13,530 ± 1300.34
Total fixed solids (mg L^{-1})	3665.83 ± 195.26	2545.33 ± 139.91
Total volatile solids (mg L^{-1})	14,943.33 ± 698.49	10,984.67 ± 57.18
Free fatty acids (%)	0.75 ± 0.031	0.51 ± 0.023
Acidity index (mgKOH g^{-1})	1.64 ± 0.689	1.11 ± 0.051
Saponification (mgKOH g^{-1})	5.38 ± 0.39	4.32 ± 0.77
Fatty acids composition (%)		
Caprylic acid—C8:0	4.30	-
Myristic acid—C14:0	4.49	-
Palmitic acid—C16:0	30.00	30.71
Stearic acid—C18:0	0.34	-
Oleic acid—C18:1	31.30	35.92
Linoleic acid—C18:2	29.56	33.37
Average molecular weight of FFAs (g mol^{-1})	273.79	265.68

The results in Table 1 highlight that the evaluated *RSWW* presented higher concentrations of solids, as previously reported in the literature [7,22]. A lower concentration of solids is evident in the effluent collected directly from the flotation tank (*SWWF*), showing a decrease in total solids of 27.29% (from 18,609.17 to 13,530 mg L^{-1}), total fixed solids of 30.57% (from 3665.83 to 2545.33 mg L^{-1}), and total volatile solids of 26.49% (from 14,943.33 to 10,984.67 mg L^{-1}). Similarly, the measurements of the free fatty acids, acidity index, and saponification also decreased due to their treatment in the flotation tank. The primary flotation treatment system is well known for separating suspended and/or fatty particles from the effluent, directly influencing its physicochemical parameters that are related to oils and fats [23].

Regarding the distribution of fatty acids within the triacylglycerols present in the lipids of *RSWW*, the raw effluent contained saturated fatty acids that were not detected in the *SWWF*, such as caprylic acid (4.30%), myristic acid (4.49%), and stearic acid (0.34%); whereas the most concentrated saturated fatty acid, palmitic acid (30%), was also quantified in the *SWWF* with similar concentrations (30.71%). Despite the low percentage of fatty acids present in the flotation tank wastewater, higher concentrations of unsaturated fatty acids were found in this sample; 35.92% and 33.57% for oleic and linoleic acids, respectively. The higher proportions of oleic (31.30–35.92%) and palmitic (30–30.71%) acids were expected, as these acids are reported to be the most abundant in food processing effluents, such as slaughterhouse effluent [13].

3.2. The Influence of Biocatalyst Mass on the Hydrolysis of Slaughterhouse Wastewater

In order to evaluate the influence of the mass of catalytic biomass added on the hydrolysis process, that is, how much hydrolytic activity will be generated, different masses of biomass were evaluated, using 0.5, 1.0, and 2.0 g of dry mycelium. The obtained results are shown in Figure 1.

The higher hydrolytic activity provided was effective for the RSSW (Figure 1A), with a maximum FFA formation of 85.34 ± 2.59 mM. However, a better performance was observed in the system with 1.0 g of biomass, showing a profile similar to the 2.0 g system up to 10 h of operation. However, after this time, the FFA formation stabilized for 1.0 g of the biocatalyst, reaching only 68.12 ± 0.36 mM, whereas the reaction with 2.0 g of biomass increased from 60.84 to 85.34 mM.

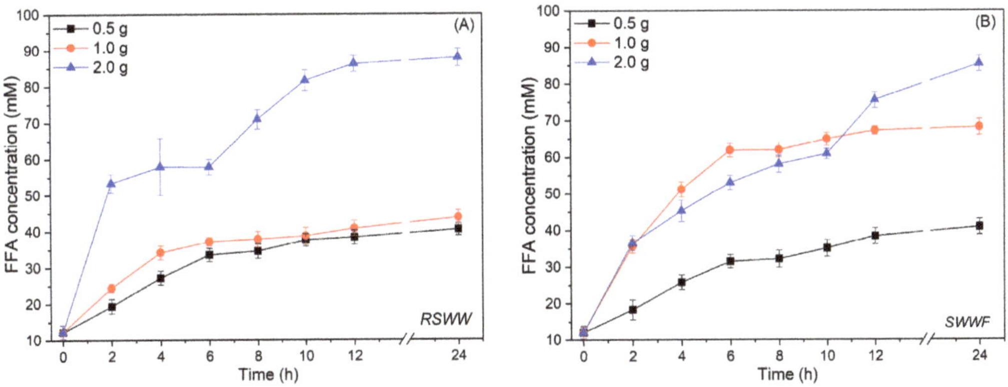

Figure 1. Evaluation of the initial mass of the biocatalyst in the formation of FFA from the hydrolysis of *RSWW* (**A**) and *SWWF* (**B**).

In the hydrolysis process of *SWWF* (Figure 1B), a higher initial supply of hydrolytic activity favored a higher formation of FFAs within the first 2 h of the reaction, with an FFA value of 53.33 ± 2.53 mM, which reached 87.85 ± 0.28 mM. For the masses 0.5 g and 1.0 g, similar hydrolysis profiles were observed, with maximum FFA formation values of 40.46 ± 0.12 mM and 43.71 ± 1.59 mM, respectively. From 8 h of reaction time onwards, the system containing 2.0 g of biomass managed to produce twice the results of the other systems (0.5 g and 1.0 g) by the end of the 24 h operation. This result was expected, due to the known influence that the mass of a biocatalyst has on the efficiency of lipase in the hydrolysis reaction of an effluent [24,25]. In a study by Valladão, Freire, and Cammarota (2007) [26], the influence of enzymatic load was also evaluated in the pretreatment of a slaughterhouse effluent using a solid enzymatic pool (SEP) for the subsequent application of an anaerobic treatment. Within the adopted conditions, it was observed that an increase in the SEP led to a higher formation of fatty acids; however, a lower SEP concentration favored organic matter removal.

3.3. Influence of the Initial pH of Slaughterhouse Wastewater on the Hydrolysis Process

A pH adjustment of the *SWW* was evaluated to determine its influence on the enzyme's performance, as the pH of the reaction medium directly affects the stability of the lipase's molecular structure and, consequently, its catalytic power and, furthermore, studies generally adjust the pH to the optimum pH for the enzyme that is to be used. The pH of the SWW was adjusted to pH 6.0, which is the optimal pH of *Rhizopus oryzae* CCT3759 whole-cell lipase [13,26,27].

Based on the results of the influence of pH shown in Figure 2, the hydrolysis profile presented by *RSWW* with an adjusted pH was slightly higher than that presented by the original pH (6.15) for up to 12 h of the reaction, but, after the first 12 h, the hydrolysis of *RSWW* without an adjustment of pH had a maximum FFA formation of 101.62 ± 0.75 mM, while the pH-adjusted system had a maximum conversion of 87.85 ± 0.48 mM. For *SWWF*, the hydrolyses without (pH 7.59) and with a pH adjustment were also similar, reaching values close to optimal FFA formation at the end of 24 h of reaction; values of 85.11 and 85.34 mM, respectively. The small differences in the hydrolysis process of the *SWWs* may have been due to the close pH values of the *SWWs* to the optimum pH of the enzyme, thus the lipase could act in a similar way in both study conditions; therefore, as the pH adjustment did not provide a considerable increase in the formation of FFAs, the other tests continued without pH adjustment.

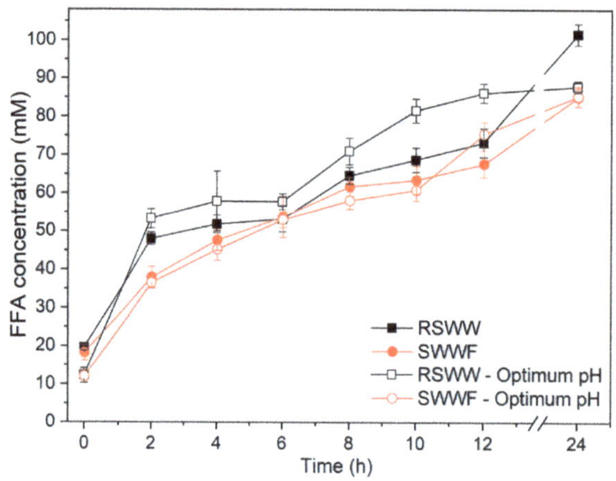

Figure 2. Influence of a pH adjustment on the enzymatic pretreatment.

3.4. *Influence of Surfactants and Emulsifiers on the Enzymatic Pretreatment*

Surfactants and emulsifiers can emulsify triglycerides, facilitating the action of lipases at the water/oil interface and thus accelerating the biodegradation process, eliminating the need for additional pretreatment processes to remove fats, which results in lower operating costs in the treatment of fatty effluents [28].

The surfactant Triton X-100 and the emulsifier arabic gum were evaluated in the enzymatic hydrolysis process of *RSWW* and *SWWF*. The formation of FFAs was evaluated during 24 h of reaction, as were the initial reaction rates of each system, and the results obtained are given in Figure 3 (*RSSW*) and Figure 4 (*SWWF*).

The results of the use of surfactant/emulsifier in the hydrolysis of *RSWW* (Figure 3A) show a higher production of FFAs with the use of Triton over 24 h of reaction. On the other hand, arabic gum was the system with the lowest FFA production among the systems evaluated, reaching 84.34 ± 0.50 mM. The hydrolysis generated only by the action of lipase linked to the mycelium of *Rhizopus oryzae* was superior to that achieved by arabic gum + lipase during the first 12 h of reaction, with a production of 88.97 ± 0.19 mM, which came close to the 24 h reaction value of FFA obtained by the arabic gum + lipase system, which was a maximum volume of FFAs of 90.14 ± 0.48 mM.

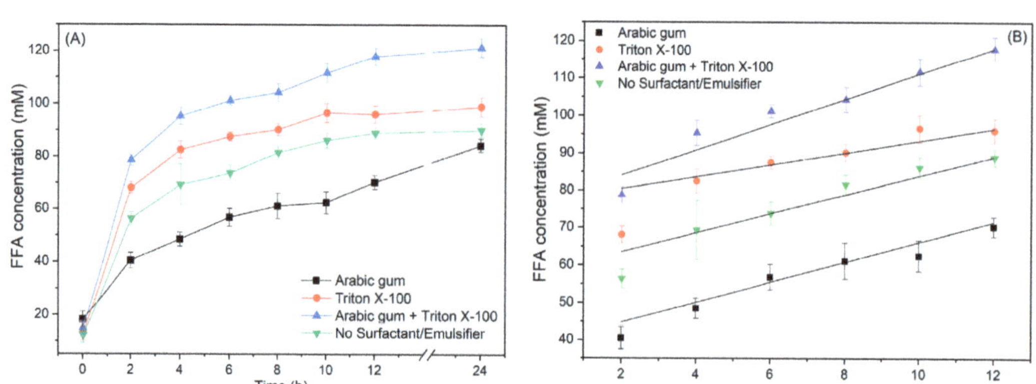

Figure 3. Influence of the use of surfactant and emulsifier on the *RSWW* pretreatment. (**A**) FFA concentration over 24 h; (**B**) FFA concentration in the first 12 h for initial hydrolysis rate analysis.

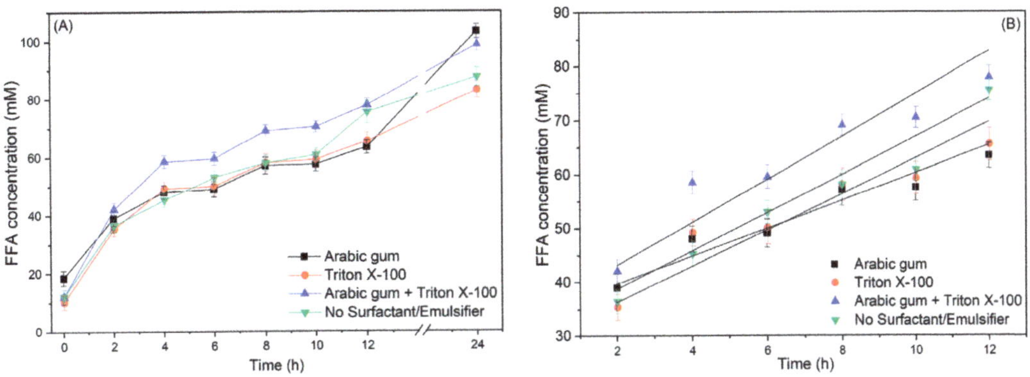

Figure 4. Influence of the use of surfactant and emulsifier on the *SWWF* pretreatment. (**A**) FFA concentration over 24 h; (**B**) FFA concentration in the first 12 h for initial hydrolysis rate analysis.

The combined action of Triton X-100 + arabic gum resulted in the highest FFA formation when compared to the use of the biosurfactant and emulsifier individually, with a maximum production of 121.38 ± 1.60 mM. This outcome may indicate that both components promoted a better stabilization of the formed emulsions, consequently enhancing the lipase-catalyzed reaction. The data also suggest that, at least within the initial 12 h of the reaction, Triton X-100 might have had a better role in stabilizing the water/lipid interface. This is supported by the fact that, when used individually, Triton X-100 led to higher FFA formation compared to the results of arabic gum alone.

The initial rates promoted in the *RSWW* (Figure 3B and Table 2) also indicate the positive effect of the combined use of Triton X-100 and arabic gum, as this showed the highest initial reaction rate (3.38 mM/h). It is worth noting that the reaction rates exhibited by the biosurfactant were the lowest obtained, with an FFA formation rate of 1.60 mM/h, possibly due to the smaller difference in FFA production over the reaction time (from 68.08 to 98.91 mM).

Table 2. Initial reaction rates of the hydrolysis of *RSWW* catalyzed by whole-cell *Rhizopus oryzae* CCT3759.

SWW—Pre-Flotator	Maximum FFA Concentration (mM)	v (mM/h)
Arabic gum	107.11 ± 0.50	2.66
Triton X-100	84.34 ± 1.60	1.60
Arabic gum + Triton X-100	121.38 ± 1.63	3.38
No surfactant/emulsifier	90.14 ± 0.48	2.55

When evaluating the action of the surfactant and emulsifier in the hydrolysis process of the *SWW* collected from the flotation unit (Figure 4A), a different reaction profile is observed. The systems containing Triton X-100, arabic gum, and the system without surfactant/emulsifier showed similar hydrolysis profiles during the initial 10 h of the reaction, differing only after 12 h of reaction, with a maximum FFA production of 82.95 ± 0.15, 103.17 ± 0.40, and 87.43 ± 2.59 mM, respectively. This result might be due to the lower complexity of the fatty acids in the *SWWF* (Table 1) compared to the fatty acids in the *RSWW*, which exhibited a higher proportion of various saturated fatty acids (C 8:0, C 14:0, C16:0, C18:0), while the *SWWF* presented only one type of saturated fatty acid (C 18:0). Despite showing higher FFA production values in the first 12 h of the reaction, the reaction system containing Triton X-100 and arabic gum also remained close in performance to the results obtained in the other assays.

Observing the results presented in Figure 4 and Table 3, it is evident that similar initial reaction rates were obtained for the use of Triton X-100, Triton X-100 and arabic gum, and without the use of surfactant and emulsifiers, which show initial reaction rates of 3.34, 3.38, and 3.53 mM/h. It is noteworthy that higher reaction rates were achieved in the hydrolysis of *SWWF* than in *RSWW*, which could be attributed to the difference in the fatty acid composition of both wastewater types. The *SWWF*, besides having lower proportions of saturated fatty acids, also exhibits a higher proportion of unsaturated fatty acids. Studies on the lipase linked to *Rhizopus oryzae* CCT3759's mycelium demonstrate its higher selectivity for substrates with higher proportions of oleic and linoleic acid [29].

Table 3. Initial reaction rates of the hydrolysis of *SWWF* catalyzed by whole-cell *Rhizopus oryzae* CCT3759.

SWW—Flotator	Maximum FFA Concentration (mM)	v (mM/h)
Arabic gum	103.17 ± 0.40	2.57
Triton X-100	82.95 ± 0.15	3.34
Arabic gum + Triton X-100	98.59 ± 0.15	3.38
No surfactant/emulsifier	87.43 ± 2.59	3.53

The obtained results align with studies reported in the literature. In Damasceno et al.'s [28] study, the combined use of a biosurfactant produced from *Pseudomonas aeruginosa* PA1 and an enzymatic pool produced by solid-state fermentation with *Penicillium simplicissimum*, in the anaerobic treatment of a high-fat content effluent from a poultry slaughterhouse, resulted in higher lipid hydrolysis and subsequently led to higher specific methane production in the anaerobic treatment.

In studies by Alves et al. [18]; Braz et al. [27]; and Ferreira et al. [30], integral cells of filamentous fungi were evaluated for pretreating wastewater from the dairy industry. The mycelium of *Penicillium citrinum* and the fungus *Mucor circinelloides* were used as enzymatic catalysts in a hybrid treatment process during anaerobic treatment. It is also worth highlighting that filamentous fungi have a versatile ability to grow on a wide range of substrates and are able to produce lipolytic cells from several low-cost substrates, such as residual vegetable oil. The combined use of lipolytic integral cells not only increased the biodegradability of dairy waste but also promoted methane generation during treatment. These results highlight the potential of the biomass produced to act in tandem with the biodigestion process of oil- and fat-rich wastewater, such as that from slaughterhouses.

4. Conclusions

Whole cells of *Rhizopus oryzae*, with high hydrolytic activity, were effective in the hydrolysis process of slaughterhouse wastewater, resulting in FFA formations ranging between 40.36 and 90.14 mM. Adjusting the pH of wastewater to the optimal pH for lipase activity did not lead to a higher efficiency in FFA formation, as the original pH of the wastewater is close to the optimal pH for lipase. The performance of the lipase in the hydrolysis of *RSWW* and *SWWF* indicates its effectiveness in both residues, contributing to FFA production and potentially enhancing the anaerobic treatment microbiota. However, the use of a surfactant might be more suitable when combined with lipase in *RSWW* hydrolysis to increase FFA production, since our results indicated that the lipase's performance without the addition of surfactant was similar to its performance with Triton X-100 in *SWWF* hydrolysis. In conclusion, whole cells of *Rhizopus oryzae* demonstrate significant potential for application as an enzymatic pretreatment for slaughterhouse wastewater, aiming to enhance the biodegradability of the residue during the anaerobic digestion stage. Future studies will assess the optimization of the enzymatic pretreatment's efficiency at hydrolyzing slaughterhouse wastewater during the biodigestion process, as well as evaluate the toxicity parameters of slaughterhouse wastewater before and after the enzymatic pretreatment. The operational stability of lipase and its reaction conditions will be vital parameters to be assessed for the feasibility of applying lipolytic cells of *R. oryzae* to the enzymatic pretreatment of wastewater with high levels of oils and fats.

Author Contributions: Conceptualization, W.S.M.R., H.B.S.B., A.K.F.C. and E.B.P.; methodology, A.K.F.C. and E.B.P.; validation, H.B.S.B., A.K.F.C. and E.B.P.; formal analysis, W.S.M.R.; investigation, W.S.M.R.; resources, A.K.F.C. and E.B.P.; data curation, W.S.M.R., H.B.S.B., A.K.F.C. and E.B.P.; writing—original draft preparation, A.K.F.C., H.B.S.B., W.S.M.R. and E.B.P.; writing—review and editing, W.S.M.R., H.B.S.B., A.K.F.C. and E.B.P.; visualization, W.S.M.R. and E.B.P.; supervision, A.K.F.C. and E.B.P.; project administration, A.K.F.C. and E.B.P.; funding acquisition, E.B.P. All authors have read and agreed to the published version of the manuscript.

Funding: This study was financed in part by the Coordenação de Aperfeiçoamento de Pessoal de Nível Superior—Brasil (CAPES)—Finance Code 001. W.S.M.R. thanks CAPES for his student fellowship.

Data Availability Statement: Data are available on request.

Conflicts of Interest: The authors declare no conflicts of interest.

References

1. Lee, S.Y.; Stuckey, D.C. Separation and biosynthesis of value-added compounds from food-processing wastewater: Towards sustainable wastewater resource recovery. *J. Clean. Prod.* **2022**, *357*, 131975. [CrossRef]
2. OECD/FAO. *OECD-FAO Agricultural Outlook 2022–2031*; OECD Publishing: Paris, France, 2022. [CrossRef]
3. Al-Gheethi, A.; Ma, N.L.; Rupani, P.F.; Sultana, N.; Yaakob, M.A.; Mohamed, R.M.S.R.; Soon, C.F. Biowastes of slaughterhouses and wet markets: An overview of waste management for disease prevention. *Environ. Sci. Pollut. Res.* **2021**, 1–14. [CrossRef] [PubMed]
4. Chowdhury, M.W.; Nabi, M.N.; Arefin, M.A.; Rashid, F.; Islam, M.T.; Gudimetla, P.; Muyeen, S.M. Recycling slaughterhouse wastes into potential energy and hydrogen sources: An approach for the future sustainable energy. *Bioresour. Technol. Rep.* **2022**, *19*, 101133. [CrossRef]
5. Bustillo-Lecompte, C.F.; Mehrvar, M. Slaughterhouse wastewater characteristics, treatment, and management in the meat processing industry: A review on trends and advances. *J. Environ. Manag.* **2015**, *161*, 287–302. [CrossRef]
6. Ramadan, L.; Deeb, R.; Sawaya, C.; El Khoury, C.; Wazne, M.; Harb, M. Anaerobic membrane bioreactor-based treatment of poultry slaughterhouse wastewater: Microbial community adaptation and antibiotic resistance gene profiles. *Biochem. Eng. J.* **2023**, *192*, 108847. [CrossRef]
7. Aziz, A.; Basheer, F.; Sengar, A.; Khan, S.U.; Farooqi, I.H. Biological wastewater treatment (anaerobic-aerobic) technologies for safe discharge of treated slaughterhouse and meat processing wastewater. *Sci. Total Environ.* **2019**, *686*, 681–708. [CrossRef] [PubMed]
8. Cheng, D.; Liu, Y.; Ngo, H.H.; Guo, W.; Chang, S.W.; Nguyen, D.D.; Zhang, S.; Luo, Y.; Liu, Y. A review on application of enzymatic bioprocesses in animal wastewater and manure treatment. *Bioresour. Technol.* **2020**, *313*, 123683. [CrossRef] [PubMed]
9. Jankowska, E.; Sahu, A.K.; Oleskowicz-Popiel, P. Biogas from microalgae: Review on microalgae's cultivation, harvesting and pretreatment for anaerobic digestion. *Renew. Sustain. Energy Rev.* **2017**, *75*, 692–709. [CrossRef]
10. Vasco-Correa, J.; Khanal, S.; Manandhar, A.; Shah, A. Anaerobic digestion for bioenergy production: Global status, environmental and techno-economic implications, and government policies. *Bioresour. Technol.* **2018**, *247*, 1015–1026. [CrossRef]
11. Bhunia, S.; Bhowmik, A.; Mukherjee, J. Waste management of rural slaughterhouses in developing countries. In *Advanced Organic Waste Management*; Elsevier: Amsterdam, The Netherlands, 2022; pp. 425–449. [CrossRef]
12. Cammarota, M.C.; Freire, D.M.G. A review on hydrolytic enzymes in the treatment of wastewater with high oil and grease content. *Bioresour. Technol.* **2006**, *97*, 2195–2210. [CrossRef]
13. Valladão, A.B.G.; Torres, A.G.; Freire, D.M.G.; Cammarota, M.C. Profiles of fatty acids and triacylglycerols and their influence on the anaerobic biodegradability of effluents from poultry slaughterhouse. *Bioresour. Technol.* **2011**, *102*, 7043–7050. [CrossRef] [PubMed]
14. Palatsi, J.; Affes, R.; Fernandez, B.; Pereira, M.A.; Alves, M.M.; Flotats, X. Influence of adsorption and anaerobic granular sludge characteristics on long chain fatty acids inhibition process. *Water Res.* **2012**, *46*, 5268–5278. [CrossRef]
15. Carrere, H.; Antonopoulou, G.; Affes, R.; Passos, F.; Battimelli, A.; Lyberatos, G.; Ferrer, I. Review of feedstock pretreatment strategies for improved anaerobic digestion: From lab-scale research to full-scale application. *Bioresour. Technol.* **2016**, *199*, 386–397. [CrossRef]
16. Nimkande, V.D.; Bafana, A. A review on the utility of microbial lipases in wastewater treatment. *J. Water Process Eng.* **2022**, *46*, 102591. [CrossRef]

17. Radha, P.; Prabhu, K.; Jayakumar, A.; AbilashKarthik, S.; Ramani, K. Biochemical and kinetic evaluation of lipase and biosurfacta assisted ex novo synthesis of microbial oil for biodiesel production by *Yarrowia lipolytica* utilizing chicken tallow. *Process Biochem.* **2020**, *95*, 17–29. [CrossRef]
18. Alves, A.M.; de Moura, R.B.; Carvalho, A.K.; de Castro, H.F.; Andrade, G.S. *Penicillium citrinum* whole-cells catalyst for th treatment of lipid-rich wastewater. *Biomass Bioenergy* **2019**, *120*, 433–438. [CrossRef]
19. Rice, E.W.; Bridgewater, L.; American Public Health Association (Eds.) *Standard Methods for the Examination of Water and Wastewate* American Public Health Association: Washington, DC, USA, 2012. Available online: https://www.standardmethods.org/doi/book/10.2105/SMWW.2882 (accessed on 1 November 2023).
20. AOCS Press. *AOCS-American Oil Chemists' Society Official Methods and Recommended Practices of the AOCS*, 5th ed.; AOCS Pres Champaign, IL, USA, 2004. Available online: https://www.aocs.org/attain-lab-services/methods?SSO=True (accessed o 1 November 2023).
21. De Castro, T.F.; Cortez, D.V.; Gonçalves, D.B.; Bento, H.B.; Gonçalves, R.L.; Costa-Silva, T.A.; Gambarato, B.C.; de Carvalho, A.K. Biotechnological valorization of mycelium-bound lipase of *Penicillium purpurogenum* in hydrolysis of high content lauric aci vegetable oils. *Process Saf. Environ. Prot.* **2022**, *161*, 498–505. [CrossRef]
22. Lima, J.A.M.; Magalhães Filho, F.J.C.; Constantino, M.; Formagini, E.L. Techno-economic and performance evaluation of energ production by anaerobic digestion in Brazil: Bovine, swine and poultry slaughterhouse effluents. *J. Clean. Prod.* **2020**, *277*, 12333 [CrossRef]
23. De Nardi, I.R.; Fuzi, T.P.; Del Nery, V. Performance evaluation and operating strategies of dissolved-air flotation system treatin poultry slaughterhouse wastewater. *Resour. Conserv. Recycl.* **2008**, *52*, 533–544. [CrossRef]
24. Duarte, J.G.; Silva, L.L.S.; Freire, D.M.G.; Cammarota, M.C.; Gutarra, M.L.E. Enzymatic hydrolysis and anaerobic biologica treatment of fish industry effluent: Evaluation of the mesophilic and thermophilic conditions. *Renew. Energy* **2015**, *83*, 455–46 [CrossRef]
25. Qiao, H.; Zhang, F.; Guan, W.; Zuo, J.; Feng, D. Optimisation of combi-lipases from *Aspergillus niger* for the synergistic an efficient hydrolysis of soybean oil. *Anim. Sci. J.* **2017**, *88*, 772–780. [CrossRef]
26. Valladão, A.B.G.; Freire, D.M.G.; Cammarota, M.C. Enzymatic pre-hydrolysis applied to the anaerobic treatment of effluents fron poultry slaughterhouses. *Int. Biodeterior. Biodegrad.* **2007**, *60*, 219–225. [CrossRef]
27. Braz, C.A.; Carvalho, A.K.; Bento, H.B.; Reis, C.E.; De Castro, H.F. Production of value-added microbial metabolites: Oleaginou fungus as a tool for valorization of dairy by-products. *BioEnergy Res.* **2020**, *13*, 963–973. [CrossRef]
28. Damasceno, F.R.; Cammarota, M.C.; Freire, D.M. The combined use of a biosurfactant and an enzyme preparation to treat a effluent with a high fat content. *Colloids Surf. B Biointerfaces* **2012**, *95*, 241–246. [CrossRef] [PubMed]
29. Matias, A.B.; de SM Reis, W.; Costa-Silva, T.A.; Bento, H.B.; de Carvalho, A.K.; Pereira, E.B. Mycelium-bound lipase as skillfu biocatalysts: Production of fatty acid concentrates from waste oils for the food industry. *Catal. Commun.* **2023**, *184*, 10678 [CrossRef]
30. Ferreira, T.F.; Santos, P.A.; Paula, A.V.; de Castro, H.F.; Andrade, G.S. Biogas generation by hybrid treatment of dairy wastewate with lipolytic whole cell preparations and anaerobic sludge. *Biochem. Eng. J.* **2021**, *169*, 107965. [CrossRef]

processes

ticle

ylanase Production by *Cellulomonas phragmiteti* Using ignocellulosic Waste Materials

ta Buda [1], Tünde Fekete [1], Ornella M. Ontañon [2], Eleonora Campos [2] and Csaba Fehér [1,*]

1 Biorefinery Research Group, Department of Applied Biotechnology and Food Science, Faculty of Chemical Technology and Biotechnology, Budapest University of Technology and Economics, Szent Gellért tér 4, H-1111 Budapest, Hungary; kata.buda.bk@gmail.com (K.B.); fek.tundike@gmail.com (T.F.)

2 Instituto de Agrobiotecnología y Biología Molecular (IABIMO), Instituto Nacional de Tecnología Agropecuaria (INTA), Consejo Nacional de Investigaciones Científicas y Técnicas (CONICET), De los Reseros y N. Repetto s/n, Hurlingham, Buenos Aires B1686IGC, Argentina; ontanon.ornella@inta.gob.ar (O.M.O.); campos.eleonora@inta.gob.ar (E.C.)

* Correspondence: feher.csaba@vbk.bme.hu; Tel.: +36-1-463-2843

Abstract: Lignocellulosic biomass holds promise as a renewable feedstock for various applications, but its efficient conversion requires cost-effective degradation strategies. The main objective of this study was to investigate the effect of the growth conditions of *Cellulomonas phragmiteti* in the production of (hemi)cellulosic supernatants. To meet this aim, different lignocellulosic residues were used as carbon sources for growth using defined mineral or nutritive culture media. Cell-free culture supernatants with xylanolytic activity were produced in all the conditions evaluated, but the highest xylanase activity (15.3 U/mL) was achieved in Luria–Bertani (LB) medium containing 1% waste paper. Under these conditions, almost negligible β-glucosidase, cellobiohydrolase, β-xylosidase, and α-arabinofuranosidase activity was detected. The xylanolytic supernatant showed tolerance to salt and displayed maximal catalytic efficiency at pH 6 and 45 °C, along with good activity in the ranges of 45–55 °C and pH 5–8. As it showed good stability at 45 °C, the supernatant was employed for the hydrolysis of birchwood xylan (50 g/L) under optimal conditions, releasing 10.7 g/L xylose in 72 h. Thus, *C. phragmiteti* was found to produce a xylanolytic enzymatic supernatant efficiently by utilizing the cheap and abundant lignocellulosic residue of waste paper, and the produced supernatant has promising attributes for industrial applications.

Keywords: bacterial enzymes; hemicellulases; enzyme fermentation; waste valorization; xylanase characterization; enzyme stability

1. Introduction

Lignocellulosic biomass serves as a vital and abundant resource for the production of renewable energy and bioproducts [1]. Industrial and agricultural residues and forestry by-products usually remain as non-utilized lignocellulosic wastes; however, they contain substantial amounts of carbohydrates and other valuable substances. In order to valorize these waste materials into energy and bioproducts in an environmentally friendly way, the efficient biodegradation of their carbohydrates is crucial [2]. However, due to the complex polymeric structure of lignocellulose, accessing the sugar components that built it up is still a major challenge [3]. Lignocellulose represents a complex highly recalcitrant structure comprising cellulose surrounded by hemicellulose and lignin. The complete deconstruction of lignocellulose requires the simultaneous action of many different enzymes, such as cellulases, hemicellulases, and lignin-decomposing enzymes [4,5]. Among hemicellulases, xylanases hold particular significance due to the abundance of xylan hemicellulose in many lignocellulosic residues having great potential for biotechnological valorization. Xylanases are hydrolytic enzymes that break xylan into smaller units [6]. These enzymes have wide applications in the food industry, animal feed production, and paper manufacturing, and in recent years, they have garnered increasing attention for their role in the production of biofuels and biochemicals [7,8].

Bacterial xylanase production using lignocellulosic waste shows great promise for cost-effective enzyme production. Various microbial strains, including *Clostridium* sp., *Cellulomonas* sp., *Bacillus* sp., *Thermomonospora* sp., and *Streptomyces* sp., exhibit the capability to produce xylanases that can be used in lignocellulose degradation [9]. *Bacillus* species such as *B. halodurans* and *B. pumilus* have been widely studied as efficient xylanolytic enzyme producers [10,11]. *Cellulomonas* strains are also promising sources of xylanolytic enzymes [12]; however, less attention has been dedicated to them so far. *Cellulomonas fimi* and *Cellulomonas flavigena* have been reported to have extracellular xylanase activity [9,13]. Fourteen genes potentially encoding xylanases were found in the *C. flavigena* genome sequence [14]. Ontañon et al. investigated *C. fimi* and *Cellulomonas* sp. B6 and their use for biomass deconstruction. Different lignocellulosic residues (e.g., sweet corn cob, waste paper, and wheat bran) were tested. Both strains showed high xylanolytic activity in culture supernatants, although *Cellulomonas* sp. B6 was more efficient [15].

The production of xylanases from lignocellulosic waste materials offers a dual advantage. On one hand, it utilizes inexpensive substrates, thereby reducing the production costs of xylanases significantly; on the other hand, it contributes to the eco-friendly management of these waste materials [16,17]. Lignocellulosic wastes such as agricultural residues, forestry by-products, and industrial remnants can serve as low-cost and efficient carbon sources for the production of xylanases and other high-value enzymes [18]. Xylanases produced from lignocellulosic wastes can have versatile applications. They can be employed in different tasks in various industries, including biofuel production, bioremediation, and food processing, making them a high-value bioproduct that can be produced from low-cost substrates [19].

In this context, this article explores the production of bacterial xylanases by *Cellulomonas phragmiteti* using lignocellulosic residues as substrates and characterizes the produced enzyme preparation (e.g., pH and temperature optima, NaCl tolerance, thermostability).

2. Materials and Methods

2.1. Microorganism

Cellulomonas phragmiteti NCAIM B.02303 was kindly donated by the National Collection of Agricultural and Industrial Microorganisms (Budapest, Hungary). *Cellulomonas phragmiteti* is a Gram-positive, facultatively anaerobic bacterium with motile rod-shaped cells. Its colonies on King's B agar plates became smooth, yellow to pale orange, and circular within 3 days of cultivation at 25 °C [20]. *C. phragmiteti* grows well at 15–37 °C (optimum: 25 °C) and pH 7.0–9.0 (optimum: pH 8.0), and in the presence of 2.0–7.0 $w/v\%$ NaCl (optimum: 5.0 $w/v\%$) [20]. *C. phragmiteti* was maintained at 4 °C on Luria–Bertani (LB) [21] agar in Petri dishes containing the following: 0.5 $w/w\%$ yeast extract, 1 $w/w\%$ NaCl, 1 $w/w\%$ trypton and 1.5 $w/w\%$ agar.

2.2. Lignocellulosic Materials

Wheat bran (WB), brewer's spent grain (BSG), rye bran (RB), rice straw (RS), distillers dried grain with solubles (DDGS), and waste paper (WP) were examined as carbon sources for xylanase enzyme production by *C. phragmiteti*. Xylan from birchwood was used in enzymatic hydrolysis tests, and it was purchased from Sigma-Aldrich (St. Louis, MI, USA). The WB was provided by Gyermelyi Ltd. (Gyermely, Hungary); the RB was kindly donated by the Research Group of Cereal Science and Food Quality, Budapest University of Technology and Economics (Budapest, Hungary); the RS was provided from Suranaree University of Technology (Nakhon Ratchasima, Thailand); the DDGS was provided from Hungarian University of Agriculture and Life Science (Budapest, Hungary); and the WP was provided from a local paper and stationery shop (Budapest, Hungary). The WP consisted of unprinted, pressed, recycled, corrugated cardboard paper sheets, which were cut into small pieces (smaller than 0.5 cm) (Figure S2), mixed with distilled water to set

10 w/w% dry matter content, homogenized with a hand blender for 10 min, and autoclaved (121 °C) for 30 min before being used to prepare culture media for cell cultivation or xylanase fermentation. WB, BSG, RB, and DDGS were mixed with distilled water to set 10 w/w% dry matter and then autoclaved (121 °C) for 30 min before being used in preparing culture media for cell cultivation or xylanase fermentation. RS was cut into small pieces (0.5 cm) and then prepared in the same way as WB, BSG, RB, and DDGS before being used in preparing culture media for cell cultivation or xylanase fermentation. The structural carbohydrates (glucan, xylan, and arabinan) and acid-insoluble solids (Klason lignin) of WP were determined according to the method of the National Renewable Energy Laboratory (DEN, USA) [22]. The structural carbohydrate analysis of WP was carried out in triplicate (Table 1).

Table 1. Relative structural carbohydrate and acid-insoluble solid contents of waste paper. Average values and standard deviations (indicated in parentheses) were calculated from triplicates.

	Percentage of Dry Matter
Glucan	56 (0.7)
Xylan	15 (0.24)
Arabinan	0 (0.0)
Acid-insoluble solid (Klason lignin)	10.5 (0.07)

2.3. Enzyme Production in Shake Flask

C. phragmiteti was grown on culture media containing LB medium (10 g/L tryptone, 5 g/L yeast extract, 10 g/L NaCl) or minimal medium (MM) (1.67 g/L K_2HPO_4, 0.87 g/L KH_2PO_4, 0.05 g/L NaCl, 0.1 g/L $MgSO_4 \times 7H_2O$, 0.04 g/L $CaCl_2$, 0.004 g/L $FeCl_3$, 0.005 g/L $Na_2MoO_4 \times 2H_2O$, 0.01 g/L biotin, 0,02 g/L nicotinic acid, 0.01 g/L pantothenic acid, 1 g/L NH4Cl, 1 g/L yeast extract), all supplemented with 1 w/w% of different lignocellulosic carbon sources (WP, WB, BSG, RB, RS, and DDGS) which were pretreated according to the method described in Section 2.2. Culture media (LB or MM media with lignocellulosic carbon sources) were sterilized in autoclave at 121 °C for 20 min. Starter cultures were obtained by inoculating colonies (from agar plates) in 10 mL LB medium and incubating them at 30 °C and 220 rpm for 72 h in 100 mL flasks closed by cotton plugs. Cultures for enzyme production (fermentations) were inoculated from the starter cultures to set an initial cell concentration that corresponded to an optical density (OD) of 0.05. Fermentation experiments were performed in 25 mL culture media poured into 100 mL shake flasks at 30 °C and 220 rpm for 72 h. Fermentations were performed in triplicate. After 72 h, the fermentation media were vacuum-filtered to separate the solids (cells and biomass) from the fermentation supernatant, which was stored at −18 °C until further use.

2.4. Enzymatic Activity Measurements

The xylanase and carboxymethyl cellulase (CMC-ase) activities of the fermentation supernatants were assayed in test tubes by using a beechwood xylan (Sigma-Aldrich, St. Louis, MI, USA) suspension (1 w/w%) or wheat arabinoxylan (arabinoxylan for reducing sugar assays, low-viscosity arabinoxylan, medium-viscosity arabinoxylan, and high-viscosity arabinoxylan (Megazyme, Bray, Ireland)) solutions (1 w/w%) and CMC solution (2 w/w%) as substrates, respectively [23]. For these assays, 0.75 mL of appropriately diluted cell-free fermentation broths were added to 0.75 mL of each substrate prepared in citrate buffer (0.1 M, pH 6). The assays were carried out at 45 °C with magnetic stirring for 10 min. Reducing sugars released during the assay were measured by the dinitrosalicylic acid (DNS) method [24] using glucose or xylose standard curves.

The β-glucosidase, cellobiohydrolase, β-xylosidase, and α-arabinofuranosidase activities were assayed using 5 mM p-nitrophenyl-β-D-glucopyranoside (pNPG), p-nitrophenyl-β-D-cellobiosid (pNPC), p-nitrophenyl-β-D-xylopyranoside (pNPX), and p-nitrophenyl-α-L-arabinofuranoside substrates, respectively, according to previously established protocols [25]. Briefly, the reactions were performed in test tubes; 1 mL p-nitrophenyl reagent was added to 0.1 mL appropriately diluted cell-free fermentation broth. The reactions were performed at 45 °C with magnetic stirring for 10 min. The reactions were stopped with 2 mL sodium carbonate (1 M), and absorbance was determined at a wavelength of 400 nm using a spectrophotometer. A p-nitrophenol (pNP) curve was used as a standard.

All enzymatic assays were conducted in triplicate, and control enzymes without a substrate and a substrate without an enzyme were included. In all cases, one international unit (U) was defined as the amount of enzyme required to release 1 μmol of product per minute under the assay conditions.

2.5. Investigation of the Time Dependence of Xylanase Production

Xylanase production by *C. phragmiteti* as a function of the fermentation time was also investigated. Enzyme production was performed on WP as a carbon source as described in Section 2.3. Xylanase activity production was monitored by daily sampling (0, 24, 48, 72, 96 h). Xylanase activity measurements were performed at each sampling time as described in Section 2.4.

2.6. Total Protein Content Assay

The total protein contents of the fermentation supernatants were quantified by the Bradford assay. The Bradford reagent contained 10 mg Coomassie blue, 5 mL 96 *w*/*w*% ethanol, and 10 mL 85 *w*/*w*% phosphoric acid, and the solution was completed to 100 mL with distilled water. The assay was performed in test tubes. Next, 5 mL of reagent was added to a 0.1 mL sample and carefully homogenized. Two minutes later, the absorbance was determined at a wavelength of 595 nm using a spectrophotometer. A bovine serum albumin curve was used as a standard.

2.7. Effect of NaCl Concentration on Xylanase Activity and Xylanase Production

The effect of NaCl concentration on xylanase activity was investigated using cell-free fermentation broth derived from fermentations containing 1 *w*/*w*% WP as a carbon source. Xylanase enzyme activity was measured according to the method previously described in Section 2.4., with small modifications. Different amounts of NaCl (25 g/L, 50 g/L, 100 g/L, 150 g/L, and 200 g/L) were added to the reaction mixtures. The NaCl stock solutions were made using citrate buffer (0.1 M, pH 6). The effect of NaCl concentration on xylanase production by *C. phragmiteti* was investigated by adjusting 100 g/L NaCl concentration during xylanase fermentation on 1 *w*/*w*% WP.

2.8. Determination of the pH and Temperature Optima of the Produced Xylanolytic Supernatant

The pH and temperature optima of the xylanase activity produced by *C. phragmiteti* on WP were investigated. Regarding pH, the experiments were carried out within a pH range of 3–11, at 45 °C. At pH 3, pH 4, pH 5, and pH 6, citrate buffer (0.1 M) was used. At pH 6, pH 7, and pH 8, phosphate buffer (0.1 M) was used, and at pH 8, pH 9, pH 10, and pH 11, carbonate buffer (0.1 M) was used. The substrate suspension (1 *w*/*w*% beechwood xylan) was made using the same buffers as the reaction mixture. Regarding temperature, 25 °C, 35 °C, 45 °C, 55 °C, 65 °C, 75 °C, and 85 °C were applied during the enzyme activity measurements in citrate buffer (0.1 M, pH 6).

2.9. Enzyme Stability Measurement

Enzyme stability tests were carried out at two different temperatures (45 °C and 55 °C) at four different pH values: pH 5, pH 6, pH 7, and pH 8. Enzymatic stability was measured in 0.05 M phosphate buffers. The produced xylanase-containing supernatant was diluted (tenfold) with buffer, and the diluted enzyme solutions were incubated at elevated temperatures (45 °C or 55 °C; 220 rpm for 72 h). During the test, samples were taken at 0, 3, 24, 48, and 72 h to perform xylanase activity measurements.

2.10. Enzymatic Hydrolysis of Xylan

An enzymatic hydrolysis experiment was performed on xylan from birchwood by using the supernatant derived from the fermentation using 1 *w*/*w*% WP as a carbon source. Five *w*/*w*% dry matter of xylan and 10 U/mL of the produced xylanases were set in the enzymatic hydrolysis. The hydrolysis reaction was carried out at 45 °C, pH 6, and 150 rpm for 72 h. Daily sampling was conducted from the reaction mixture. The supernatants were separated by vacuum filtration through a nylon filter (0.2 μm pore size), and they were analysed by high-performance liquid chromatography (HPLC) for xylose. HPLC analysis was performed by using a BioRad (Hercules, CA, USA) Aminex HPX-87H (300 × 7.8 mm) column equipped with a Micro-Guard Cation H+ Refill Cartridge (300 × 4.6 mm) pre-column at 65 °C and a refractive index detector. The eluent was 5 mmol/L sulphuric acid at a flow rate of 0.5 mL/min. The injection volume was 40 μL. To determine the total solubilized xylose content (including the xylose liberated in monomer and oligomer forms), an oligomer hydrolysis step was also carried out with the 72 h samples. They were mixed with sulphuric acid solution (8 *w*/*w*%) at a volume ratio of 1:1 and treated at 120 °C in an autoclave for 15 min to decompose oligosaccharides prior to HPLC analysis.

3. Results and Discussion

3.1. Effect of Different Media and Lignocellulosic Culture Substrates on the Production of a Xylanolytic Enzymatic Supernatant

The use of lignocellulosic residues and by-products as substrates for microbial growth has the advantage of being an inexpensive strategy for inducing the production of enzymes [26]. Thus, *C. phragmiteti* was cultivated on LB and MM media supplemented with different lignocellulosic residues as carbon sources, which were WP, WB, BSG, RB, RS, and DDGS. After 72 h cultivation, the xylanase activities were measured from each cell-free fermentation broth. The results of the xylanase activity measurements are shown in Figure 1.

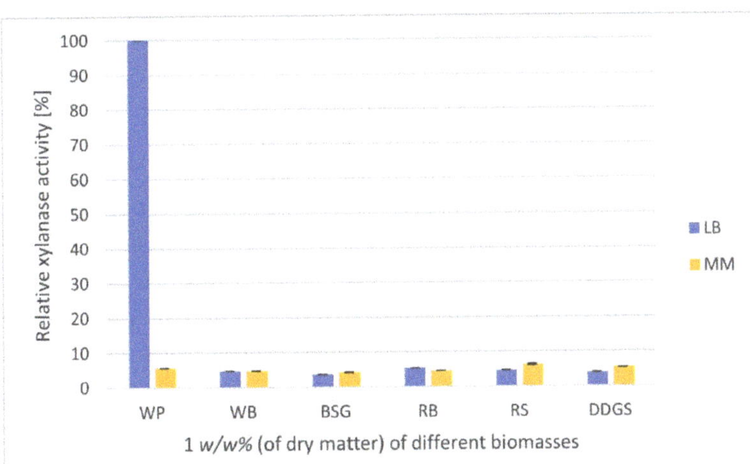

Figure 1. Relative xylanase activities [%] produced by *C. phragmiteti* on different carbon sources (1 *w*/*w*% of dry matter) in LB and MM media. WP—waste paper; WB—wheat bran; BSG—brewer's spent grain; RB—rye bran; RS—rice straw; DDGS—distillers dried grains with solubles. The average values of relative xylanase activity are presented with error bars representing the standard deviations of triplicate cultures in the case of WP and WB and duplicate cultures in the case of RB, RS, BSG, and DDGS.

The highest xylanase activity (referred to as 100% relative xylanase activity) was obtained using WP in LB medium. The relative xylanase activities were between 3.6–5.4% and 4.1–6.2% for the other biomasses (WB, BSG, RB, RS, and DDGS) in LB and MM media, respectively. The xylans of RB, RS, WB, DDGS (corn), and BSG are complex xylans highly decorated with side chains that frequently contain arabinofuranosyl units [27–30]. The complex structure of these xylans hinders the action of xylanases in the absence of accessory side chain-hydrolysing activities [10], which might have contributed to their limited potential for inducing xylanase enzyme production by *C. phragmiteti*. In contrast, the waste paper used in our study contained xylan (15% in terms of dry matter) without arabinose substitutions. In addition, during the process of paper production, the complex structure of its lignocellulose is disintegrated to decrease the lignin content, which could make the remaining cellulose and hemicellulose fractions of paper materials more accessible for hydrolytic enzymes. These factors could play a role in making waste paper an efficient substrate to induce the xylanase production of *C. phragmiteti*. Thus, LB medium containing WP was chosen for the following fermentations for xylanase activity production by *C. phragmiteti*. The use of *Cellulomonas* sp. B6 [31], *C. fimi* [32], *C. flavigena* [14], and *C. biazotea* [33] for the production of xylanases has also been reported. *Cellulomonas* sp. B6 and *C. fimi* showed high xylanase production on wheat bran and pre-treated waste paper, respectively [15], while xylanase production was mainly induced by sugarcane bagasse in the cases of *C. flavigena* and *C. biazotea* [14,33].

3.2. *Effect of the Amount of Waste Paper on Xylanase Production*

As WP was found to be the most appropriate substrate, the effect of WP concentration on the xylanolytic activity was investigated. The experiments were performed by using 0.5 w/w%, 1 w/w%, 1.5 w/w%, 2 w/w%, 2.5 w/w%, and 3 w/w% WP in LB medium. The highest xylanase activity (15.3 U/mL) was measured when 1 w/w% dry matter of WP was used for fermentation (Figure 2). Also, high xylanase activities were detected using 0.5 w/w% and 1.5% w/w% of WP. Between 1.5 w/w% and 2 w/w% of WP, a large decrease was observed in the produced xylanase activity (from 15 U/mL to 2.2 U/mL). Low xylanase activity values were measured in the case of 2 w/w% (2.2 U/mL), 2.5 w/w% (1.3 U/mL), and 3 w/w% (0.3 U/mL) of dry matter of WP (Figure 2). The supernatant derived from the fermentation using 1 w/w% WP showed the highest xylanase activity, so it was chosen for our further investigations.

C. fimi and *Cellulomonas* sp. B6 were also cultivated on pretreated waste paper (1 w/w% dry matter) by Ontañon et al. during an investigation of their xylanases enzyme production [15]. The highest xylanase activities achieved were 1.3 U/mL and 1.9 U/mL in the case of *C. fimi* and *Cellulomonas* sp. B6, respectively [15]. Thus, WP seems to be much more suitable for inducing the production of xylanolytic enzymes in *C. phragmiteti* than in the other two strains.

The decrease in the activity of the enzyme extract when the substrate concentration is above the optimal value has been related to the increase in viscosity and nutrient content in the medium. This inhibits microbial growth, lowering enzyme production. Some authors have reported that a lower substrate concentration is more effective for enzyme induction than higher concentrations [34,35]. This could also be an economic advantage in the large-scale production of hemicellulases at low substrate loads.

The xylanase activity of the supernatant derived from fermentation on 1 w/w% WP was measured by using different substrates, namely xylan from beechwood (BX) and wheat arabinoxylans with different viscosities (WAX-RS—arabinoxylan for reducing sugar assays; WAX-L—low-viscosity arabinoxylan; WAX-M—medium-viscosity arabinoxylan; WAX-H—high-viscosity arabinoxylan) (Figure 3). Relative activity values are displayed compared to that measured with beechwood xylan (100%). Higher xylanase activities were measured using WAX-RS and WAX-L (129% and 131%) compared to BX. Verma et al. indicated that enzymatic activity can vary significantly with the nature of the xylan used [36]. For example, the choice of the type of xylan is critical for obtaining positive clones during a functional screening. This phenomenon may be related to the good solubility and low viscosity of the listed arabinoxylan substrates, in contrast with xylan from beechwood, which is an insoluble substrate. In addition, BX contains glucuronic acid substitutions instead of arabinose. Regarding WAX-M and WAX-H, slightly lower xylanase activities were detected (102% and 108%) compared to WAX-RS and WAX-L. This is probably because the viscosity of the substrates can affect the enzyme activity [37]. Thus, the higher viscosity values of WAX-M and WAX-H could have caused the lower xylanase activities [35].

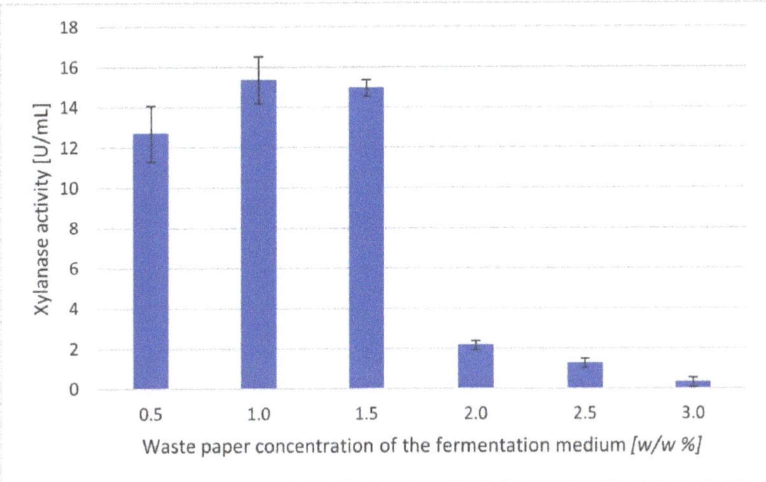

Figure 2. Xylanase activities [U/mL] obtained in LB medium containing different amounts of waste paper (*w*/*w*% of dry matter). The average values of xylanase activity are presented with error bars representing the standard deviations of triplicate cultures.

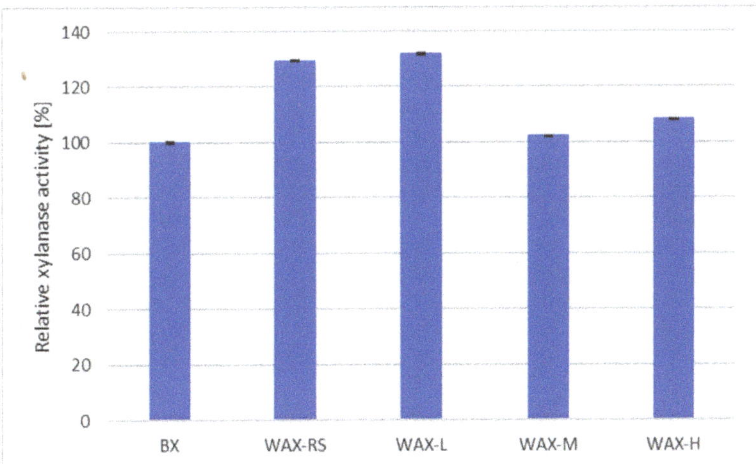

Figure 3. Relative xylanase activities [%] obtained from fermentation by using *C. phragmiteti* in LB medium containing 1 *w*/*w*% of dry matter waste paper. Xylanase activity measurements were performed using different xylan substrates: BX—xylan from beechwood, WAX-RS—wheat arabinoxylan for reducing sugar assays, WAX-L—low-viscosity wheat arabinoxylan, WAX-M—medium-viscosity wheat arabinoxylan, WAX-H—high-viscosity wheat arabinoxylan. Average values of xylanase activity are presented with error bars representing standard deviations of triplicates.

Side enzymatic activities (Table 2) were also measured from cell-free supernatants produced by *C. phragmiteti* on 1 *w*/*w*% WP, such as β-glucosidase, β-xylosidase, cellobiohydrolase, CMC-ase, and α-arabinofuranosidase. β-xylosidase had the highest side activity (0.61 U/mL) (Table 2). β-xylosidase activity was around six times higher compared to that of β-glucosidase (0.11 U/mL), cellobiohydrolase (0.12 U/mL), and CMC-ase (0.15 U/mL). Arabinofuranosidase had the lowest side activity (0.007 U/mL). These results prove that the most dominant enzyme, in terms of activity, in the extracellular extracts of *C. phragmiteti* is xylanase, and other lignocellulolytic enzyme activities are also present. Similarly, Akermann et al., Mayorga-Reyes et al., and Ontañon et al. reported a mainly xylanolytic activity in extracts of *Cellulomonas uda*, *C. flavigena*, *Cellulomonas* sp. B6, and *C. fimi* B-402 obtained by growth on lignocellulosic biomass [14,15,38]. These authors related this activity to the large amount of xylanases secreted by the bacteria under appropriate culture conditions.

Table 2. β-glucosidase, β-xylosidase, cellobiohydrolase, carboxymethyl-cellulase, and α-arabinofuranosidase enzyme activities (U/mL) of a fermentation supernatant obtained by *C. phragmiteti* on 1 *w*/*w*% waste paper in LB. The average values and standard deviations (indicated in parentheses) were calculated from triplicates.

Enzyme Activity	U/mL
β-glucosidase	0.11 (0.010)
β-xylosidase	0.61 (0.013)
Cellobiohydrolase	0.12 (0.005)
Carboxymethyl-cellulase	0.15 (0.032)
α-arabinofuranosidase	0.007 (0.002)

In comparison, *C. biazotea* showed higher cellulolytic activity than xylanolytic activity by growing on CMC and sugarcane bagasse in a study by Saratale et al. [33]. CMC and sugar cane bagasse induced cellulase (endoglucanase, exoglucanase, and cellobiase) production [33]. In our study, *C. phragmiteti* growing on WP showed much lower cellulase (CMC-ase) (Table 2) activity than the reported activity of *C. biazotea* on sugarcane bagasse and CMC. Thus, future investigations could focus on investigating whether other carbon sources would induce preferable cellulase production in *C. phragmiteti.*

3.3. Investigation of the Time Curve of Xylanase Activity Production

An investigation of the produced xylanase activity as a function of fermentation time was carried out for 96 h (Figure S1). Relative activity values at all sampling times are displayed compared to the values measured after 96 h (100%). Xylanase activity was barely observed after one day (1.5%). The production of xylanases started after 24 h. The relative activity of xylanase increased from 1.5% to 67.5% and 91.8% after 48 and 72 h, respectively. The production rate of xylanase activity greatly slowed down between 72 and 96 h; so, 72 h fermentation time was selected. Amaya-Delgado et.al. studied the induction of xylanase activity by sugar cane bagasse in *C. flavigena*, and they found that the maximal xylanase activity was reached after 100 h, but the most significant increase in the xylanase activity occurred between 60 and 82 h [39], which is in line with our results.

3.4. Effect of NaCl Concentration on Xylanase Activity

According to Rusznyák, *C. phragmiteti* is a salt-tolerant bacterium [20], so xylanase activity production might also be affected by the NaCl content of the medium, and the produced xylanolytic supernatants might have a salt-tolerating attribute. In order to investigate these hypotheses, xylanase activity was examined by setting different concentrations of NaCl in the test tubes during the measurement of xylanase enzyme activity, and xylanase enzyme production was measured in the presence of a high concentration of NaCl (100 g/L) in the fermentation medium.

The effect of NaCl concentration on the measured xylanase activity is represented in Figure 4. The xylanase activity slightly decreased by increasing the concentration of

NaCl. Using 25 g/L (0.43 M) NaCl, 13 U/mL xylanase activity was measured, which is slightly lower compared to that measured without NaCl (15.3 U/mL). Similar values were obtained by using 50 g/L (0.86 M) and 100 g/L (1.71 M) of NaCl; these values were 12.4 U/mL and 12.2 U/mL, respectively. The xylanase activity further decreased to 11.6 U/mL and 10.3 U/mL by using 150 g/L (2.56 M) and 200 g/L (3.42 M) of NaCl, respectively. The lowest activity was 10.3 U/mL (achieved by using 200 g/L NaCl), which is approximately 32.7% decrease compared to the highest (15.3 U/mL) activity measured without NaCl. The presence of high salt concentrations can negatively influence xylanase activity; however, our results suggests that the xylanases produced by *C. phragmiteti* are quite resistant against high NaCl concentrations, which might be useful in specific applications. An important challenge of industrial biotechnology is the high consumption of fresh water. A practical solution is the replacement of fresh water with abundant seawater in water-intensive industrial settings such as lignocellulosic biorefineries. In this context, a halophilic xylanase has the potential for application in the enzymatic decomposition of plant biomass in seawater [40].

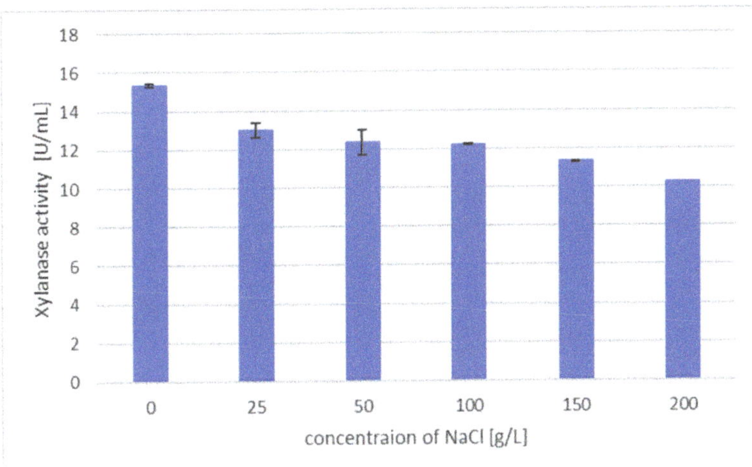

Figure 4. Xylanase activity values (U/mL) using different concentrations of NaCl (25 g/L, 50 g/L, 100 g/L, 150 g/L, and 200 g/L) during the xylanase assay (performed using cell-free fermentation broth of *C. phragmiteti* cultivation in LB medium containing 1 *w*/*w*% of waste paper).

Fermentation was also performed in the presence of high concentrations of NaCl to investigate the influence of salt on the enzyme production of *C. phragmiteti*. The xylanolytic activity dropped to 0.77 U/mL in the medium containing 100 g/L of NaCl despite the fact that *C. phragmiteti* can grow in a salty environment [20]. Rusznyák et al. stated that 5–7 *w*/*v*% NaCl concentration is optimal for its growth. Our measurements prove that xylanase production by *C. phragmiteti* is greatly inhibited by high salt concentrations. However, the xylanolytic supernatant seems to have salt-tolerant attributes. Since, in this study, only the use of 100 g/L NaCl was investigated during enzyme production, further experiments are needed to explore how the concentration of NaCl influences the xylanase production of *C. phragmiteti*.

3.5. Investigation of the pH and Temperature Optima of the Produced Xylanases

The determination of the operating range and optimal conditions of an enzyme of interest is crucial to specify its possible fields of application. Thus, the effect of pH and temperature on the xylanase activity produced by *C. phragmiteti* on 1 *w*/*w*% WP were investigated (Figure 5).

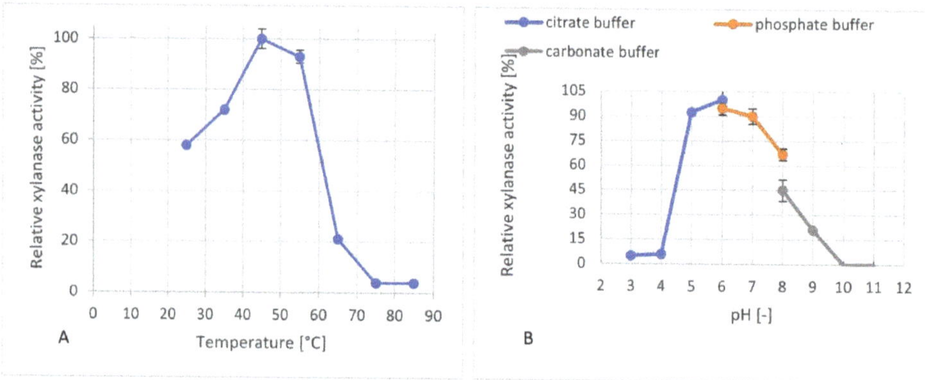

Figure 5. Relative xylanase activities at different temperatures (**A**) and pH values (**B**) measured in fermentation supernatant of *C. phragmiteti* cultivated in LB medium containing 1 *w*/*w*% of waste paper. Average values of relative xylanase activity are presented with error bars representing standard deviations of triplicates.

The results in Figure 5A,B represent the relative xylanase activity compared to the maximal activity, which was reached at 45 °C and pH 6 in citrate buffer. At 55 °C, an activity nearly as high as at 45 °C was detected (93%). At 25 °C, the relative xylanase activity was 58%. The xylanase activity experienced extreme decreases at higher temperatures (65 °C, 75 °C, 85 °C). Almost zero xylanase activity was measured at over 70 °C (Figure 5A).

The effect of pH on the xylanase activity was investigated by changing it between pH 3 and pH 11 and by using three types of buffers: citrate, phosphate, and carbonate (Figure 5B). At the pH values where a buffer change was necessary, xylanase activity was measured by using both buffers in order to monitor the effect of the type of buffer on the measured xylanase activity.

The maximal activity was detected at pH 6 (0.1 M) using citrate buffer (100%). The appropriate pH range for the produced xylanolytic supernatant was found to be pH 5–pH 8, which is a relatively wide range. A considerable effect regarding the type of buffers was observed between the phosphate and carbonate buffers at pH 8; higher xylanase activity was reached using the phosphate buffer (67%) compared to the use of the carbonate buffer (45%). At pH 10 and pH 11, xylanase activity was not measurable. Lisov et al. investigated the temperature and pH optima of xylanase enzymes derived from *C. flavigena* [13]. The optimum activity occurred at pH 7–7.5 and 40–50 °C, which is quite similar to the results observed for the xylanolytic supernatant of *C. phragmiteti*, whose optimal conditions were 45 °C and pH 6 (Figure 5).

3.6. Enzyme Stability Test

The stability of the xylanolytic supernatant of *C. phragmiteti* was evaluated during incubation at elevated temperatures and under different pH conditions. According to the previous results, the highest xylanase activities were detected between pH 5 and pH 8 and at 45 °C and 55 °C. Thus, the supernatant derived from fermentation on WP in LB medium by *C. phragmiteti* was incubated under these conditions for 72 h, and its residual activity was measured at different times. The results obtained at 45 °C are represented in Figure 6.

Relative activity values at all pHs are displayed compared to that of measured at pH 6 (100%) without previous incubation (0 h). The highest xylanase activity was detected at 0 h at each pH value. The most marked loss of activity, between 22 and 26%, was observed for all the evaluated pHs in the first 3 h. Then, the activity remained almost constant. After 72 h of incubation, 57%, 62%, 56%, and 53% of the original xylanase activity were remained at pH 5, pH 6, pH 7, and pH 8, respectively. Thus, all pH values applied in the experiments resulted in similar decreases in xylanase activity at 45 °C.

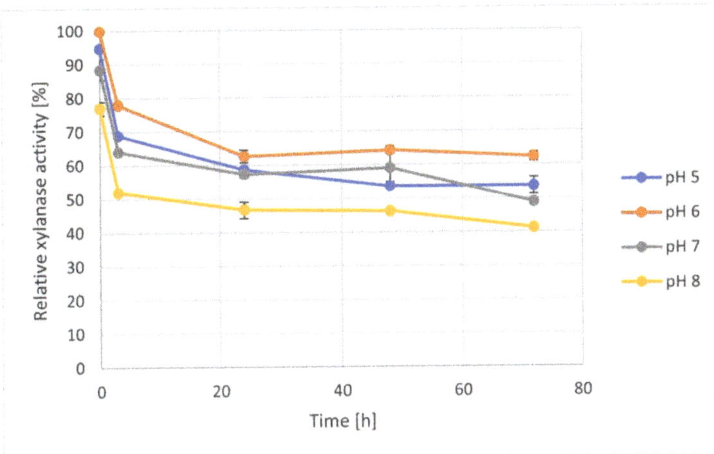

Figure 6. Results of the xylanase enzyme stability test at 45 °C and pH 5, 6, 7, 8 using the fermentation supernatant of *C. phragmiteti* cultivated in LB medium containing 1 *w*/*w*% of waste paper. The average values of relative xylanase activity are presented with error bars representing the standard deviations of triplicates.

The xylanase activity decreased faster and to a greater extent at 55 °C compared to 45 °C (Figure 7). In the first 3 h, the activity decreased by 44%, 35%, 36%, 43%, and 68% at pH 5, pH 6, pH 7, and pH 8, respectively. After 72 h, only 4%, 8%, 15%, and 3% of the original xylanase activities remained at pH 5, pH 6, pH 7, and pH 8, respectively. Thus, xylanases produced by *C. phragmiteti* on 1 *w*/*w*% WP seem to be more stable at 45 °C compared to 55 °C. In comparison, a greater thermostability was reported for the xylanolytic extracts of *Cellulomonas* sp. B6, which retained almost 80% activity after 48 h at 45 °C, although their specific activity was significantly lower than the extract from *C. phragmiteti* [31]. Our results suggest that the extracts of *C. phragmiteti* can be used in long-term reactions at 45 °C with good catalytic efficiency [41].

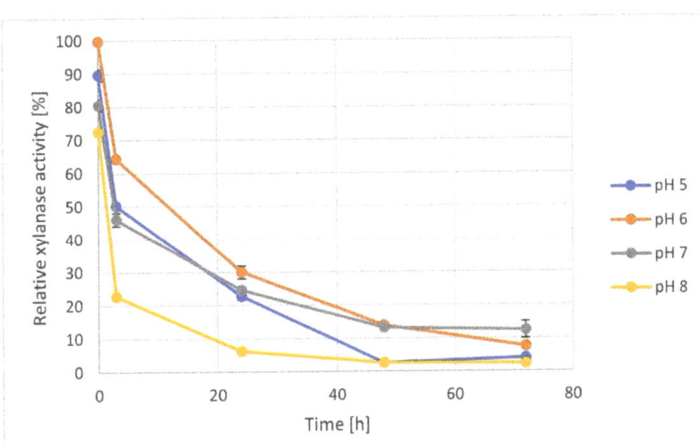

Figure 7. Results of the enzyme stability test at 55 °C and pH 5, 6, 7, and 8 by using the fermentation supernatant of *C. phragmiteti* cultivated in LB medium containing 1 *w*/*w*% of waste paper. The average values of relative xylanase activity are presented with error bars representing the standard deviations of triplicates.

3.7. *Enzymatic Hydrolysis of Xylan*

The xylanolytic supernatant of *C. phragmiteti* grown on WP was employed to hydrolyse birchwood xylan in a 3-day reaction at 45 °C, taking into account the stability results reported in the previous section. The xylose released from the reaction was quantified daily. Increasing values were measured after each day: 4.7 g/L, 7.2 g/L, and 10.7 g/L xylose was liberated after 24, 48, and 72 h, respectively. The 72 h supernatant was also subjected to sulphuric acid treatment in order to decompose oligosaccharides and determine the amount of total solubilized xylose (monomers and oligomers). The total solubilized xylose content was similar to the released monomer xylose concentration, indicating that the solubilized fraction of the xylan substrate was completely hydrolysed until reaching monomer form by the xyalnolytic supernatant of *C. phragmiteti*.

4. Conclusions

In this study, *C. phragmiteti* was found to be a promising candidate for the production high-value xylanase enzymes from the abundant and cheap lignocellulosic residues of WP. Producing enzymes using low-cost lignocellulosic wastes could reduce the price of the enzymes, which is usually a critical point in biotechnology, and could also contribute to mitigating waste handling issues. The most suitable culture medium and WP concentration to enhance xylanase production by *C. phragmiteti* was determined, and the obtained xylanases were characterized in terms of substrate specificity, pH and temperature optima, thermal stability, and salt tolerance. Water-intensive industrial areas might take advantage of the xylanase produced by *C. phragmiteti* because it can tolerate high salt concentrations. Thus, seawater might be used instead of fresh water in bioprocesses applying this enzyme. In contrast, using high concentrations of salt in the production of xylanases via *C. phragmiteti* should be avoided. Xylanases produced by *C. phragmiteti* show high activity at a wide pH range (from pH 5 to 8) and between 45 and 55 °C, which could provide them with a versatile portfolio of industrial applications, including biofuel, feed, and food production. These xylanases also have great thermal stability, preserving more than half of their activity after 3 days of incubation at 45 °C, making them great candidates for bioprocessing techniques that require long residence times (e.g., second-generation biofuel production) and allowing for them to be recycled multiple times. Thus, cultivating the novel bacterium *C. phragmiteti* on waste paper offers a great alternative for xylanase production, as *C. phragmiteti* shows promising attributes that could be useful in many industrial applications.

Supplementary Materials: The following supporting information can be downloaded at: https://www.mdpi.com/article/10.3390/pr12020258/s1, Figure S1. Relative xylanase activities [%] obtained from fermentation by using *C. phragmiteti* in LB medium containing 1 *w*/*w*% of dry matter waste paper as a function of fermentation time. Average values of relative xylanase activity are presented with error bars representing the standard deviations of triplicates. Figure S2. Appearance of the waste paper used in the experiments.

Author Contributions: K.B. conducted experiments, analysed data, and wrote the manuscript. T.F. conducted experiments and analysed data. O.M.O. and E.C. analysed data and made corrections to the manuscript. C.F. conceived and designed the study, was responsible for funding acquisition, and corrected the manuscript. All authors have read and agreed to the published version of the manuscript.

Funding: Project no. TKP2021-EGA-02 has been implemented with the support provided by the Ministry of Culture and Innovation of Hungary from the National Research, Development and Innovation Fund, financed under the TKP2021-EGA funding scheme. Project no. RRF-2.3.1-21-2022-00015 has been implemented with the support provided by the European Union. Financial support from the Foundation of József Varga, Faculty of Chemical Technology and Biotechnology, BUTE, within the project of Mihály Somogyi is acknowledged. This article is based on work from COST Action (CA18229, Yeast4Bio), supported by COST (European Cooperation in Science and Technology, www.cost.eu).

Data Availability Statement: The data presented in this study are available from the corresponding author upon request. The data are not publicly available due to privacy restrictions.

Acknowledgments: The authors are grateful to Gyermelyi Ltd. (Gyermely, Hungary), Suranaree University of Technology (Thailand), National Collection of Agricultural and Industrial Microorganisms (Budapest, Hungary), Research Group of Cereal Science and Food Quality, Budapest University of Technology and Economics (Budapest, Hungary), and Hungarian University of Agriculture and Life Science (Budapest, Hungary) for kindly providing research materials. The authors also thank Kinga Kóder for providing technical support.

Conflicts of Interest: The authors declare no conflicts of interest. The funders had no role in the design of the study; in the collection, analyses, or interpretation of data; in the writing of the manuscript; or in the decision to publish the results.

References

Saini, J.K.; Saini, R.; Tewari, L. Lignocellulosic Agriculture Wastes as Biomass Feedstocks for Second-Generation Bioethanol Production: Concepts and Recent Developments. *3 Biotech* **2015**, *5*, 337–353. [CrossRef]

Bomble, Y.J.; Lin, C.Y.; Amore, A.; Wei, H.; Holwerda, E.K.; Ciesielski, P.N.; Donohoe, B.S.; Decker, S.R.; Lynd, L.R.; Himmel, M.E. Lignocellulose Deconstruction in the Biosphere. *Curr. Opin. Chem. Biol.* **2017**, *41*, 61–70. [CrossRef]

Andlar, M.; Rezić, T.; Marđetko, N.; Kracher, D.; Ludwig, R.; Šantek, B. Lignocellulose Degradation: An Overview of Fungi and Fungal Enzymes Involved in Lignocellulose Degradation. *Eng. Life Sci.* **2018**, *18*, 768–778. [CrossRef] [PubMed]

Den, W.; Sharma, V.K.; Lee, M.; Nadadur, G.; Varma, R.S. Lignocellulosic Biomass Transformations via Greener Oxidative Pretreatment Processes: Access to Energy and Value Added Chemicals. *Front. Chem.* **2018**, *6*, 141. [CrossRef] [PubMed]

Balan, V. Current Challenges in Commercially Producing Biofuels from Lignocellulosic Biomass. *ISRN Biotechnol.* **2014**, *2014*, 463074. [CrossRef] [PubMed]

Saldarriaga-Hernández, S.; Velasco-Ayala, C.; Leal-Isla Flores, P.; de Jesús Rostro-Alanis, M.; Parra-Saldivar, R.; Iqbal, H.M.N.; Carrillo-Nieves, D. Biotransformation of Lignocellulosic Biomass into Industrially Relevant Products with the Aid of Fungi-Derived Lignocellulolytic Enzymes. *Int. J. Biol. Macromol.* **2020**, *161*, 1099–1116. [CrossRef]

Gonçalves, G.A.L.; Takasugi, Y.; Jia, L.; Mori, Y.; Noda, S.; Tanaka, T.; Ichinose, H.; Kamiya, N. Synergistic Effect and Application of Xylanases as Accessory Enzymes to Enhance the Hydrolysis of Pretreated Bagasse. *Enzym. Microb. Technol.* **2015**, *72*, 16–24. [CrossRef] [PubMed]

Woldesenbet, F.; Virk, A.P.; Gupta, N.; Sharma, P. Effect of Microwave Irradiation on Xylanase Production from Wheat Bran and Biobleaching of Eucalyptus Kraft Pulp. *Appl. Biochem. Biotechnol.* **2012**, *167*, 100–108. [CrossRef] [PubMed]

Sharma, H.K.; Xu, C.; Qin, W. Biological Pretreatment of Lignocellulosic Biomass for Biofuels and Bioproducts: An Overview. *Waste Biomass Valorization* **2019**, *10*, 235–251. [CrossRef]

Bhardwaj, N.; Kumar, B.; Verma, P. A Detailed Overview of Xylanases: An Emerging Biomolecule for Current and Future Prospective. *Bioresour. Bioprocess.* **2019**, *6*, 40. [CrossRef]

Alokika; Singh, B. Enhanced Production of Bacterial Xylanase and Its Utility in Saccharification of Sugarcane Bagasse. *Bioprocess. Biosyst. Eng.* **2020**, *43*, 1081–1091. [CrossRef]

Robinson, R.K.; Batt, C.A.; Patel, P.D. Rajoka1999. In *Encyclopedia of Food Microbiology*; Elseiver: Amsterdam, The Netherlands, 1999; pp. 365–371.

Lisov, A.V.; Belova, O.V.; Lisova, Z.A.; Vinokurova, N.G.; Nagel, A.S.; Andreeva-Kovalevskaya, Z.I.; Budarina, Z.I.; Nagornykh, M.O.; Zakharova, M.V.; Shadrin, A.M.; et al. Xylanases of *Cellulomonas flavigena*: Expression, Biochemical Characterization, and Biotechnological Potential. *AMB Express* **2017**, *7*, 5. [CrossRef]

Mayorga-Reyes, L.; Morales, Y.; Salgado, L.M.; Ortega, A.; Ponce-Noyola, T. *Cellulomonas flavigena*: Characterization of an Endo-1,4-Xylanase Tightly Induced by Sugarcane Bagasse. *FEMS Microbiol. Lett.* **2002**, *214*, 205–209. [CrossRef]

Ontañon, O.M.; Bedő, S.; Ghio, S.; Garrido, M.M.; Topalian, J.; Jahola, D.; Fehér, A.; Valacco, M.P.; Campos, E.; Fehér, C. Optimisation of Xylanases Production by Two *Cellulomonas* Strains and Their Use for Biomass Deconstruction. *Appl. Microbiol. Biotechnol.* **2021**, *105*, 4577–4588. [CrossRef] [PubMed]

Goyal, M.; Kalra, K.L.; Sareen, V.K.; Soni, G. Xylanase production with xylan rich lignocellulosic wastes by a local soil isolate of trichoderma viride. *Braz. J. Microbiol.* **2008**, *39*, 535–541. [CrossRef]

Elisashvili, V.; Metreveli, E.; Khardziani, T.; Sokhadze, K.; Kobakhidze, A.; Kachlishvili, E. Review of Recent Advances in the Physiology of the Regulation of Cellulase and Xylanase Production by Basidiomycetes. *Energies* **2023**, *16*, 4382. [CrossRef]

Blasi, A.; Verardi, A.; Lopresto, C.G.; Siciliano, S.; Sangiorgio, P. Lignocellulosic Agricultural Waste Valorization to Obtain Valuable Products: An Overview. *Recycling* **2023**, *8*, 61. [CrossRef]

Santibáñez, L.; Henríquez, C.; Corro-Tejeda, R.; Bernal, S.; Armijo, B.; Salazar, O. Xylooligosaccharides from Lignocellulosic Biomass: A Comprehensive Review. *Carbohydr. Polym.* **2021**, *251*, 117118. [CrossRef] [PubMed]

Rusznyák, A.; Tóth, E.M.; Schumann, P.; Spröer, C.; Makk, J.; Szabó, G.; Vladár, P.; Márialigeti, K.; Borsodi, A.K. *Cellulomonas phragmiteti* sp. Nov., a Cellulolytic Bacterium Isolated from Reed (*Phragmites australis*) Periphyton in a Shallow Soda Pond. *Int. J. Syst. Evol. Microbiol.* **2011**, *61*, 1662–1666. [CrossRef] [PubMed]

21. Bertani, G. Studies on lysogenesis I: The mode of phage liberation by lysogenic *Escherichia coli*. *J. Bacteriol.* **1959**, *62*, 293–3 [CrossRef]
22. Sluiter, A.; Hames, B.; Ruiz, R.; Scarlata, C.; Sluiter, J.; Templeton, D.; Crocker, D. Determination of Structural Carbohydrates a Lignin in Biomass. *Lab. Anal. Proced. (LAP)* **2008**, *1617*, 1–16.
23. Ghio, S.; Sabarís, G.; Lorenzo, D.; Lia, V.; Talia, P.; Cataldi, A.; Grasso, D.; Campos, E. Isolation of *Paenibacillus* sp. and *Variovo* sp. Strains from Decaying Woods and Characterization of Their Potential for Cellulose Deconstruction. *Int. J. Biochem. Mol. B* **2012**, *3*, 352.
24. Miller, G.L. Miller1959. *Anal. Chem.* **1959**, *31*, 426–428. [CrossRef]
25. Ontañon, O.M.; Ghio, S.; Marrero Díaz de Villegas, R.; Piccinni, F.E.; Talia, P.M.; Cerutti, M.L.; Campos, E. EcXyl43 β-Xylosid Molecular Modeling, Activity on Natural and Artificial Substrates, and Synergism with Endoxylanases for Lignocellul Deconstruction. *Appl. Microbiol. Biotechnol.* **2018**, *102*, 6959–6971. [CrossRef] [PubMed]
26. Lopes, A.M.; Ferreira Filho, E.X.; Moreira, L.R.S. An Update on Enzymatic Cocktails for Lignocellulose Breakdown. *J. A Microbiol.* **2018**, *125*, 632–645. [CrossRef] [PubMed]
27. Sárossy, Z.; Tenkanen, M.; Pitkänen, L.; Bjerre, A.B.; Plackett, D. Extraction and Chemical Characterization of Rye Arabinoxy and the Effect of β-Glucan on the Mechanical and Barrier Properties of Cast Arabinoxylan Films. *Food Hydrocoll.* **2013**, *30*, 206–2 [CrossRef]
28. Coelho, E.; Rocha, M.A.M.; Moreira, A.S.P.; Domingues, M.R.M.; Coimbra, M.A. Revisiting the Structural Features of Arabino lans from Brewers' Spent Grain. *Carbohydr. Polym.* **2016**, *139*, 167–176. [CrossRef] [PubMed]
29. Appeldoorn, M.M.; Kabel, M.A.; Van Eylen, D.; Gruppen, H.; Schols, H.A. Characterization of Oligomeric Xylan Structu from Corn Fiber Resistant to Pretreatment and Simultaneous Saccharification and Fermentation. *J. Agric. Food Chem.* **2010**, 11294–11301. [CrossRef] [PubMed]
30. Scheller, H.V.; Ulvskov, P. Hemicelluloses. *Annu. Rev. Plant Biol.* **2010**, *61*, 263–289. [CrossRef] [PubMed]
31. Piccinni, F.E.; Ontañon, O.M.; Ghio, S.; Sauka, D.H.; Talia, P.M.; Rivarola, M.L.; Valacco, M.P.; Campos, E. Secretome Profile *Cellulomonas* sp. B6 Growing on Lignocellulosic Substrates. *J. Appl. Microbiol.* **2019**, *126*, 811–825. [CrossRef]
32. Wakarchuk, W.W.; Brochu, D.; Foote, S.; Robotham, A.; Saxena, H.; Erak, T.; Kelly, J. Proteomic Analysis of the Secretome *Cellulomonas fimi* ATCC 484 and *Cellulomonas flavigena* ATCC 482. *PLoS ONE* **2016**, *11*, e0151186. [CrossRef]
33. Saratale, G.D.; Saratale, R.G.; Lo, Y.C.; Chang, J.S. Multicomponent Cellulase Production by *Cellulomonas biazotea* NCIM-2550 a Its Applications for Cellulosic Biohydrogen Production. *Biotechnol. Prog.* **2010**, *26*, 406–416. [CrossRef] [PubMed]
34. Sudeep, K.C.; Upadhyaya, J.; Joshi, D.R.; Lekhak, B.; Chaudhary, D.K.; Pant, B.R.; Bajgai, T.R.; Dhital, R.; Khanal, S.; Koirala, et al. Production, Characterization, and Industrial Application of Pectinase Enzyme Isolated from Fungal Strains. *Fermentat* **2020**, *6*, 59. [CrossRef]
35. Palaniyappan, M.; Vijayagopal, V.; Viswanathan, R.; Viruthagiri, T. Screening of Natural Substrates and Optimization of Operati Variables on the Production of Pectinase by Submerged Fermentation Using *Aspergillus niger* MTCC 281. *Afr. J. Biotechnol.* **2009** 682–686.
36. Verma, D.; Satyanarayana, T. Xylanolytic Extremozymes Retrieved from Environmental Metagenomes: Characteristics, Gene Engineering, and Applications. *Front. Microbiol.* **2020**, *11*, 551109. [CrossRef] [PubMed]
37. Engel, P.; Mladenov, R.; Wulfhorst, H.; Jäger, G.; Spiess, A.C. Point by Point Analysis: How Ionic Liquid Affects the Enzyma Hydrolysis of Native and Modified Cellulose. *Green. Chem.* **2010**, *12*, 1959–1966. [CrossRef]
38. Akermann, A.; Weiermüller, J.; Chodorski, J.N.; Nestriepke, M.J.; Baclig, M.T.; Ulber, R. Optimization of Bioprocesses wi Brewers' Spent Grain and Cellulomonas Uda. *Eng. Life Sci.* **2022**, *22*, 132–151. [CrossRef]
39. Amaya-Delgado, L.; Vega-Estrada, J.; Flores-Cotera, L.B.; Dendooven, L.; Hidalgo-Lara, M.E.; Montes-Horcasitas, M.C. Inducti of Xylanases by Sugar Cane Bagasse at Different Cell Densities of *Cellulomonas flavigena*. *Appl. Microbiol. Biotechnol.* **2006**, 477–481. [CrossRef]
40. Ghadikolaei, K.K.; Sangachini, E.D.; Vahdatirad, V.; Noghabi, K.A.; Zahiri, H.S. An Extreme Halophilic Xylanase from Cam Rumen Metagenome with Elevated Catalytic Activity in High Salt Concentrations. *AMB Express* **2019**, *9*, 86. [CrossRef]
41. Garrido, M.M.; Piccinni, F.E.; Landoni, M.; Peña, M.J.; Topalian, J.; Couto, A.; Wirth, S.A.; Urbanowicz, B.R.; Campos, E. Insigh into the Xylan Degradation System of *Cellulomonas* sp. B6: Biochemical Characterization of RCsXyn10A and RCsAbf62 *Appl. Microbiol. Biotechnol.* **2022**, *106*, 5035–5049. [CrossRef]

MDPI AG
Grosspeteranlage 5
4052 Basel
Switzerland
Tel.: +41 61 683 77 34

Processes Editorial Office
E-mail: processes@mdpi.com
www.mdpi.com/journal/processes

www.ingramcontent.com/pod-product-compliance
Lightning Source LLC
Chambersburg PA
CBHW062054220926
51850CB00010B/2765